DATE DUE

NOV - 9 2005		
GAYLORD		PRINTED IN U.S.A.

CONTROLLING DRUGS

International Handbook
for Psychoactive Drug Classification

UNDER THE AUSPICES OF UNITED NATIONS
SOCIAL DEFENCE RESEARCH INSTITUTE, ROME

PREPARED BY THE INTERNATIONAL RESEARCH GROUP
ON DRUG LEGISLATION AND PROGRAMS, GENEVA

Richard H. Blum

Daniel Bovet

James Moore

& Associates

CONTROLLING

DRUGS

Jossey-Bass Publishers
San Francisco · Washington · London · 1974

CONTROLLING DRUGS
International Handbook for Psychoactive Drug Classification
by Richard H. Blum, Daniel Bovet, James Moore, and Associates

Copyright © 1974 by: Jossey-Bass, Inc., Publishers
615 Montgomery Street
San Francisco, California 94111
&
Jossey-Bass Limited
3 Henrietta Street
London WC2E 8LU

Library of Congress Catalogue Card Number LC 73-9070

International Standard Book Number ISBN 0-87589-203-5

Manufactured in the United States of America

JACKET DESIGN BY WILLI BAUM

FIRST EDITION

Code 7405

The Jossey-Bass
Behavioral Science Series

Published under the auspices of the

United Nations Social Defence
Research Institute (*Rome*)

Prepared by the

International Research Group
on Drug Legislation and Programs (*Geneva*)

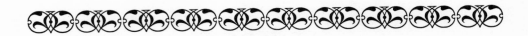

PARTICIPANTS IN THE WORK OF THE GROUP

(Participants are not responsible for the positions taken by any Group member writing in this volume. The contents of each chapter reflect solely the work and opinions of its author(s).)

DAVID H. ARCHIBALD, *director, Addiction Research Foundation, Toronto*

MAUREEN BAILEY, *Scientific Staff, United Nations Social Defence Research Institute, Rome*

GUIDO BELSASSO, *general director, Centro Mexicano de Estudios en Farmacodependencia, Mexico City*

BRIT BERGERSEN-LIND, *director of research, Department of Health and Social Affairs, Oslo*

J. P. BERTSCHINGER, *head, Pharmaceutical Section, Public Health Service, Berne*

EVA M. BLUM, *codirector, Joint Program in Drugs, Crime and Community Studies, Center for Interdisciplinary Research, Stanford University*

RICHARD H. BLUM, *director, Joint Program in Drugs, Crime and Community Studies, Center for Interdisciplinary Research, and consulting professor of psychology, Stanford University*

DANIEL BOVET, *professor of psychobiology, University of Rome, and director, Laboratory of Psychobiology, Rome*

KETTIL BRUUN, *research director, Finnish Foundation for Alcohol Studies, Helsinki*

DALE C. CAMERON, *chief, Drug Dependence and Alcoholism, World Health Organization, Geneva*

H. DANNER, *minister counsellor, Ministry of Youth, Family Affairs and Health, Bonn*

JOSEPH DITTERT, *secretary, International Narcotics Control Board, Geneva (Observer)*

GIUSEPPE DI GENNARO, *legal consultant, United States Social Defence Research Institute, Rome, and Justice, Supreme Court of Italy*

HARRY GREENFIELD, *president, International Narcotics Control Board, and chairman, Institute for the Study of Drug Dependence, London*

HANS HALBACH, *professor of pharmacology, University of Munich*

KOKICHI HIGUCHI, *director, Research and Training Institute, Ministry of Justice, Tokyo*

LAWRENCE HOOVER, *special counsel, Bureau of Narcotics and Dangerous Drugs, Washington, D.C.*

SUSANNE IMBACH, *legal adviser, Hoffmann La Roche, Ltd., Basle*

C. R. B. JOYCE, *vice-director, Medical Department, Ciba-Geigy, Ltd., Basle*

JOHN KAPLAN, *professor of law, Stanford University*

A. M. KHALIFA, *director, National Centre for Social Research and Criminology, Cairo*

PEIDER KÖNZ, *director, United Nations Social Defence Research Institute, Rome*

VLADIMIR KUSEVIC, *former director, United Nations Division of Narcotic Drugs, Zagreb*

EMIL LANG, *vice-director, Ciba-Geigy, Ltd., Basle*

WILLIAM LANOUETTE, *senior staff member,* The National Observer

ROBERT C. LIND, *professor, Graduate School of Business, Stanford University*

JAMES MOORE, *research expert, United Nations Social Defence Research Institute, Rome*

SATYANSHU MUKHERJEE, *Scientific Staff, United Nations Social Defence Research Institute, Rome*

LYNN PAN, *coordinator, International Research Group on Drug Legislation and Programs, Geneva*

INGEMAR REXED, *secretary, Swedish Narcotics Commission, and magistrate, Svea Appellate Court, Stockholm*

MAX TAESCHLER, *deputy director, Sandoz, Basle*

JARED TINKLENBERG, *professor of psychiatry, Stanford University*

JASPER WOODCOCK, *assistant director, Institute for the Study of Drug Dependence, London*

Consulting Editors

Sven Arndt
Peter Beedle
Philip Berger
T. H. Bewley
Dale C. Cameron
E. Carlini
H. O. J. Collier
Gerald A. Deneau
Ed Fujii
Sylvio Garattini
Giuseppe di Gennaro

Donald W. Goodman
Harry Greenfield
Lars N. Gunne
David Hawks
Harris Isbell
Sanford Kadish
P. Kielholz
Vladimir Kusevic
Gerald Le Dain
W. H. McGlothlin
Jorge Mardones

Patricia L. Murphy
M. J. Rand
N. H. Rathod
Walton T. Roth
Charles R. Schuster
Maurice Seevers
Reginald Smart
Walter P. von Wartburg
E. Leong Way
Jonathan Wolfe
Tomoji Yanagita

Preface

Controlling Drugs provides information useful to lawmakers, officials, professional people, and citizens whose duties or interests have to do with the control of psychoactive drugs. Special emphasis is placed on how drugs are or can be classified and on what kinds of data, logic, and analysis are useful aids for drug classification and for related public action program decisions—including those bearing on governmental controls. Particular attention is paid to methods and problems that arise in connection with drug evaluation, subsequent classification schemes, and the evaluation of programs for control. Special interest is taken in the international aspects of drug control.

The volume introduces the reader to the issues and considerations that ought to be kept in mind as one tries to choose the methods and programs, especially those involving the development and application of international collaborative agreements, which best fit the needs and realities of individual groups and nations.

Since most laws and programs rest on estimates of drug effects, particularly dangers and benefits, our attention focuses on classification schemes, first looking at the kinds of data that assist in predicting or assessing drug outcomes and drug use correlates. Following an overview and the consideration of basic pharmacological and medical approaches to psychoactive drug classification, the role of clinical data and the logic of scientific experimental design are set forth. These chapters are followed by an examination of what epidemiology and the behavioral sciences can contribute. Next the advantages of economic models and of benefit-cost concepts applied to classification are shown. Subsequently the legal framework in and for which drugs are categorized is analyzed, and then the administrative structures and processes of international operations are described so that one sees how these realities affect classification decisions. In the final chapter major issues are identified and recommendations for action are offered.

Several major themes recur in *Controlling Drugs*. The reader is invited to keep these in mind from the outset. One theme is the state of *uncertainty* that characterizes estimates of drug effects and the consequent judgments which systems for classification and proposals for control entail. That uncertainty arises from the nature of scientific inquiry itself as well as from the variety of standards used in evaluating those drug effects that can be demonstrated. Uncertainty also occurs because drug effects vary depending on the circumstances of use—that is, as a function of drug-person-environment interaction, as a result of drug-drug interactions within a person, or as a person is himself different from one occasion of use to another. Uncertainty also arises from the fast-changing nature of psychoactive drug use today, from the fact that new drugs—or new uses for known drugs—are rapidly being introduced, and because new knowledge about the outcomes of drug laws, about institutions and actions, and about other forms of response is rapidly accumulating. Uncertainty also occurs because political, social, moral, religious, health, and other interests dictate changes in both laws and programs. These changes in turn alter forms of drug distribution and use; thus the bases for evaluation of the effects of laws and programs are themselves undergoing change. Uncertainty means that one must expect that today's drugs and drug effects may not be tomorrow's, that today's minimum needs for information on drug users or program impact may be insufficient by tomorrow, and that classification schemes and legislative apparatus are inevitably temporary. The orientation that is common today with regard to drug production, use, and control or toward standards for evaluating either drug users or programs for affecting drug use is likely also to change. The fact of uncertainty as an element in science and in policy suggests that the positions nations or international bodies adopt as an immediate response to current needs should incorporate mechanisms for adapting to change.

Another theme is that policy-makers in the field of drug legislation, control, and programs should consider as many *alternatives* as possible. Because of the complexity of scientific information, of drug applications, of user populations, and of the social and political circumstances in which programs are applied, simple or singular approaches cannot adequately meet diverse needs. Knowledge of alternatives is a requirement for the international lawmaker as well as for the local community-based professional or official. At the least, the policy-maker will want to know about the many different treatment programs available, about the several ways in which education can be introduced, about the alternatives within the administration of justice (informal disposition, referral to nonjudicial agencies, probation, disposition to different correctional or rehabilitation settings, sentencing variations, parole, after-care, and so forth), and about community programs. Knowledge of how various alternatives best fit the capabilities and requirements of a given situation—be that the medical needs of a patient or the law enforcement apparatus of several nations working together to reduce illicit traffic—allows policy-makers to create and implement activities that are likely to be effective in particular circumstances.

A third theme is *evaluation*. We should be committed to learning as much as possible about how different drugs affect individuals in various settings, over differing time periods, or when used at differing life stages; how various laws work in diverse locales or nations; and how alternative programs for preventing or treating drug-related problems turn out in practice. Evaluation implies knowledge of the various standards that can be used to judge drugs, people, programs, and laws. These standards are themselves diverse, embracing concepts of health, efficiency, economics, and morality. Evaluation implies systematic information-gathering about impact and, for wise policy-making, the use of what is learned in revising concepts, policies, and programs. The theme of evaluation, like uncertainty, like alternatives, implies that all public action in the drug field be designed as a continuing cycle: (1) information-gathering before action; (2) action in response to immediate knowledge, needs, and pressures; (3) mechanisms for assessment of the consequences of the immediate action; and (4) mechanisms for revision in policies and programs to fit them to new knowledge and to better-understood future needs.

A fourth theme arises from the third but is implicit throughout: the expectation that *policy be based on knowledge*. One must acknowledge that much, perhaps most, national and international policy-setting in the social-problem arena rests on moral views, untested assumptions, political necessity or opportunism, and other powerful but not necessarily reasoned or factually based decisions. Our assumption is that lawmakers will best serve their people, the international community, and themselves if they fit their work in the drug field to the facts about drugs, about users, and about the impact of various programs. Ignoring evidence about the impact of laws and programs is costly not just in terms of immediate fiscal waste or the pain introduced into human lives by programs that either are ineffective or produce more trouble than they prevent, but because future efforts must undo the tangle of administrative apparatus, vested interests, and misinformed partisans before these revised corrective endeavors can be of any assistance. Today's error, based on failure to use the admittedly limited information that does exist, creates trouble for tomorrow's citizens, professionals, and lawmakers. All those with public responsibilties for drug legislation or programs at any level (local, national, international) must seek out, consider, and—insofar as they are free to be rational in their own political circumstances—act on facts rather than emotion, guesses, or short-run political interests. Scientists, administrators, and other professionals have the obligation to gather information and make it available to lawmakers. Because it is to the advantage of lawmakers and program administrators to attend to what has been learned, we hope that the reader will adopt as his own the theme of *alertness to facts* in using this volume.

The United Nations Social Defence Research Institute (UNSDRI) has followed with great interest the preparations for this handbook. While it may not subscribe to all the opinions formulated in it, it is convinced that this new and at times critical look at the problems and objectives that underlie the classification of psychoactive drugs for control purposes meets a real need. Undoubtedly the contributions made by the various authors will help policy-makers—national and international—in their efforts to devise controls that are both effective and consistent with fundamental human rights.

The International Research Group on Drug Legislation and Programs (also known as the Consortium), which prepared this volume, exists because its participants believe it should, and its projects are under way because their shoulders are to the wheel. However, these personal commitments could not be carried out without the support, in funds and facilities, of others who also believe that international collaboration in the drug field is worth while and can be improved. Toward that end the Consortium or its individual projects have received the support of nations, institutions, foundations, and industry. A list of acknowledgments of persons to whom we are grateful could not be complete, so we shall not begin. Even a list of nations is incomplete, although if a nation has not supported the work of a participant, granted facilities, or given funds, it may well have joined in assisting in the birth of the Group or in persuading others to assist that inquisitive child. We acknowledge among the original "midwives" in Geneva delegates from Australia, Canada, Denmark, Hungary, Iran, Finland, Sweden, the United Kingdom, and the United States. In the support of Consortium participants and participation, we happily attest to the assistance of Canada, Egypt, Finland, Italy, Japan, Mexico, Norway, Sweden, Switzerland, the United Kingdom, the United States, West Germany, and Yugoslavia. Associated with UNSDRI in its country studies project, in collaboration with the Consortium and with the support of the United Nations Special Fund, are Iran, Singapore, Hong Kong, Brazil, Panama, Lebanon, Afghanistan, Indonesia, Egypt, Yugoslavia, Mexico, Italy, Norway, Japan, and Puerto Rico; all deserve our respectful thanks for their cooperative efforts. Among international organizations, special appreciation must be expressed to the United Nations Narcotics Commission, the International Narcotics Control Board, the World Health Organization, the United Nations Division of Narcotic Drugs, the United Nations Social Defence section, and the sponsor of this work, UNSDRI itself. Among government-affiliated agencies offering special fiscal support are the Finnish Foundation for Alcohol Studies, the Swedish National Board of Health and Welfare, and the United States Bureau of Narcotics and Dangerous Drugs. Among private institutions, thanks are especially due to Stanford University (California) and the Institute for the Study of Drug Dependence (London). The research reported here was supported in part by a grant from the Drug Abuse Council, Inc., Washington, D.C. A grant from the European pharmaceutical industry is also gratefully acknowledged.

Because each person participates in the Consortium as an individual, even though he may simultaneously be an official elsewhere, no participant, consultant, editor, affiliated agency, or any institution or national government can take responsibility for what an individual author has written in *Controlling Drugs*. The views expressed here, however much the authors have benefited from the help of others, are individual views. The chapters, however, are integrated because of each writer's previous commitment to the overall plan of the project. Integration was also assisted by each writer's willingness to respond to the suggestions of editors and consultants and by our efforts to make a solid structure.

Rome   PEIDER KÖNZ
September 1973

Contents

Contributors

RICHARD H. BLUM, *director, Joint Program in Drugs, Crime and Community Studies, Center for Interdisciplinary Research, and consulting professor of psychology, Stanford University*

DANIEL BOVET, *professor of psychobiology, University of Rome, and director, Laboratory of Psychobiology, Rome*

P. H. CONNELL, *director, Drug Dependence Clinical Research and Treatment Unit, Maudsley Hospital, London*

HANS HALBACH, *professor of pharmacology, University of Munich*

C. R. B. JOYCE, *vice-director, Medical Department, Ciba-Geigy, Ltd., Basle*

HAROLD KALANT, *professor of pharmacology, University of Toronto*

JOHN KAPLAN, *professor of law, Stanford University*

KEITH F. KILLAM, *professor and chairman, Department of Pharmacology, School of Medicine, University of California, Davis*

A. EUGENE LeBLANC, *scientist, Addiction Research Foundation, Toronto*

xix

ROBERT C. LIND, *professor, Graduate School of Business, Stanford University*

JAMES MOORE, *research expert, United Nations Social Defence Research Institute, Rome*

N. H. RATHOD, *Horsham & Crawley Psychiatric Service, St. Christopher's Day Hospital, Horsham, England*

JARED TINKLENBERG, *professor of psychiatry, Stanford University*

JASPER WOODCOCK, *assistant director, Institute for the Study of Drug Dependence, London*

CONTROLLING DRUGS

International Handbook
for Psychoactive Drug Classification

UNDER THE AUSPICES OF UNITED NATIONS
SOCIAL DEFENCE RESEARCH INSTITUTE, ROME

PREPARED BY THE INTERNATIONAL RESEARCH GROUP
ON DRUG LEGISLATION AND PROGRAMS, GENEVA

Classification and
Drug Control

Richard H. Blum

I

Psychoactive drugs* are ordered by a variety of classification schemes linked to scientific and practical purposes. Classification schemes contained in systems of control measures are of paramount interest to policy-makers and to citizens, for these classifications are the building blocks upon which national and international legislation and programs are built. That legislation, through the criminal law and through provisions for education, treatment, agricultural quotas, and other intervention, attempts to deal with what many people worldwide view as an urgent social matter, one usually referred to as the drug problem or drug abuse.

BASES OF CLASSIFICATION

Basic to classifications schemes used in legislation for drug control, including law enforcement, problem prevention, or individual treatment, are the following questions. What are drugs? What do they do? Under what conditions do given outcomes of use occur? Who uses which substances and in what ways? How are judgments arrived at about the advantages and disadvantages of given drugs, outcomes, situations of use, and kinds of users? What plans and require-

---

* The term *psychoactive drug* is used to refer to all chemical substances that affect primarily the central nervous system and, in consequence, the moods, sleep–wakefulness cycles, tension levels, and thought processes of humans. This definition embraces all the drugs identified in the Single Convention and the Protocol on Psychotropic Substances. It includes many other mind-altering materials as well (for example, alcohol, tobacco, aspirin, antihistamines, and coffee).

ments for control develop? When stated and when implemented, what are the functions and the objects of control? What organization is imposed on these assembled facts, inferences, assumptions, and intentions so as to construct a classification-and-control scheme?

The questions that are answered—even if not necessarily explicitly asked —in the development of classification schemes are by no means trivial. They require an analysis of the spectrum of data and beliefs about drugs, about people, and about laws and programs addressed to people who use drugs. For those concerned with international legislation, the understanding of the bases for classification systems is critical. These interests on the part of a few leaders with international responsibilities ought by no means to be restricted to the international leaders, for international treaties once acceded to become binding on national law and policy. Moreover, multilateral collaboration, even when not codified through international conventions, also has dynamic effects on the nations and the people of the world. It is a two-way street, for national interests, experience, and legislation form much of the basis for constructing international legislation and/or multilateral programs. It is a two-way street in one world. No one who cares about drug production and use, the outcomes and correlates of that use, the adequacy and propriety of the means that societies take either to assess drug phenomena in their midst or to respond to and control those events that they define as drug problems, can afford not to be profoundly interested in international classification efforts.

Drug classification as such has not been widely recognized by the public as central to drug control endeavors. Yet the public has its own drug classification schemes even if not called that. Anyone who knows about psychoactive substances, who makes judgments as to when and when not to possess and use them, and who has any views as to the drug-using predilections or claims of others does have his own drug classification scheme. Probably such popular systems are least practical and potentially most mischievous when the drugs, settings, and users involved are believed important by, but are little known personally to the citizen making the judgment. Insofar as the policy-maker has constituents with strong opinions he will be under pressure to make their classification system his own. The leader's alternative—to create a more extensive and more adequate system that is to be imposed on the popular one—requires that he be fortified by time, patience, an abiding interest, competent help, and, at some point in time, the means by which to educate the public at least to accept, if not fully to comprehend the elements and the goals of the more adequate system.

Present Dissatisfaction

Among those personally involved in fact-finding about drugs or drug users and those responsible for drafting legislation or planning and executing programs, the processes, elements, and goals of drug classification are already important. Among these persons there is much dissatisfaction with these processes, elements, and goals as they now stand. The reasons for dissatisfaction vary greatly, ranging from that which a scientist feels when his curiosity is whetted but his theories and facts are inadequate, to the practical man's compelling sense of the need for action accompanied by a sense of terrible practical frustration. Others have a deep conviction that current or proposed practices are faulty, either on scientific, practical, or moral grounds. Thus, among those who ponder the faults of existing systems are those who believe these represent serious misconceptions, pose threats to cherished interests or values, exact unnecessary costs in their execution, or provide insufficient strength and protection.

However diverse these reasons for dissatisfaction, present mechanisms and/or efforts have given rise to serious misgivings on the part of some, if not many, of those who are involved in their planning, operation, or evaluation. Dissatisfaction also exists among those who are on the receiving end of services and efforts, be these farmers, manufacturers, policemen, or drug users and offenders. Given this diversity of viewpoints and interests, one can understand that there are great differences, too, in the focus of attention and in the direction of criticism or proposed change. Understandably, there are conflicts among those with responsibilities in the international arena, as well as among the national or local folk who are objects or citizen observers of efforts of the existing mechanisms.

In spite of this dissatisfaction and disagreement, there is, we believe, welcome agreement on at least two points. One is that the classification process, elements, and objectives are crucial to international action. The other is that they can be improved. We believe further that there is general agreement that such improvements are urgent as well as feasible and that they will work to the benefit of mankind. We believe that there is also agreement that one of the means by which improvement can be furthered is through the application of scientific procedures. Thus, the principles set forth in the Preface (accepting uncertainty, developing alternatives, requiring evaluation, valuing rational policy, and being alert to new information) constitute a partial basis for achieving further agreement in the development of drug classification and control systems.

One should recognize that these principles are by no means only positive in their impact. It is difficult, sometimes painful, to live with uncertainty, to doubt programmatic endeavor to the point of requiring its constant evaluation, to suppress the simple and the emotional in favor of rational policy, and always to remain on the alert to novelty, assuming revelation of new data that will require revision of legislation and programs that one has set up with such difficulty. Understandably, people can resent such a difficult path, among them scientists and policy-makers themselves. For the sake of tranquility as well as common sense, one had best not argue that such principles ought to preempt other considerations. It is a real world as well as one world; and, in the future as in the past, drug classification will be influenced by that which is held to be simple, gratifying, permanent, absolute, and thereby, of course, at least temporarily practical.

To those responsible for or seriously interested in drug legislation and programs, both optimism and pessimism attach to the present state of affairs. There seems little question that scientific attention and methodology and administrative experience have brought to the drug arena great increases in knowledge and in sophistication. There is greater awareness of the facts pertaining to drug use and effects, more understanding of how legislation bears on these, and an appreciation of the alternatives that exist: alternatives in science, in commerce, and in social response—alternatives that can be complementary rather than exclusive. There are a greater governmental and institutional capability, probably a greater public sensitivity, and certainly more personnel who are expert in drug matters. Very importantly, there is apparent commitment on the part of many governments to thorough and conscientious striving after information, evaluation and flexibility, and program efficacy.

At the same time, there is pessimism. Pronouncements and programs, laws and law enforcement, treaties and treatment, new edifices and education have not appeared to reduce production and consumption of potentially unhealthy substances, the proliferation of myths and romance surrounding drug experiences, the rate of arrests in connection with drug crimes, or the distress of the ordinary citizen viewing those drugs and those forms of drug use that tempt, frighten, or anger him. Nor have our efforts to date created an international mechanism or community joined in full and harmonious enterprise. In consequence, we have not yet reason to be pleased with what has been accomplished. This holds for drug legislation and programs in general and for drug classification in particular.

One of the bedeviling aspects of the situation is that the tools one uses to move forward also turn back upon one. Language is such a tool. So many misunderstandings are conveyed or generated by it just as one is intent on clarification. It is a time in need of more semantic sense. Wise observers speak of a famine in language (P. Beedle, personal communication, 1973), others of fat words (Christie and Bruun, 1969); all refer to the inadequacies of terms such as *drug abuse, the drug problem, addiction, control, public health,* and the like. Famine or feast, the classification of drugs, of settings for use, of users, and of outcomes suffers from the confusion engendered by words that are well intentioned but are without clear referents. As the poverty of one term is acknowledged, abuses of its replacement spring up. It is not hopeless. Most are learning to qualify as they speak, to be as operational in definitions as circumstances warrant, and to specify the referents. Even so, communication is not always either clear or easy.

In language, in law, in administration, in treatment, in science, in social programs, and in international endeavor generally, this is a period of transition from things well conceived in their time but now believed inadequate. Yet transition in the drug arena—for instance, in the methods used for classification for purposes of control—should not be assumed itself only to be temporary, like a quick jump from a sinking ship to solid ground. No, for this century at least, we are in a state of permanent change, of chronic impermanence. If so, no language will be enduringly sound; no scientific method solidly right; no viewpoint unassailable; and no method or system of classification for control anything but an endeavor to adjust, temporarily and as best one can, to the changing world and our changing understanding of it.

That implies that the methods for evaluating drugs, settings, and people— plus whatever new objects are revealed to be relevant as work goes on—must themselves be undergoing constant evaluation of their contribution to practical affairs. This by no means demeans the role of basic science as it contributes to the satisfaction of curiosity, but it does suggest that, in the business of international legislation, scientific curiosity should be directed to practical affairs. A caution is in order as well. Dissatisfaction with existing devices should not become synonomous with irritability. We shall all be dissatisfied with any drug-classification system because in an age of great expectations we sense that we can and should do better. Yet if we are doing the best we can, then the sharing of methods and problems, rather than annoyance or harsh accusations, is a good rule. If international legislation and programs are continually to be reconstructed based on fleetingly sound classification systems, one can see how immense good will will be required.

We may thus summarize and characterize our state of affairs as simultaneous progress and retrogression, as transition only to further transition, as curiosity serving practicality and practicality encouraging curiosity, as ever more narrowly qualified views of more and more facts placed in ever more encompassing unified perspectives, as feast-and-famine words waxing and waning but never firm enough to achieve the golden meaning. We should strive for international-national legislation as a two-way street, with neither legislative nor drug traffic ever quite controlled and with easily irritated partners in politics, law, administration, medicine, and science committed to good humor in spite of themselves, thereby not spiting each other.

Given this characterization, our mission is to acquaint the reader with the methods and problems of drug classification as these are linked to issues of control. Although we strive for objectivity, any neutrality on our part is pretense, for we believe that classification systems now need reworking. We present here, not a new classification of drugs but rather a perspective that should contribute facts about drugs, about settings, about users and correlates of use, about laws, and about the outcomes and correlates of laws. We are proposing a more complex matrix of data for decision-making, a much more explicit range of procedures for fact-finding, clearer standards for judgment and inference, and a broader representation of views in the classification-and-control process. Other contributors to this volume do their part to open up alternatives—in science, medical practice, administration, law, and economics. From it all, we hope that national and international lawmakers as well as others responsible for or interested in drug legislation and programs will see new doors that have opened, new ways of gathering information, and new questions to ask before and after policy decisions on control are made. Our good news is that there are many people with many skills, each of whom is willing to contribute to a common task.

One question remains, one raised by a reader of a draft of this section. He put it gently, but it translates into colloquial American as "If you're so smart, why ain't you rich?" Since we pretend to some knowledge of drug classi- fication methods and problems and to an inkling of how controls might be linked, why stop with a presentation of the problems and issues? Why not con- struct a scheme that others can put to use? There are three reasons why. One was mentioned above: our emphasis at this point is on perspectives and process, a consideration of what might go into system construction, not what should go into it. As a group, we are opting to sit on the fence a while longer while we mull over what it is we have just said. Perhaps that looks like abdication of responsi- bility. In reply we would say that even transitional systems are too important to be proposed for international legislation without many people having time to think about them. This is a "think about it" book, a handbook of methods and problems, not a "this is it" set of tables. We want people to think about it, using this volume as a stimulus, perhaps as a guide, but not as *the* answer. Thirdly, we ourselves, as an international research group, as collaborators, or as participants in professions, governments, or UN agencies, are not yet sure how to put our thinking into its fleetingly final shape. We need to talk with each other further, and we need to talk with many others, all those who share with us an interest in international legislation and programs. So ours is not a permanent evasion, just a transitory one. The Group's participants do have on their agenda the con- struction of a process, the outline of a system, the formulation of a design, that would be adaptable to international collaboration. Like the contents of this volume, that is something to think about.

APPROACHES TO CLASSIFICATION

Historical Considerations

Classifications for psychoactive drugs are probably as old as man's use of these substances to achieve an altered mental state or to change his physical sensations. Certainly the use of psychoactive drugs is historically old as well as nearly universal among humans.* Archaeological and historical research, as well as observations on contemporary nonliterate tribes, indicate four major purposes for such drug use (Blum and Associates, 1969a). These are religious (to achieve mystical or trance states, or as part of ceremonies to commune with the divine); medical (to alleviate pain or to improve or cure defects and illnesses); social (to

---

* Seevers states (World Health Organization, 1970), "Over indulgence in drugs appears to be a biological necessity for a sizable fraction of the population" (p. 54). The findings from cross-cultural studies (Blum and Associates, 1969a) show that almost all human societies employ psychoactive drugs for nonmedical purposes.

make social relations easier or more pleasant); or private (to achieve individualized effects, for example, to dull or heighten sensations, to escape emotional distress, to experience new feelings, and the like).

Early records from China, Greece, India, Egypt, and other centers of civilization describe drugs and drug effects. In reviewing these, one finds explicit classifications related to practical purposes, that is, the efficacy of drugs for treating various illnesses, for magical employment, or for achieving sleep or wakefulness. Classifications relating to drug dangers are also apparent; for example, drugs that produce mental disturbance, abortion, or death.

Insofar as drug effects were recognized and either desired or undesired, the nature and manner of use was recommended or constrained. Such attempts to influence the nature of drugs used, how they are used, by whom, under what conditions, and with what outcomes constitute controls. Controls as such must have been introduced prehistorically. Some of the earliest written records pertaining to drug use speak of these measures, which vary from advice on the production and preparation of materials, the manner and amount of administration, designations for the setting of use or who might properly use, to prohibitions on and sanctions against forms of use or associated behavior. In some cultural situations, the available drugs were limited to plants and plant preparations, the free choice of drug use by people in a relatively stable and homogeneous society was restricted, the means to supplementary knowledge were meager, and the scope and interests of governing authorities were limited. In such situations, there was likely to be but limited attention to drug classification and control. Early laws and early pharmacopoeias demonstrate these limits. Yet we recognize that modern life has in common with ancient times the major purposes for use, some of the problems, and a few of the social responses.

The differences between early and modern times are certainly many. Our current state of affairs is unique. Were that not so, there would be neither that optimism about new knowledge, sophistication, and capabilities nor that pessimism about rising rates of troublesome statistics and failures to achieve what one aspires. What is both modern and important are scientific classification as such and the possibility of constant improvement using modern methods. Improvement is measured by the relevancy of the classification system for the purposes to which it is put—in the present instance, drug legislation and drug programs.

Scientific Taxonomy

Scientific taxonomy has grown as part of science itself. An accurate description of nature and interest in discovery necessarily lead to the development of ideas and concepts, to the identification of underlying processes and structures, and to the definition of classes of objects and events whose relationships to one another are, or are hypothesized to be, understandable and predictable. Classifications for psychoactive drugs have been and are used as part of the scientific process. Since the number of drugs known to affect the mind and moods has, until recently, been relatively small—and their applications, however important, few—scientific psychopharmacological taxonomies have been late in developing. Most of that work has been done in the twentieth century.

With further discoveries of drugs that are useful in psychiatry, there have been rather dramatic improvements in the treatment of patients and, as part of general developments in related fields (neurophysiology, biochemistry), in understanding of drug action. This understanding, coupled with expanding endeavors in psychiatry, psychology, and sociology has led, not just to increasingly sophisticated and complex ways for classifying drugs, but also to the development of several perspectives on scientific classification. This means that one can approach classification through several doors and can develop systems that are internally consistent. Nevertheless, these are likely to represent differing levels of interest or of observation.

Sources of Conflict

Differing levels of scientific observation do not conflict unless it is argued that one level is pertinent to the exclusion of others or a theory engendered by or appropriate to one level of observation is expanded and forced upon another level. On the other hand, when interests and views external to any level of factual inquiry are brought to bear on the evaluation of drugs, outcomes, users, and the like (as, for example, positions arising from moral, economic, or political interests), then conflict among these is likely. Insofar as legislative purposes arise that reflect such interests and these purposes require a classification system linked to legislative (or other programmatic) objectives, then the system will serve other than scientific uses. This fitting of scientifically derived information to interests and purposes that are likely to be both diverse and strongly practical constitutes a source of basic conflict. If the classification system used is one that is borrowed, that has not been specifically tailored for the legislative and programmatic purposes for which it is to be employed, there will be trouble.

Consider some uses of drugs, each of which may entail a practical system of classification:

> The practice of medicine or folk medical care to alleviate distress or improve an undesirable condition

> The production and sale of drugs for profit, the drugs to be employed for medical, religious, social, or private purposes

> The application of drugs for purposes of social control, that is, their use to suppress undesirable conduct (defined by the controller) or even, as in warfare, to disable or kill

> The religious use of drugs (as in the Navajo peyote cult, the Jamaican Rastafarian ganja, or wine in Christian Mass)

The social use of drugs occurring as interpersonal recreation, to facilitate interaction and to celebrate occasions whether informal or ritualized

The private use of drugs in the service of varying sensations or altered states of consciousness, relief, or escape from unpleasant environmental or inner states, the pursuit of personal values and goals

Consider the major forms of public action that are part of control efforts:

General interventions to restrict or prevent disapproved use (ranging from rules for production or sales through mass education)

Individual interventions to affect selected persons, as in arrest or treatment

Within most countries of heterogeneous populations that have access to manufactured as well as naturally occurring drugs, most of the foregoing uses and actions will be present. Whenever a classification system developed and formalized for any one of these is put in the service of another use or action, there is likelihood of trouble as far as the requirements of its application differ from the functions for which it was developed.

To the degree that the application in legislation and programs of a classification system affects the beliefs or interests of those engaged in a form of use, then a borrowed system or a maladapted system will be seen as at least inappropriate if not threatening or actually harmful to those whose interests were not considered in the system's development. Potentials for conflict are generated in such circumstances. Since control efforts may be even broader in their impact—constraining drug activities, specifying required conduct, and threatening sanctions for violations—interests of many persons will be affected by control systems. Furthermore, values and interests may differ widely even among those who favor controls as such. One may distinguish, quite roughly, separate medical, moral, commercial, and law enforcement views.

Because of such conflicts, struggles for power occur. These center on *who* has the right to classify drugs, *what effects* according to *what criteria* shall be described, and *which purposes* will take precedent in national or international action. Struggles also center on *what methods* are to be used to achieve purposes, as for example, to influence drug production, distribution, and regulated use.

What at first glance is said to be a problem of *drug* classification is rarely really that. It is not a matter of describing chemicals—but of the reactions of people and societies to chemicals. In some places, drugs grow as botanical products; in others, drugs are manufactured and exported. In some societies, people using one drug are considered abusers, those using another are criminals, those using a third are accepted as normal or perhaps admired or even venerated. In their commerce and use of drugs, people behave in various ways, being influenced by the social definitions of drugs themselves and their uses of them. People seek to influence one another in regard to their drug preferences, amounts and styles of use, and outcomes of use. We shall see that, for these reasons, some modern approaches to classification rest on the description of several components interacting, for example, the drug, societal definitions and reactions to drugs and uses, the person, and the situation of use. Indeed, some sociologically based classifications limit themselves almost exclusively to the characteristics of the people who use the drug—their expectations of drug effects, their styles of use, and the significance of that use for them—paying little attention to the chemical structure and pharmacodynamics that have in the past ordinarily constituted the basis for classification. In any event, unless the real elements and objects of classification are understood, trouble can arise.

LIMITATIONS ON ACCURACY

When any complication is introduced into a prediction system, increased chances for error are introduced. Today, any drug classification scheme that includes statements about the likely effects of drugs on people or that implies the ability of one or another system of control to influence how humans have access to, use, and respond to groups of drugs, will not be exact. Thus, all drug classifications that go beyond straightforward descriptions of the chemical structure of substances to estimate drug effects will be, at best, estimates as to what is likely to happen when someone takes a certain drug given certain conditions. The conditions that actually affect how people respond to psychoactive drugs are many and include, at the very least, the purity and form of the drug; how it is administered and how often; what time elapses between administrations; what other drugs are also present in the body; the state of the person's health, nutrition, metabolism, and the like; his expectations of the drug effects; the setting in which he takes the drug; how he evaluates the specific effects of the drug on his mind, mood, biological cycles, and the like; and how others respond to his drug use and to any changes that the user shows.

Those who are interested in drug classification and control systems should appreciate how many different factors do contribute to what are called drug effects in the normal range of dosage. The dose-response function means that with very heavy doses the prediction of effects for many psychoactive substances becomes easier as toxic outcomes are encountered and people become sick, unconscious, or dead. These extreme responses are the unusual ones simply because most people take or are given psychoactive drugs in those lesser amounts—and frequencies—that allow them some happier outcomes and a range of choice in behavior even though they are under "the influence of a drug." At these lesser dosages, social and personal factors are influential.

Drug classifications that imply prediction of effects must be understood as sets of estimates or statements of probability, the accuracy of which depends on the adequacy of information about drug effects under the conditions of use for which the prediction is made. Accuracy also depends on the excellence of the logic and the acumen of those who are constructing the classification system. Insofar as the effectiveness of one or another system for control (that is, for influencing drug access, use, or reactions) is part of a categorization scheme, accuracy in classification depends on the knowledge of how these various influence mechanisms affect various people under a variety of real-life conditions.

The foregoing limitations on accuracy mean that those who use or construct drug classification systems for practical purposes (that is, for public action with, for, or against kinds of drugs, drug use, or drug reactions) must accept the tentativeness of any category and prediction scheme. The responsible policy-maker, official, professional, or citizen realizes that in the drug arena, as with most human affairs, he is dealing with unknowns. Although it is possible to make reasonably accurate predictions as to the effects of psychoactive drugs on groups of persons (most drinkers can estimate quite well what one shot of whiskey will do to them as compared with six shots), prediction becomes more difficult for a given individual. The best estimate in the absence of additional information is the group or average response; however, there are individual variations in preferences for drugs and for styles of use, as well as for responses. This state of affairs requires one to think in terms of probabilities, not certainties.

The more immediate and actual control one has over a drug (its forms, purity, and the like), over its manner of administration (for example, by a physician or a priest) or the setting in which it is taken (a hospital, a family meal), over the learned expectations of the user, and over the environment of the user following as well as during drug use, then the more accurately one can say what bodily changes and behavior will occur. These highly controlled conditions are the situations least likely to lead to unexpected, disapproved, or physically dangerous outcomes. Situations in which drugs, their administration, and drug-related environmental conditions are controlled have not given rise to worldwide concern over drug abuse; indeed, one definition of *abuse* is "uncontrolled use." Consequently, it is likely that, under the conditions least controlled (for some), there arises the strongest pressure (by others) for control. One assumes that the very novelty of the observed behavior as well as its function in signifying social differences and social changes contributes to uncertainty—if not worry or anger in certain publics—which contributes to these pressures for control. When pressures for control exist, one assumes that accuracy is necessary to any classification scheme that seeks effectively to influence the availability of these drugs or their styles of use and outcomes in people. Yet the very conditions helpful in developing accurate classification incorporating the diversity of real-life conditions are least associated with the varied, disapproved, unexpected, or dangerous forms of private or noninstitutional social use (for example, heroin self-administration among slum youth, cannabis-smoking among commune hippies, alcoholism in a disorganized tribal society). This bedeviling paradox faces persons who are interested in classification for purposes of control.

Semantic Confusion

A number of terms are employed that lead to difficulties in the field of practical psychopharmacology. *Drug abuse* is a term charged with moral and emotional loadings. It has diverse referents and is a semantic quagmire. It may refer to any illicit drug acquisition, possession, use, or distribution; to any compulsive ingestion; to any use that has untoward health or social outcome. It may refer to use that the viewer considers overfrequent or by means of a disapproved manner of administration. It can mean use of a drug from a disapproved source or in the company of disapproved others. It can imply improper motives for use, a disapproved substance or form of drug, or use in settings that are not acceptable. It may be taken as a symbol for membership in groups or causes that are not liked by the viewer. References to drug abuse may also serve to express personal feelings, for instance, anxiety about what someone fears in his environment—be that changing youth, lack of old-fashioned self-discipline, the prevalence of deviants from drunkards to acid heads, or the risk of being robbed by a criminal. Use of the term may also be symbolic or propagandistic, for instance, when it is used by a speaker to coalesce his audience. The very diffuseness of the term can be its temporary advantage; it allows all manner of worrisome or disapproved matters to be subsumed together and obviates any immediate need for quarrelsome debate over definitions, sources of concern, or diverse positions.

Another difficult word is *control*. It often implies an effect that is being achieved rather than, as in most legislation and programs, an objective. Sometimes it connotes the exercise of authority, at other times an efficient mechanism. Control can mean efforts such as passing laws and providing punishment, restraint, education, treatment, or moral admonitions. Optimism is inherent insofar as the exercise is confused with the result; and, should the result not be the one sought, there are those who believe that virtue lies in trying. Others would judge control by its costs and effectiveness.

Drug problem is another phrase that is conducive to misunderstandings. As a replacement for the term *abuse,* it may offer the promise of objectification, but unless one is clear about what is being referred to, who decides that it is a problem, and by what criteria of judgment, the promise may not be kept.

Misconceptions

A number of misconceptions, most of them oversimplifications or unmodified acceptance of earlier medical or scientific concepts, hinder policy-making in the drug field. The standard for judging these to be misconceptions arises from the relatively recent work that has been done with real-life populations.

One misconception has to do with *physical dependence and/or addiction.* It seems widely believed that drugs that in the laboratory show dependence liability (that is, the capability under some conditions, for example, repeated administration at certain dosages, to produce tolerance and withdrawal syndrome) will inevitably lead to such dependence if taken socially or privately. Heroin is most often discussed in this manner. Yet dependence liability, like all other drug affairs, is a matter of probability that varies with circumstances. Alcohol, tobacco, barbiturates, some tranquilizers (anxiolytic-sedatives), and the opiates all have such liability. Studies in normal populations demonstrate that many if not most of the people who are exposed to any of these substances do not use them with such frequency or in such doses as to develop physical dependency. Even when physical dependency does occur, it is pharmacologically reversible. When it is not reversed, that is, when a treated user returns to compulsive use, the drug is only one factor—albeit an important one—accounting for that behavior.

The recent history of public concern about drugs—reflected in late-nineteenth- and early-twentieth-century United States and Canadian legislation, in United Kingdom and European writings and investigations, and in parallel international legislation beginning about 1912 with the Hague Convention—focused on opium, morphine, heroin, and, later, other opiates (opioids). Since these drugs do have the capability of producing physical dependency, which once was termed addiction, this latter term, for some, came to be synonymous with drug abuse. Several consequences followed. One was—and is—the tendency not only to see nondependent users of opiates as addicts, but also to see any illicit or disapproved drug user as an addict, even if the drug he employs (cannabis, LSD, cocaine) is not likely to produce physical dependency. This confusion has not been abated by those laws—the Single Convention, for example—that, perhaps reflecting the same confusion, lumped a variety of differently acting drugs together as "narcotics" and that have encouraged certain police statistics that count any person arrested on a narcotics charge as an addict. Probably many people still consider any drug user an "addict" regardless of the existence or absence of physical dependency.

Evidence for the dominance of the opiate concept is found, not only in the Single Convention, in which nonaddicting drugs are placed under the narcotics umbrella (keep in mind that pharmacologically defined, a narcotic is a drug capable of producing both sleep and analgesia, that is, a soporific or stupefacient), but also in the extension to additional drugs (listed in the Vienna Psychotropic Convention) of those control measures originally devised for and represented in the narcotics classification. This reliance on precedent in constructing later international treaties—and in parallel national laws—represents a typical process of lawmaking, for precedent is important in judicial decisions and in legislative language. Yet doubts must be expressed about the generalizability of the opiate model. Past pharmacological research serving international classification was, of necessity, preoccupied with "morphine-type" drugs (WHO terminology) because of the Single Convention, yet there is a carryover of the "morphine model" in current classification efforts for nonopiate drugs, that can be seen whenever there is exclusive focus on "dependency" phenomena to the exclusion of other drug-and-behavior phenomena. Research as well as law, insofar as these derive from the morphine model, may have suffered from constriction, forced adjustments, conceptual error, and retardation in the development of research methods better suited for estimating the consequences associated with the many nonopiate substances.

Misconceptions also arise from the belief that the use of one drug inevitably leads to the use of anther more potent one. The typical idea of this progression is that marijuana use leads to heroin. Evidence from user populations makes it clear that no such inevitable sequence occurs. Involvement in illicit use definitely can be associated with centering one's life on drugs. In the United States a marijuana user does have a greater risk of trying heroin than someone who has not used illicit drugs. Drug interests do evolve over time; and some who find drugs very satisfying will become multiple users and further, if deprived of one substance, will readily substitute another in its place. Such processes do occur and observation of them may account for the misconception. Yet the facts—as best we know them today—are that no commonly employed psychoactive drug used in normal dosage range compels complex social behavior nor does it compel a step from one particular drug to another. The principle may therefore be stated more generally than what one sees drug users do is likely to be only partly attributable to the pharmacological action of the drug.

The more common misconceptions take the form of confusing observed behavior in association with drugs with specific pharmacological effects. Within the normal dosage range, certain predictable physiological processes are likely to occur with a given drug. However, their expression in conduct, especially in social behavior, is limited. Many other drug effects can be traced to variables of person, expectation, and environment. Consequently, what may be interpreted as drug-caused behavior is very likely to be complex social behavior influenced by factors that are not just pharmacological. Usually, potent pharmaceutical preparations are operating (interacting) with these other features to produce observed conduct. Classification systems that focus on drugs alone cannot predict what drug outcomes will be nearly as well as do classification systems that augment their prediction of effects with other knowledge about the person, his expectations, and the environment in which he uses a drug. The higher the dosage the more accurate the predictions based on drug knowledge alone become, but this accuracy is possible because the available repertoire of behavior is severely restricted by chemical dominance so that little ordinary behavior is possible. Thus a heavy dose of heroin can be predicted to lead to drowsiness, a heavier one to coma, and a massive one to death. But heroin behavior on the street—drug-selling, conversation, prostitution, eating dinner, whatever it is—must be accounted for by factors beyond heroin use per se.

Specific to General Effects

Particularly difficult is the transition from descriptions of specific drug effects (as derived from experiment, clinical observation, or population studies) to general categories. Classification-and-control systems can rest on inclusive judgments such as public health danger, risk, psychic dependence, danger of abuse, abuse potential, medical utility, therapeutic benefit, and the like. Let us say that, in 50 percent of the cases in controlled trials, drug X is found to make subjects who take it feel dulled, reduces their performance on learning tasks by 10 percent efficiency, and aids in sleep production by potentiating secobarbital. Another 30 percent of the subjects who take it show no behavioral changes. Ten percent who take it report euphoria, show performance deficits of 20 percent in simulated auto driving, and prefer X over barbiturates and alcohol to facilitate either sleep or sociability.

Further investigation might reveal that these are dose-related effects; for example, if one increases the dose, the previously unaffected persons could feel dull too, and, with further increases, those who felt dulled might show driving performance deficit. On the other hand such a dose-response curve may not appear so clearly, making the characterization of the effects of the drug more difficult. In either case one would require a probability statement, with the average response for a given dose set forth and driving disability also given as a function of dose. Yet, how would one translate these observations into a general statement about risk, danger, or benefit? The translation problem is faced whenever one would build from a body of discrete experimental findings (which almost always show differences among people taking drugs) to a higher level of semantic abstraction, that is, a prediction of population effects implying control needs. Poisons and thoroughly ineffectual substances do not offer that difficulty, but then neither are they likely to be widely employed medically (at least not by informed physicians) or enjoyed socially (at least not by informed citizens). Most psychoactive drugs in use today—from alcohol and aspirin to LSD and heroin—do offer those difficulties. Anyone tempted to generalize from specific data on effects without bothering to qualify or to attempt to specify dangers and benefits for whom, how defined, under what conditions, with what probability, is likely to do a disservice to classification and control endeavors. Those who are ready to base their thinking and recommendations on a recognition of the complexity of drugs are likely to render a most welcome service in public policy-making.

LEVELS OF OBSERVATION

The approach in this book is to consider classification schemes as these arise from differing methods and levels of data. We progress from physical sciences through the biological to medical-psychiatric, behavioral-psychological and then social-cultural observations to legal schemes; from a restricted (laboratory) to a broad (environmental) data base; and, perhaps, from more easily to less easily objectified observations. Although observations at all levels are complex, insofar as a succeeding level incorporates a preceding one (for example, if behavioral classifications take into account chemical, biological, and clinical pharmacological features) then complexity is multiplied. On the other hand, one will see that classification systems at any one level give primacy to observations at that level.

Each level of classification serves a function within its own discipline, that is, provides a framework for thinking, research, and practice by professionals in that—and related—fields. Therefore, our assumption about classification systems is not that one kind or level is, in principle, better or worse than another, but only that one may fit a particular purpose better than another. The more restricted systems, even if more exact in methodology and fully appropriate for applications within a field, do not work well if they are applied too broadly. A biologically based pharmacological system may be excellent for therapeutic research purposes, but it may fail miserably if used to predict what forms of social drug use will occur or which young persons will undergo debilitating or disapproved lifestyle changes in connection with multiple drug use.

Way (1969) illustrated a typical difficulty that occurs when the level of observation does not fit the practical goal. He noted that preoccupation with heroin as the basis for opium dependence diverted attention from the emotions, personality, and conduct of the user. Physical dependence was easy enough to treat; treatment cooperation and relapse prevention were the obstacles: The heroin user "relapses because of our inability to cope. . . . Hence we keep changing our approaches in the hope of finding a solution for the recidivist— from uncontrolled free clinics, to imprisonment, to narcotic farms, to civil commitments, to half-way houses, to pharmacological blockage." Change of this sort is not an illustration of progress but of its lack. Some of the present appeal of new disciplines working on the drug field will also be found to be unwarranted. But we trust that shall not always be the case, and so here we do opt for multidisciplinary awareness.

Decisions and Data

Richard H. Blum

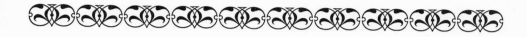

II

In this chapter the major levels of data bearing on psychoactive drug classification systems are considered. Although scientific information plays a role in classifying drugs, perspectives about science, about people, and about which substances are to be called drugs are also critical determinants of decisions.

INITIAL CLASSIFICATION AS A DRUG

The initial classificatory act is the definition of what is a drug. To identify a substance as a drug is the beginning of scientific and legislative classification and all that follows therefrom. Many chemical substances, either naturally grown or manufactured, can produce problems in or for those who use or who are exposed to them but are not handled under most classificatory schemes. Poisonous plants or household poisons, automotive or industrially derived pollutants in air or water are illustrations. So too are those thousands of herbs (possibly only botanically classified) that are used around the world in folk medicine and those other substances (industrial or household) used (misused) explicitly for mind-altering effects—glue, gasoline, paint thinner, hair spray, and dozens of other volatile solvents. These latter are not ordinarily studied pharmacologically and, although toxicologists may work on them, are likewise excluded from most extant "drug" legislative measures. The latter is sometimes true for certain psychoactive substances that are self-administered and are studied pharmacologically but are used almost exclusively socially rather than medically, for instance, tobacco, alcohol, coffee, tea, soft (cola) drinks, and the like.

17

The foregoing serve to illustrate how important the initial decision is as to whether a substance primarily affecting the central nervous system is considered a drug or not. Widely employed substances producing dangers and pleasures are excluded, even from those embracing classificatory systems that purport to regulate chemicals that may be subject to abuse. The history and practical considerations that account for the definitions that emerge are of considerable interest. It is beyond our scope here to examine these important matters at any length except to offer the impression that existing classifications —as, for example, those in various national and international drug control laws—focus almost exclusively on substances that have had and do have use in medicine, whether in research or in treatment. Therefore, psychopharmacology, legislative acts, and public interventions (enforcement, treatment, prevention, and the like) are directed toward a very limited class of substances, most members of which are produced through pharmaceutical manufacture and, theoretically at least, dispensed through pharmaceutical-medical channels. There are, of course, important exceptions—cannabis and opium, for instance—whose Western medical uses are limited (although they are widely used in Asian traditional or folk medicine). Why are classifications and controls limited mostly to substances studied and used medically?

The Canadian (Le Dain) Commission of Enquiry into the Non-medical Use of Drugs (1970), commented on John Stuart Mill's *Essay on Liberty* to consider the principle of whether the criminal law should be used in the field of nonmedical drug use, holding Mill's to be the classic exposition of nonintervention by government except when there is damage or injury to another person resulting from one person's conduct (for example, drug use).

> Mill indicates the general tenor of his thinking in certain observations concerning government policy with respect to poisons and the consumption of alcoholic beverages. Always making exception for the protection of the young, his policy with respect to poisons is that where they have legitimate uses the government must limit its intervention, despite the risks of harm, to assuring that people are suitably warned of the dangers by proper labelling. His reasoning is that, assuming such poisons have useful purposes, people should not be deprived completely of access to them. . . . He goes further . . . that people should not be put to the inconvenience and expense of having to obtain a special permission, such as a doctor's prescription, to obtain them. This is, in fact, the general approach which is adopted by present legislative policy to a wide variety of substances with a potential for harm. . . . It is felt that they cannot be removed entirely from the market because of their necessity or usefulness. Such is the case with drugs having a medical value, . . . and . . . with a wide variety of industrial and household products containing volatile substances, gases and solvents. Despite their potential for harm, especially to young people, as a result of their chemical properties, it is not practicable to consider their removal from the market because of their

utility. . . . Occasionally it may be necessary . . . [as] with cyclamates. With drugs having therapeutic value the requirement of a prescription must for the reasons indicated by Mill—inconvenience and cost—be applied very judiciously.

With respect to the consumption of alcoholic beverages, Mill is . . . against prohibition, and he sees the prohibition of sale as an attempt to prohibit use, as an infringement not only of the liberty of the seller but the liberty of the user as well. . . . Mill is . . . ambivalent . . . as to how far and upon what principles society is justified in interfering with the operations of the seller or purveyor of goods or services of which it disapproves. . . . The reasoning . . . seems to be . . . that it is not right to subject the majority who do not abuse (alcoholic beverages) to inconvenience simply because of those who are liable to do so.

The Canadian Commission, while itself rejecting Mill's thesis, offers his arguments in accounting for those actions by governments that have not subjected either poisons or substances in social use (for example, alcohol and tobacco) to drug classification for purposes of control. Although this may well be the case, the arguments of necessity, inconvenience, cost, and infringement on liberty and commerce do not necessarily account for why those substances that are classified as drugs and subject to control tend also to be those with a history of development for and applications in medicine. The arguments for controls of any kind are embodied in many forms—the Le Dain Commission sets them forth clearly—but whether or not those mostly medicinal substances are in fact best classified and controlled as drugs when other substances are not deserves further consideration.

Emphasis on the control of substances used medically occurs, as Bovet points out in Chapter Six, because those that are psychoactive are remarkable in their capacity to produce multiple effects depending upon the conditions of use. Certain effects are sought by physicians and patients in prescribing, whereas other effects are sought in self-administration. Barbiturates, for example, are prescribed to aid in sleep, to control anxiety, as cardiovascular medicaments, and so on. Youthful drug-takers, however, may take them to achieve a sense of euphoria (intoxication, a high). Medical dosage may be exceeded by a factor of 4 in street use, and the controlled frequency of a prescription regime is likely to be ignored entirely by street users, leading to very serious problems including the risk of convulsions and death upon withdrawal as well as aggressivity when "under the influence." Similar instances of quite different intentions associated with the selection of effects and the variation in dosage, frequency, and manner of administration to obtain such effects occurs in the case of street use of the amphetamines and other substances.

Neither can one overlook the ubiquity with which modern humans ingest a variety of psychoactive substances, many of which are likely to be unfamiliar to them. One thing that may be said for alcohol is that our cultural education in its use is long-standing; and, for most people, its benefits and dangers are known. This is not the case for newly developed pharmaceutical products, which are complex in nature; whose ingredients are known only to chemists and pharmacologists; and whose actions and outcomes, until testing over time occurs, may not be understood.

The readiness of modern man to employ pharmaceuticals coupled with a range of products so broad as to confuse physicians plus the aforementioned risky complexity does create a sense of uncertainty and of danger. Testing and control seem reasonable responses to this state of affairs, which does not hold for most of the industrial and household products, for which temptations to ingest are fortunately low. It is among the young, whose protection Mill championed, that such ingestion occurs most often, either accidentally, as in the case of household poisons, or in the pursuit of "kicks" among those aged ten to sixteen who sniff glue, gasoline, and other volatile compounds.

H. Kalant and O. Kalant (personal communication, 1973) ask if a further feature might not bear on the understanding of the law's nearly exclusive concern with medicaments. They ask, in a historical-anthropological vein, if there is not still magic in the role of the physician with his medicaments still held sacred and consequently taboo for the laity? Might not a sense of awe be perpetuated in the modern law because of that substrate of magic? Industrial materials are not now touched with the sacred (although once they may have been, as inferred from the punishment conferred upon Prometheus by Zeus for giving fire to man and the godly role of the smith Hephaestus) and so receive less awe-inspired attention. The Kalants observe that opium, for a short time available in patent medicines, was withdrawn from profane use and restored to its magical role in the hands of physicians. Toluene, which is employed widely as an industrial solvent and an ingredient in glues sniffed by the young, is not so controlled. If attention to medicaments is linked to the magical powers of healing, then the roots of the initial acts of drug classification for control are deep in the mind indeed.

The questions that surround the initial decision as to what is or is not a drug open up major issues from which classification systems devolve:

1. If several substances are considered as drugs, shall there be classification beyond the initial one, that is, shall there be groups or subclasses ordered by one or several known or presumed qualities, for example, effects?

2. If ordering by subgroups is done, what standards for the identification and assessment of qualities (effects) shall exist?

3. If classification implies or is embodied in legislation, must the aim be control of the substances themselves, or are there other alternatives, for example, (a) aims other than control or (b) objects of control other than drugs (for example, social institutions or individual behavior)?

4. If classification and controls are decided upon, how shall the effects

of drugs be measured against the effects of controls and what standards (economic, moral, or political) shall be used in determining and judging the balance of effects so that optimal policies may be defined and may prevail?

Such issues are by no means readily resolved, even if extant classification and control systems represent implicit decisions already made. It is our position that such implicit decisions are insufficient as policy for modern problems and that satisfactory public policy requires a frank approach to these issues and their further explication.

MEDICINAL CHEMICAL CLASSIFICATION

A straightforward classification system in psychopharmacology, one that appeals to physical scientists, is based on the chemical structure of drugs. It is the province of the discipline of chemistry. In this approach, drugs are classified according to similarities in their molecular structure. New drugs developed or discovered are compared with existing ones and placed in the category their structure most resembles. If the new drug is judged unlike an existing class of drugs, it may be labeled "transitional," or a new category may be invented for it. Some of the categories for psychoactive drugs are new, having come into being after the 1940s with the development of hundreds of new compounds intended for the treatment of agitation, anxiety and depression, and other emotional distress.

Berger (1960) offers the argument for chemical classification: "The main purpose of classifying is to bring order where previously there was chaos. A desirable system of classification would divide the drugs into groups that are easily distinguishable from each other and are few in number. Classification should be such that introduction of new drugs, and of new designations for old ones, would not add to the confusion in this important field. It appears that at present classification of tranquilizers according to their chemical structure is the most useful and practical method of differentiation among the drugs used in this field" (p. 89).

Although Berger contends that the aesthetic-cognitive goal of bringing order is the only one operative, he does in fact introduce the more complex goal of linking classification to clinical usefulness. Clinical usefulness or function refers primarily to effects on humans. As with many others who are oriented to chemistry, Berger finds ordering by effects on humans unsatisfactory (1) because different (chemical) classes of drugs can have similar effects (for example, tranquilizers, opioids, and anticholinergics can all have the same effect on, for instance, sleep induction or slowed learning in animals); (2) because there is no one test of effects that can be used to create ordered categories; (3) because drugs such as tranquilizers are associated with a wide variety of effects some of which (the nonspecific ones) not only vary by person and situation but also are a matter of the individual's own reaction to the primary or specific effects, the subjective experience, produced by the drug (or in association with the conditions of its being used); and (4) because effects linked to psychiatric disease entities suffer from the inadequacy of the psychiatric description systems.

Complex priorities and assumptions underlie chemical classification schemes that appear straightforward. In Berger's case, one reason for rejecting classification on the basis of clinical effects is the lack of knowledge about how these are linked to chemical structure. The implicit expectation is that a relationship between chemical structure and biological response should occur and that, in selecting one as a basis for constructing order, the value of the chemical component has priority. Once that decision is made, the level of data used for constructing the system is set and so are their limits. Berger confines himself in his classification to tranquilizers. In so doing, he accepts a clinical, not a chemical, criterion as defining and setting the limits for his entire system.

Scientific interest in relating one level of events or structure to another persists. Berger's scientific spirit is an example. It leads him, after he rejects chemical/clinical relationships, to seek to link chemical classifications to sites of action in the brain: "Ultimately it would be desirable to define and classify tranquilizers as substances that affect certain well-defined functional units of the brain."

Berger selects, on a priori grounds, four brain areas (centers, systems) as particularly important for classes of human behavior in which he is interested (thinking and judgment, autonomic functions, emotion, and sleep–wakefulness). He then links the chemical classifications of tranquilizers to kinds of effects (stimulation or depression) on these brain systems. Chemical structure is thus linked by a classifying system to drug effects. In this instance, the system invoked ties certain demonstrable effects on the functional neuroanatomy of the brain to much broader nondiagnostic conceptual categories of behavior and biological process. Scientists examining either the mediating (functional neuroanatomical), directional (stimulating, depressing), or outcome (behavior) categories might well point out that these identifications are also imperfect and vary with the concepts and measurements employed.

As Berger noted, different chemical classes can produce similar effects. For instance, Lovetrup (1967, p. 39) notes: "Drugs belonging to quite diverse groups have been observed to have very similar actions in biochemical systems. One of the essential problems in neuro-chemistry is, therefore, to establish some kind of chemical specificity of action for the various groups of the psychopharmaca. However, little of the sort has been achieved so far." Further, even simple descriptions of effects, as for example Berger's (1960) "stimulating" or "depressing" action require qualification. Amphetamines, for instance, in monkeys reduce high levels of certain kinds of activity while the same drug in the same animal increases low levels of that same activity, thus "the effect of psychotropic drugs seems to depend on the behavioral base level on which they are introduced" (Dureman, 1967, p. 18). This is a statement of the axiom that the action (effect) of a drug depends on the actual state of the system with which it interacts. One must also be reminded how inhibitory action can lead to stimulation or vice versa, for instance, a drug that depresses an inhibitory center in the brain releases inhibited behavior so that the observed effect is stimulation.

Further, effects (depending on what is measured) may vary with slight molecular differences among drugs within the same classification. For example, consider Petracek's comments, quoted by Clark and del Giudice (1970, pp. 166–167) with regard to the chemical and physical properties of a drug as these affect action at the receptor site (in a nerve cell), events that "are of key importance" to the understanding of drug action:

> A receptor site is very likely a discrete arrangement of atoms which forms a complex with the drug molecule in a precise manner by utilizing several types of weak bonding forces. Even slight changes in the structure of the drug molecule would be expected to affect the balance of the drug-receptor complex, and changes in one part of the molecule could be more critical than in others. . . . In addition, these receptor sites, which interact with the drug molecule, are themselves only a part of the extremely complex anatomical, chemical and electrical systems comprising the central nervous system. Therefore, extrapolations and conclusions based on structure—activity studies must be viewed with more caution in the case of the central nervous system than in other areas [of the body].

To complicate matters further, differences in action at receptor sites do not necessarily lead to different effects elsewhere in the central nervous system or in behavior and differing modes of action (aside from receptor sites, as, for example, effects on neurotransmitter substances or on enzyme systems that affect transmitters) can lead to apparently identical changes. As Jacobsen (1967, p. 14) says, "The same gross effect is obtained by agents acting on different sites or having different modes of action . . . [and] agents having a different mode of action or acting on different receptor sites may have apparently identical gross pharmacological effects."

By now it should be apparent that there are considerable problems in those straightforward "simple" classification systems, if there is any effort to link a description of drug classes to effects at any level (for example, molecular receptor sites, brain centers, specific behavior, general conduct). These difficulties in classification are not particular to Berger or any other scientist whose work is used here to illustrate difficulties. The problems arise from the present state of knowledge—and sometimes from our logic. Given inadequate information, the temptation to overgeneralize, and perhaps the allure of levels and concepts taken from a scientific discipline or profession other than one's own as hopefully being sounder, it is in order to warn the nonscientist that the apparent rigor or certainty of chemical, neuroanatomical, physiological, or behavioral concepts used even in simple (for example, chemical) and limited (for example, tranquilizers) systems can be misleading. Any drug classification system that leads from the apparently simple to the obviously complex broad classes of human conduct is, at present, inexact.

Berger's classification was limited to the functional category of tranquilizers. A much more complex chemical scheme is encountered if one moves beyond a limited class of compounds to embrace a greater variety of psychoactive drugs. An illustration of a wider classification of the psychopharmaca is that of Usdin (1970). The system presented is limited to phenothiazines (and related compounds), indoles, other heterocycles, aromatic compounds, and aliphatic compounds. Considering these groups, Usdin observes (p. 193), "There are no universally accepted definitions of terms and there are no clear-cut lines of demarcation between the various classes of drugs with psychotropic action." Usdin's system excludes, without comment, the opiates and synthetic analogues, the alcohols, the cannabinols (from cannabis), and a variety of other substances known to affect the central nervous system, producing altered moods and states of mind. Usdin's category of inclusion appears to be manufactured compounds employed primarily in Western medicine for the purpose of treating conduct diagnosed as a psychiatric disorder. Clearly, the group of drugs termed psychopharmaca or psychotropic can exclude compounds with known medical-psychiatric use (for example, opium and cannabis in Ayurvedic medicine) and may include compounds (LSD) without known medical applications. That substances widely used socially but not medically (tea, coffee, alcohol) are also excluded illustrates how unstated standards define chemical classifications. This point is made not in any sense to criticize Usdin (or Berger) whose careful work is used only illustratively and fully follows conventional procedures, but to show that classification systems that are straightforward and simple themselves are likely to be influenced by the operation of the orientation, interests, and values of given professions or, as anthropologists can show us, of cultures. Even within the rules of the chemical classification system, order may have to be imposed arbitrarily for—as Usdin implies—it is the judgment of the classifier as to whether one chemical structure is to be termed analogous to or different from another.

PHARMACOLOGICAL CLASSIFICATION

As soon as one moves from descriptions of chemical structure into classifications that are openly based on probable effects, one is involved within physiologically based pharmacological estimates. Some systems refer primarily to effects; some marry chemistry and pharmacology. Biochemistry, physiology, and related disciplines contribute strongly to work at this level. The pharmacological classifications now in use—embracing biochemical, neurophysiological, and clinical data—are widely accepted by pharmocologists as accurate and useful. Pharmacological considerations have been widely employed over recent decades in the development of classification systems that form the basis for recommended or actual legislation for control. The predominance of biochemically-physiologically based pharmacological systems integrated into psychiatric nomenclature and treatment goals constitutes the core of psychopharmacology today.

Insofar as these same medical concepts are applicable to uses of drugs that are considered drug abuse (that is, the disapproved, unsupervised, or uncontrolled social or private use of psychoactive substances), there can be hope that present classification systems will be applicable in the social (and psychological, moral, and political) sphere. There is, however, much dispute as to whether the medical model, with the associated public health approach, should be the primary one used in thinking about social and private drug use. The dispute, which bears directly on who should be given responsibility for classifying drugs and for proposing control measures, involves fundamental issues, for different groups have quite different ideas about the reasons for which drugs are used and about the nature and significance of the associated conduct or resulting effects.

An illustration of the marriage of chemical and pharmacological classification is found in a World Health Organization publication, *Dependence Liability of "Non-Narcotic" Drugs* (Isbell and Chrusciel, 1970). This work limits itself to drugs and herbs used socially and privately, for which there is evidence of the effects of stimulation, depression, hallucinations, or distortions in perception, thinking, or judgment and, additionally, which may produce dependence. The authors stipulate that drugs already under international narcotics control (opioids, coca leaves, cocaine, and cannabis) are excluded. Being careful to define the terms they employ (a drug, for example, is "any substance that, when taken into the living organism, may modify one or more of its functions" and drug abuse is "persistent or sporadic excessive drug use inconsistent with or unrelated to acceptable medical practice"), the authors proceed to set up the major pharmacological categories of effect (namely, central nervous system depressants and stimulants), plus the subjective (human) effect of the hallucinogens. Major categories that are derived from source and chemistry are, respectively, crude plant drugs and precursors. The authors exclude from their classification a number of substances with mind-altering effects that are used medically but that "do not appear to cause dependence or abuse," for example, many tranquilizers and antidepressants. Within their five major categories, these authors then classify by chemical description. For example, there are thirteen chemical types within their central nervous system depressant category. Their classification lists likely effects based on reports derived primarily from the scientific literature of chemistry, pharmacology, and, to a much lesser extent, psychiatry. Effects linked to classification are symptoms of intoxication, tolerance, psychic dependence, physical dependence, major dangers of abuse, and, as a rating by the authors, abuse potential.

This scholarly work demonstrates some of the hidden dilemmas in classification that are linked to outcome predictions. These are in no sense the fault of the classifiers but are built into probably all category-making endeavors in the drug field, which suffer the earlier noted problems of insufficient scientific information, diverse public standards for social and private drug use, and the pressure to make very limited scientific classification systems applicable to very broad social and moral issues. One sees, for example, that these authors, like most recognized authorities, emphasize drug evaluations based on chemical analysis, laboratory studies, and clinical reports. A search of their bibliography reveals very few studies that could be termed psychological, sociological, or epidemiological in nature, and none that address the problem of evaluation of effects from the standpoint of social or moral issues. For instance, only one investigation that bears on the conduct of marijuana users in a real-life population is included; it is from a study of the 1940s that was conducted in a restricted population.

Aside from the problem of the level of scientific data that is employed in making predictions as to drug effects—or to those more general predictions for "abuse potential" that bear direct implications for control—this classification scheme can be seen to employ quite different criteria for its major categories (precursors, crude plants, central nervous system effects, and subjective effects in humans are each a basis for a category). The effect classes are crude since depression and stimulation occur pharmacologically but are not necessarily visible behaviorally in normal dose ranges and the subjective effect of hallucination is, in fact, an unusual outcome in humans (Blum and Associates, 1964; Hollister, 1968).

Existing drug-effect evaluations are incorporated into building the classification for the authors and exclude the majority of psychotropics, since these are deemed to have less abuse potential. In this the classifiers commit no fault, for they set forth what they have done. One might assume the resulting scheme is essentially a listing of drugs that are not defined legally as narcotics and that, on the basis of primarily chemical and pharmacological studies, are deemed to have high probability of ill effects when used under unspecified conditions. This is not the case, for many of the substances included are also rated by the classifiers as having few ill effects and a low abuse potential. This occurs inevitably because the chemical categories to which the authors commit themselves include compounds that have little reported activity or that, since they appear useless, have not generated research as to their effects. One observes, however, that some psychoactives that are not narcotic but are not unknown to have ill effects are excluded—alcohol and tobacco most notably.

A major feature in the definition of abuse requires comment. The standard of abuse relies on a judgment of "excessive use . . . unrelated to acceptable medical practice." We take this to mean that drug use outside of medical practice is "abuse" if a physician considers it excessive. "Excessive" may refer to dosage exceeding ordinary therapeutic ones or possibly to the production of those toxic symptoms, signs of dependency, or "abuse dangers" that are ascribed to the drugs. If the former, one would need studies on the normal distribution of dosages by prescription and patient ingestion. The definitions of each of these phenomena, while certainly referring to real symptoms or behavior, are also subject to debate by persons who do not readily adhere to the conventional Western medical-psychiatric descriptions and inferences. The level of adequacy of the scientific literature is also such that scientists themselves debate the extent of these dangers. The nonscientist reader who relies on a table of classifications linked to outcomes may have a false sense of assurance if he is not sensitive to the practical considerations, cultural and professional bias, and matters of personal judgment that can intrude on the construction of the scheme. Most classifiers themselves know this; and, as Isbell and Chrusciel do, they give warning. However, the reader in search of certainty may not understand the full significance of the abbreviated cautions offered or of the magnitude of uncertainty inherent in honest definitions set forth.

As noted, pharmacological evaluations are the predominant current ones for evaluating psychoactive drugs for purposes of social control. The categories based on most probable clinical effects vary with the nosological bias of the classifier and with his assumptions about the most pertinent levels of data. As Jacobsen (1958) observed with regard to central nervous system depressants and classifications alone, "The whole field is becoming confusing for many pharmacologists and bewildering for many clinicians." Jacobsen, trying to clarify, listed classes of actions deemed pertinent and then sought mutual relationships among compounds producing like actions. This procedure leads to the construction of functional categories that may be unrelated to similarities/dissimilarities in chemical structure. Functional categories constructed in this manner depend entirely on the kind and level of information available about effects. Jacobsen limits himself to the pharmacological level, incorporating data on gross behavior in animal laboratory studies, spinal reflexes, effects on (brain) medullary and meso-diencephalic centers, on the extrapyramidal motor and reticular arousing systems of the brain and various electroencephalographic effects. At higher levels, his data base includes drug effects on the unlearned reactivity, on learned and stress-induced behavior, on self-stimulation of the brain, and on observations of several drugs acting together. When all these data are integrated, profiles of action (see also Jacobsen, 1964) emerge, which lead to the following classes: major tranquilizers, minor tranquilizers, hypnosedatives and tranquilosedatives, centrally acting antiacetylcholines and less clearly classified compounds that are called older compounds (for example, lithium salts) and transitional compounds (for example, azacyclonal). These functional categories are based on relatively "hard" evidence. The prediction problem occurs because these are primarily derived from animal studies. As Jacobsen says, when one wants to move to classifications based on clinical effects in humans, the adequacy of information is much less, and it is quickly found that either the estimates of action for new compounds or even knowledge of old ones is not very satisfactory. Progress, Jacobsen comments, requires that one "correlate as many as possible of the relevant biochemical, physiological, pharmacological, pathophysiological, and clinical facts and then hope that we or those who come after us may make something out of them."

At the level of pharmacological classification, one can add but little to Jacobsen's hopes. If one is interested in the broader field of nonmedical drug use, it is apparent that data from levels different from clinical-medical observations would also have to be employed.

Jacobsen's system and remarks are illustrative. Other pharmacologists offer slightly different functional categories that need not be reviewed here except to note that their nature depends on the data of interest to and available to the classifier and on how his logic works. However excellent the data and the logic, no classification system has been developed that, with regard to the psychoactives, successfully marries chemical structure to pharmacological action.

Particular problems in pharmacological classification are apparent when one focuses on cannabis. The Report on Cannabis of the Canadian (Le Dain) Commission of Enquiry into the Non-Medical Use of Drugs (1970, pp. 16–17) states:

> The pharmacological classification of cannabis is still the subject of much controversy. . . . Hollister voiced the opinion that "attempts to force it into some pharmacological cubby-hole are doomed to failure." . . . Domino argued that cannabis has ". . . only superficial relationships with other drugs." Cannabis has been compared to, and apparently has characteristics in common with a wide variety of drugs including alcohol, LSD and mescaline, nitrous oxide, amphetamines, atropine, opiate narcotics, barbiturates and the minor and major tranquillizers. Under various conditions and doses cannabis has been shown to have stimulant, sedative, analgesic and psychedelic effects. Some argue that marijuana should be classified as a sedative-hypnotic-general anesthesic like alcohol and nitrous oxide; others feel that it is a mixed stimulant-depressant; still others describe it as a mild hallucinogen . . . many feel it should be listed in a separate category. Paradoxically, cannabis has been shown to potentiate both the stimulant effects of amphetamines and the sedative effects of barbiturates in animals. Legally, cannabis has traditionally been classified with the opiate narcotics, and while they may share some euphorogenic and analgesic properties, they are otherwise quite distinct pharmacologically. . . . It is clear that any attempt to completely specify a pharmacological classification for cannabis must include a clear delineation of dose, as well as the time and setting of use. The Commission, for the purposes of this report, classified cannabis with the psychedelic-hallucinogenic compounds.

Paton (1972), reviewing the cannabis evidence, concludes, "There seems no rational basis for drawing a line between cannabis and LSD, the amphetamines or the less potent opiates."

The Commission's insistence that there must be a "clear delineation of dose" calls attention to another feature of pharmacological classification that, while very apparent to pharmacologists, can be overlooked by laymen. It is that dose, along with potency, frequency, and manner of administration (along with many other variables) determines effects. Thus, the effects upon which pharmacological classifications are based usually reflect experimental work over a wide dosage range, with standard doses being specified as likely to achieve particular effects.

When classification schemes move away from the laboratory to encompass social and private drug use, the estimate of effects suffers from lack of knowledge of how users will employ the substance—in what doses, forms, in combination with what other drugs, and how often and how administered. As Way (1969) said, "A lot of caffeine can be more harmful to the individual than a bit of heroin." Given these problems, Birdwood (1972), noting that street use "is seldom played by pharmacological rules," proposes that pharmacological classifications intended for the description of social use—if not for public action— be based on the mode of administration of any drug or of particular groups of drugs; sniffing, smoking, by mouth, or by injection. Such a suggestion does not deal with a drug such as amphetamine, which can be swallowed, inhaled, or injected with similar results. Furthermore, one must be concerned with the identity of the drug; injection of physiological saline is hardly the same matter as heroin injection.

EXPERIMENTAL BEHAVIORAL CLASSIFICATION

At the next level, extending beyond internal bodily analysis, are behavioral measures either in animals or in man. Experimental psychology is the major discipline involved. In the laboratory it is possible to combine observations of internal processes or events with behavioral data, for surgical and other interventions allow this with animals (see, for example, Delgado, 1962). Necessary surgical or pharmacological interventions may also allow limited observations on humans. At any level at which data are obtained, it is possible to construct classes of drugs based upon their similar or dissimilar effects under experimental conditions.

A wide range of controlled observations have been made; the focus of attention and the sophistication of the method are limited only by the interests and resources of the research workers. Drug effects have been measured in animals by a variety of methods, some of which are by now both standard and sophisticated (see Tedeschi and Tedeschi, 1968). Otis and Crisman (1966) stated that in humans there have been measures of information-processing, psychomotor function, vehicle driving, vision, attention, memory, learned behavior, stress behavior, moods, interpersonal and group interaction (for example, aggression, affection, reliance on others for help), dreaming and dream content, drive states, and so forth. Variations in behavior during such experiments are related to a variety of factors other than drugs; these include physiological states, the subject's attitudes and expectations, environmental conditions, personality, and so forth. Not the least of these influencing variables are genetic. In consequence, behavioral measures, in animals, tied to genetic features, are likely to figure in the more sophisticated drug classifications tied to specific experimental effects.

Insofar as behavior is shown to be affected in the direction of reduced or distorted performance, measured from a normal base line, the concept of behavioral toxicity may be employed (Cole, J. O., 1960). In some instances, that which to the psychologist is behavioral toxicity is characterized by the clinical observer as an adverse, untoward, or side effect (Shader and DiMascio, 1970). As earlier noted, a side effect in one treatment may be a desired outcome in another. A psychoactive drug that produces impairment in normal humans can reduce impairment in persons who are mentally ill or functioning badly because of fatigue or worry, and the like. The folk wisdom that "one man's poison is another man's pleasure" applies here.

For the most part, classification systems based on behavioral experiments are limited to the comparisons of several drugs on a given psychological function. One learns, for example, that meprobamate improves stress performance on tasks requiring motor skills, eye-hand coordination, and persistence in normal humans, whereas chlorpromazine depresses that performance (Holliday and Dillie, 1958). The amphetamines improve some types of cognitive performance (Hurst and Weidner, 1966), whereas most other drugs do not. No extant classification system for all psychoactive substances is based on the systematic (weighted or algebraic) combination of the major psychological laboratory tests for behavioral toxicity. Any such discussion necessarily would have to deal with features such as dosage, time, frequency and manner of administration, and the like. For example, many drugs are polyphasic: low doses of amphetamine improve psychomotor performance by preventing fatigue (or even lead to an increment before fatigue), while large doses impair as flight of ideas of behavior stereotypy occurs. With sufficiently complex data it is theoretically possible to state the probabilities that, for any given group of subjects, particular effects are the most likely under given conditions of testing. Since subgroups are likely to experience unique responses, as for example those with genetic idiosyncracies, the overall accuracy of estimate is increased as general predictions for undifferentiated populations are refined into discrete statements for homogeneous subgroups.

CLINICAL PHARMACOLOGICAL CLASSIFICATIONS

Clinical classifications are those made by physicians as they evaluate their patients and the responses patients show to drugs given. The orientation is medical; psychiatrists predominate. Just as the line between physiological, pharmacological, and behavioral levels is arbitrary, so our classification of clinical pharmacology as distinct from behavioral is arbitrary. At the human behavioral level, the emphasis is on experiments and controlled measures by means of tests and objective ratings. At the strictly clinical level, evaluation is by expert judgment, impressions, and other more subjective (in the observer) measures. The systematic application of both clinical diagnostic and objective measures characterizes research that has been of particular value not only in assessing drug classification by effects but in patient classification based on drug response.

An illustration can be found in the extensive drug evaluations done in experiments in U.S. Veterans Administration (VA) hospitals (Goldberg, Cole, and Klerman, 1966), and by the U.S. National Institute of Mental Health (NIMH). These large-scale programs examined antipsychotic agents, linking treatment outcomes not only to drugs but to individual patient characteristics. The emerging classifications were not of drugs alone but of kinds of drugs working best on kinds of people. For example, comparison of three phenothiazines and placebo yielded a finding that one drug was as ineffective as no drug (placebo) whereas a second phenothiazine (chlorpromazine) was particularly useful in patients who before treatment were very agitated. The third was useful in patients who had been hallucinating and were delusional. Overall, chlorpromazine was most effective; therefore, ordering these drugs by efficacy, one emerges with a classification scheme of most and least useful for given patient syndromes. (Caffrey, Hollister, and others, 1970, pp. 429–449). A more complex interactional experiment illustrates how a prediction can gain better accuracy if data on the physician or physician-patient interaction are included in the matrix. For example, Rickels and Cattell (1969, pp. 126–140) found that improvement on some drugs depended on the type of psychiatrist and the amount of time under his care as well as on the kind of patient and kind of drug. Balint, Hunt, and others (1970) also found it useful to look at doctor characteristics better to understand what patients would receive repeat prescriptions of psychoactive drugs. Attention to the drug administrator or prescriber suggests (Blum and Wolfe, 1972) that there are in the physician consistent traits that allow one to estimate the kind and amount of drugs he prescribes and, consequently, the drug use of his patients.

There is very widespread use of psychoactive compounds in medical care. Reduction in the number of hospitalized psychiatric patients has occurred in those regions where drugs have been available (usually, such reductions are most marked when medication has been used in conjunction with modern patient management methods, for instance therapeutic communities and community mental health care). Clinical psychiatrists have tended to utilize existing psychiatric diagnoses and not to develop new nosologies based on the predictability of response to particular drugs among patients with well-defined characteristics as measured by carefully applied ratings or tests. Therefore, classification based on drug effects on psychiatric populations has not been as specific as the kind of work seen in the VA and NIMH evaluations, nor has it taken advantage of sophisticated clinical observations and statistical analysis of interaction effects to develop more accurate drugs-with-people categories of drug effects by type of person (Schou, 1967, pp. 457–463).

The weaknesses in clinical estimations either of diagnosis or of drug effects are considerable. These occur because of the low reliability of diagnosis per se and of nonobjective measures of drug effects. For instance, it has been shown (Ash, 1949; Terris, 1959) that psychiatrists looking at the same patient are likely not to agree on the diagnosis. Further, patients sharing the same diagnostic label can have widely differing traits. As Okun (1970, p. 386) states:

> In the design of psychopharmacologic trials, clinicians have become involved with therapeutic labels and classification, for example antipsychotic drugs, antianxiety drugs, antidepressants, etc. The psychoactive drugs available for clinical trial and for clinical use do not appear selective and surely cannot distinguish between a neurosis and a psychosis or between such symptoms as anxiety and depression.* Such terms defy precise definition. Patients with the same diagnosis may be quite heterogeneous and their symptoms and disabling features may require different therapy. Psychiatric nosology in its present state leaves much to be desired.

When a classification scheme designates a drug as a tranquilizer or antidepressant, these labels imply effective action on agitated anxious or depressed patients respectively. Yet even if such action occurs, it may not be the only action of the drug. Consider Usdin's (1970) remarks: "Five (psychotropic) actions have been stressed: antipsychotic, antianxiety, antidepressant, stimulant and hallucinogenic. There is no intent to imply that this action is either the only action which the compound has or even that it is necessarily the major action resulting from administration of the compound. . . . The author has been compelled . . . to interpret reported results into one of the broad classes."

Also, the functional classification of a drug may be dose dependent; for example, a minor tranquilizer in ordinary doses may calm but at higher doses may sedate. As Hordern (1968, p. 117) notes, "The difference between a hypnotic and a sedative is purely one of degree and in practical terms usually depends on the dose that is administered." Effects depend, too, on when in a patient's life, disease course, or emotional cycle a drug is given.

In the development of psychoactive substances, some of the unexpected or undesired effects (side effects) of early compounds were capitalized upon to form the basis for new drugs utilizing these effects (Hordern and Caldwell, 1970). The major tranquilizer, chlorpromazine, developed this way from earlier drugs used as antiparasitics and derivatives used as antihistaminics and to reduce shock in surgery. Yet this same multiplicity of effects—some of which are specific pharmacological consequences of the drug and some of which are due to other influences—means that a given nomenclature may be but a key word emphasizing one among many probable as well as possible outcomes. Rickels (1969) accommodates to this by providing multiple classification of the same psychoactive drug depending upon the functional category of interest.

---

* Judging by personal communication (1973), the Kalants would disagree, pointing out that drugs can have differential effect either on different patients or the same patient in different states. They note that amphetamine, for example, can decrease depression and increase anxiety in the same patient.

Furthermore, the drug effect in a person varies with the period following administration (time-action), as one sees when the very active drunk goes to sleep. Paradoxical effects also occur; for instance, some people are put to sleep by antidepressants, and amphetamines (stimulants) may quiet hyperactive children. This latter feature of drug action suggests differences in effects by age and is of special importance when considering how drug control measures may have to be tailored to distinct age groups in the population.

The unanticipated or multiple effects that in one case lead to new medical uses can in others account for the attractiveness of a drug for nonsocial and private uses. Morphine or heroin used medically for reducing pain awareness also produces, in a small portion of the population (Beecher, 1959), a euphoric state, which is so appealing that further such experiences are sought and, afterward, in some, (physical) dependency (addiction) ensues. That process of nonmedical use of opiates is a complicated one and cannot be attributed to the drug alone, for certainly special characteristics of a person contribute to his undertaking such activities. From the standpoint of classification for purposes of public action, the side effects found in medical use may become central features for drug categories applied to social and private use. For instance, there are no known cases of addiction to phenothiazine, presumably because the side effects—"chemical straitjacketing"—are so unpleasant.

Jaffe's work (1970) illustrates one such system. His classification is based on observations of users and of drugs self-administered for subjective effects in a compulsive fashion. Observing that "the relationship between the pharmacological and the behavioral phenomena is not entirely clear" (that is, some of the compulsively employed drugs produce tolerance and physical dependency and others do not), he creates four categories: hallucinogenic agents, central nervous system stimulants, central nervous system depressants, and narcotic analgesics (morphinelike drugs). Jaffe employs two definitions of abuse: "unsanctioned" use and addiction. He discriminates between addiction, in which drug-related conduct dominates lives, and physical dependence, which can occur without a life being centered about drug-getting and drug-taking. Resting part of his classification scheme not on the effects of use but on the consequences of withdrawal (what happens when a drug on which one is physically dependent is no longer available), he places a diverse group of chemicals into a single category (central nervous system depressants) because withdrawal symptoms and subsequent medical management are similar. His central nervous system depressant group thus includes alcohol, barbiturates, meprobamate (and other tranquilizers), anesthetic gases, and the like. Pharmacologically, one could argue that the narcotic analgesics (for example, morphine and heroin), are also central nervous system depressants. However, not only is withdrawal different but also there is crosstolerance only within this category. People suffering withdrawal from alcohol will be relieved when given barbiturates, but opiate addicts will receive only that relief associated with nonspecific reduction of alertness. Cross-tolerance as such does not exist between opiates and barbiturates.

This classification addresses, not the probable effects on psychiatric patients, but the appeals of a drug to nonmedical users. The criteria for the scheme are diverse: withdrawal symptoms, cross-tolerance, medical management of withdrawal, unsanctioned use, addiction, and physical dependence. The scheme embraces almost all the potent psychoactive substances and attributes to them all an "abuse" potential, although Jaffe's hallucinogenic category (in which he includes cannabis) excludes addiction and physical dependency. This conceptual broadness poses a problem and a reminder; the problem is that specificity is limited to the recommended medical management of withdrawal. The reminder is that most psychoactive drugs can be used socially and privately. When that occurs, some individuals become so drug-involved that their lives center around obtaining and using these substances and being with other people likewise engaged.

Jaffe also approaches the business of categorization systems with the drug user in mind. He comments that "drug users are a heterogeneous group . . . which uses different drugs for different reasons with widely differing social, psychological and physical consequences." Such observations herald the classification of users according to their persons, motives, lifestyles, and reactions. One finds that the greater the interest of the scientist or official in social and private use, the more likely it is that his classification system will focus on the user as much as or more than on the drugs. As the chemist classifies by drug structure and the psychiatric clinician by drug function in relationship to the primary symptoms of his patient, so the person with responsibilities for influencing private and social drug use tends to classify by kind of user and setting for use. This latter orientation is encouraged by the facts that most humans who do use psychoactive substances use a variety of them and that, at least in these times and in Western countries, those who use any drug in a disapproved way are likely to use a variety of drugs in disapproved or sometimes dangerous ways.

Classification according to "danger" may be found in simplified schemes used in legislation, as for example, in education by means of warning or recommendations for restraints on distribution. Pharmacologists giving an overall rating by degree of hazard or danger usually do so with many reservations, knowing they are mixing risks of toxicity, dependency, withdrawal severity, and the like. However, persons hearing or reading such ratings may take them to be absolute. One attempt to summarize the pharmacological and social evidence is offered by Irwin (1970). He ranks in this global way from the most to the least dangerous for self-administration, in order, glue (sniffing), methamphetamine, alcohol, cigarettes, barbiturates and hypnotics, heroin and related narcotics, LSD and other hallucinogens, and, as least hazardous, marijuana.

Irwin's system has the advantages of simplicity, inclusiveness, and audacity. His classification, based on clinical estimates of effects under self-administration, does not, as many other systems do, exclude very common private or social psychoactive uses, for it addresses itself to reported practices among youth as the basis for selection, thus glue, cigarettes, and alcohol are

included. The disadvantages rest in the usual lack of standard criteria by which
to create such orders and, as noted, the likelihood that qualifications by the
scientist are lost as the level of sophistication of the reader or controller is reduced. Indeed, one can conceive of (and recommend!) a study of classification
systems on the basis of their practical impact, that is, the extent to which nonscientists understand the criteria and definitions employed and accept the
reservations inherent.

With regard to such general schemes, the remarks of the Kalants (1971,
pp. 98, 99) might be kept in mind: "The classification of any drug effect as
either 'beneficial' or 'harmful' depends on the scale of values of the person who
is making the classification. . . . We are unlikely ever to agree completely on
a uniform scale of classification of various drug effects as either beneficial or
harmful. However, even if this were possible, there would still remain the problem of estimating the total amount of good and the total amount of harm resulting to a whole society from drug use by its members."

The Kalants also observe, with regard to all classification schemes for
drugs which rank substances on any scale of danger or harm: "This ranking or
hierarchy of drugs is quite inaccurate because it is not based on a single set of
criteria. . . . Besides being incorrect, this ranking of drugs tends to confuse
issues by focusing attention primarily upon the drugs rather than the people
who use them. . . . The point to be emphasized is that the degree of risk is
related not so much to the specific drug which is used as to the amount, frequency and manner of its use."

The interests of the classifier influence what he does. If the clinical or
practical concern is more with patients or others coming for help—or with
people who are noticed for their troubles—the classifier is likely to emphasize
the user and his traits. In this fashion, Bowman and Jellinek (1942) identified
twenty-five separate categories of problem drinkers. Jellinek reordered these
into a five-part classification reflecting what he believed to be the major types
of drinking associated with identifiable problems. His classification rested on
the presumed motives for drinking or drinker traits (including dependence and
compulsive use), the dangerous results to the user, symptoms of overuse, and
style of drinking (frequency, amounts). The particular form of the drug (beer,
wine, spirits) does not figure at all in this approach. What is emphasized is the
classification of drinkers by the (presumed) developmental history of their
alcohol use, a system that is useful etiologically and in clinical practice.

CLASSIFICATIONS BASED ON SUBJECTIVE STATES

There are two kinds of classifications based on subjective states. One
rests on cognition, that is, on the fund of information a person has; the other
rests on a person's feeling and awareness. The cognitive classification, information, is modified psychologically by how an individual gathers information
that is available to him and how he interprets it. Since information tends to
vary with a person's environment, the subjective classification state that is

cognitive anticipates some of the criteria for drug user classification in the next section on social classifications. Sociology and psychology contribute the methods for work in this area.

The other kind of subjective state rests on such states of mind and feeling as, for example, euphoria, despair, alertness, mystical experiences, and felt insights. These are close to clinical effects of the sort considered in the previous section, except that some classifiers insist that such experiences are not in the biological domain but are, rather, religious matters or expressions of human potential for insight, aesthetic experience, and the like. Since users of cannabis and hallucinogens are themselves likely to adhere to the latter view, proposals for classifications of drugs and persons based on their joint capabilities for producing such states probably reflect sensitivity to user's beliefs and experiences. Since such classification may be proposed by anyone experiencing drug effects, no methodology from a professional discipline is required. If, however, one wishes to create a science of such states the methods are derived from the discipline of psychology.

Information

Feldman's (1972) system includes subjective knowledge of drug effects as one component that allows the ranking of persons-with-drugs according to their most likely forms of use, its significance to them, and the risk entailed. In other work (Chein, Gerard, and others, 1964), subjective knowledge of possibly dangerous outcomes was one factor associated before onset of use with the risk of beginning heroin; for instance, youngsters with less knowledge of heroin risks and less contact with a family figure capable of transmitting such information were more likely to experiment with the drug.

Sensations

Subjective effects may be used more extensively as the basis for classification. The continuing Lexington work of Haertzen and colleagues (1963) provides examples. They use a research instrument that is completed by narcotic addicts working as experimental subjects in the hospital. The use of these scales allows one to discriminate drugs by their being like or unlike one another as sensed by the user. Special effects can also be categorized so that one has the choice of placing a drug in an existing category—one like existing substances—or creating a new class.

Preferences

The careful laboratory work of Haertzen and others is paralleled in real life when users themselves compare the effects of one drug with those of another. Their preferences, whether or not the user is aware of them, allow researchers to construct classification systems based on preferred drugs that "go together," as opposed to those that do not have common styles of use. For instance, studying large samples of college students in the United States, Blum and his associates (1969b) conducted a factor analysis to reveal communalities and substructures linking drug use. There was, first, a general disposition toward psychoactive drug use as such—a willingness to use a variety of drugs for many different reasons. More precise were subsets of dispositions. One factor is of drug use by source with separate components identified as conventional social-drug use, illicit-exotic use, and reliance on prescription drugs. Self medication and home remedy preferences appeared linked to prescription uses. A second factor was one of preference for similar drug effects; particularly strong were preferences for anxiety and activity reduction. A third was preference based on manner of administration, that is, oral, sniffing, injection, or smoking. Other factors, apparently not related to subjective preference as were the first three, included correlational factors bearing on the degree of immersion in use (for example, drug involvement, a feature discussed as classificatory under social classification), a typology of membership in distinct user groups (being an acid head, speed freak, junkie, or the like).

In another preference study, Blum and his associates (1972b) took case histories, including lifetime drug use, of (mostly young) California illicit drug dealers. Creating a four-component index of preference based on changes in use over time, the lifetime favorite drugs of these dealers were found to be, in order: in Class I, tobacco, cannabis, and opiates (mostly heroin); in Class II, tranquilizers, alcohol, cocaine, hallucinogens, amphetamines, and sedatives. Least preferred on the index measure were special substances such as glue sniffing, nitrous oxide, paint thinner, and the like. The authors propose that this index of preference, if verified, would lead to estimations (classifications) of which drugs are most attractive over time for drug-involved young people.

Awareness

A less empirical scheme in which subjective experience alone defines drug classifications is proposed by Weil (1972b, pp. 330–331).

> What we need is a new science of consciousness based on subjective experience rather than objective physiology. . . . I predict that from an experiential viewpoint, many unifying principles of drug states will become visible. In the pharmacological model, there is some unity. . . . But pharmacology offers no clue why the psychological changes of a marijuana high have much in common with those of an LSD trip or why heroin users may be able to satisfy their needs for a certain experience by inhaling nitrous oxide, a general anesthetic.

Weil believes that

> The desire to alter consciousness is an innate psychological drive. . . . Such practices appear to be universal. . . . They seem to be door-

ways to the next stages of evolutionary development of the human nervous system. . . . Altered states of consciousness appear to have potential for strongly positive psychic development.

Weil proceeds to outline a classification system that combines physiological effects and dangers, social circumstances of use (including the effect of the control system on observed styles of use and outcomes; for example, effect of the criminal law on narcotics users), measurable behavioral effects, pain levels, and the capability for inducing euphoria and altered states of consciousness. He classes marijuana by itself, stating (pp. 335–336) it has

> virtually no significant* pharmacological actions. . . . It provides a high with minimal physiological accompaniments. . . . It is useless to study marijuana in the pharmacological laboratory, because there is no physiological handle on the phenomenon under consideration. Except for the possibility of lung disease related to chronic inhalation, there is no evidence that marijuana is physically harmful. . . . It seems wise to think of marijuana as a class unto itself, no more closely related to the hallucinogens than to the sedative-hypnotics. Its unique chemical structure is consistent with this idea.

Weil (p. 344) proposes:

> Provision for the experience of altered states of consciousness in growing children.
> Incorporation of the experience into society for positive ends.
> Encouragement of individuals to satisfy their needs for altered consciousness by means that do not require external tools. . . .
> The first step need be nothing more than to stop what we are now doing to prevent us from reaching that goal. And that is nearly everything we are doing in the name of combating drug abuse.

As a position paper rather than carefully documented scheme, Weil's classification and control measures necessarily lack scientific documentation. Any system that explicitly excludes objective evidence as necessary criteria in favor of subjective evaluations cannot logically be asked to adhere to objectivity rather than subjectivity in its construction. One basic assumption is testable: it is that the seeking of mind-altering experience is universal. Weil's proposals are in the direction of reducing controls (see also Weil, 1972a). He proposes a reverse stepping-stone theory; that use of marijuana will lead to the abandonment of drugs in favor of other means to produce mind-altered states. His hypothesis is

---

* What Weil means by "significant" is unclear, for cannabis has many measurable pharmacological actions.

testable. As with other control proposals that affect the lives of billions of people, one hopes that objective evidence would be sought before public action would be taken.

SOCIAL CLASSIFICATIONS

Social classifications are those based on the social behavior and environmental setting of the drug user rather than, as previously, on a drug's clinical effects and the limited behavior that is of interest to clinicians in constructing classifications based on drug-person interaction for the purposes of estimating therapeutic risks or planning treatment. Social classifications rely on information about what people in real life really do and act with drugs, and how and why they employ them, and how drug use is intertwined with their personalities and lifestyles. The contributing disciplines are, primarily, social psychology, sociology, and anthropology.

Birdwood (1972) sets forth definitions of use and effects basic to a social classification system, which must be "comprehensive enough to encompass what goes on in the real world [and] based on how people actually behave and the circumstances in which they do it." Under his scheme, there is no estimate of benefit or harm, and no distinction is made between medical and nonmedical consumption. Further, *abuse* is defined by local values only, that drug use which is neither medically approved nor socially acceptable in a particular society. It is Birdwood's intent to specify culture context as carefully as dosage and manner of administration when categorizing.

A simple example of a social classification can be taken from the work of Tinklenberg and Woodrow (1974). Young delinquents using barbiturates (secobarbital) on the streets (without social control, in gang settings) are more likely to show violent aggressive behavior than those same young delinquents using the same drug in a laboratory under different controls and expectations, than those same young delinquents in either setting taking amphetamine instead of barbiturates, and than medical students taking the same barbiturate in the laboratory setting. Another illustration comes from criminal statistics (Molof, 1967; K. Roberts, personal communication, 1969), which, without information on setting, show that teen-age delinquents who are violent (assaultive) are more likely to be drinkers than are youths who are arrested for nonviolent acts. Opiate-using delinquents had a life history of violence greater than nonopiate arrested illicit users. If one is interested in likely drug effects, he must know the characteristics of the person using the drug and the nature of the setting in which he uses it. Both features are contained in social classifications.

Another example of a person and setting scheme comes from the work of Feldman (1972), who made careful observations on street gangs in a large city in the United States, attending to which young men began to use which illicit drug, which ones continued to use which drug, and what reputations they developed in connection with their social and drug use status. He identified as important for prediction each person's subjective knowledge of available illicit drugs (including awareness of feeling states induced), his estimates of risk (specifically as physical harm, addiction potential, danger of parental discovery, danger of police discovery, and danger from like-drug-using companions), and his social role or status (in the street jargon of users in the community studied: least admired are the faggots, ass-holes or jerks; then solid guys; then tough guys; and, most admired, crazy guys). All these elements were tied together by con- gruity or consonance, that is, the extent to which effects, risks, and group status were compatible or incompatible. From these, Feldman constructed a classifica- tion of drug preferences for likely use, both present and future, linked to sustain- ing or enhancing a street reputation. Feldman's logic—and its predictive utility— links illicit drug availability, effects, social and health dangers, preferred activities, and actual and desired group roles into a sociological drug classification system. In the form presented, it is limited to the setting studied.

Brotman and Freedman (1970) outline social categories by describing the lives of heroin users with respect to their involvement in conventional as opposed to criminal activities and the degree of overlap of these. Another user typology, found in Preble and Casey (1969), attends to the kind of involvement in the heroin life on New York City streets. There the classification proceeds according to the heroin buying and selling activities. Following Preble and Casey, Hughes (1972) and his colleagues (Hughes, Barker, Crawford, Jaffe, 1972; Hughes and Crawford, 1972; Hughes, Senay, Parker, 1972) elaborated a system that shows interrelationships among social position in a heroin "copping" com- munity, drug buying and selling, honest work levels and capability, interpersonal adequacy, psychiatric appraisal, and likelihood of entering and staying in drug treatment programs. Their results show how much predictable individual varia- tion occurs in traits and behavior within that which is elsewhere (Eddy, Halbach, Isbell, Seevers, 1965) considered a single drug-person category, that is, "drug dependency of the morphine (heroin) type." Again one sees that social criteria add predictive power and complexity so that the real-world correlates of use can be specified.

Folk Typologies and Street Pharmacology

Information on drugs and people that is derived from user groups, as in the work of Feldman, Hughes and his colleagues, and also Preble and Casey allows one to begin to look at the world from the viewpoint of the user. The social world seen from the inside is likely to be more differentiated and more complex than is ordinarily seen from the outside (Kosviner, Mitcheson, and others, 1968). Consider adult social drinkers who from experience know that there are many different alcoholic beverages, many ways to prepare them, quite different effects obtainable, and a wide range of short-term and long-term behavior among their acquaintances in association with alcohol. Among those who use alcohol socially the simple fact that another person is known to have taken a drink does not tell us much about that person; no stereotypes are involved. In consequence, that information about simple use is considered insignificant and does not lead either to major characterization of the person or to recommendations for urgent government action on his or society's behalf.

Among cannabis users, as Goode (1970) and also Zinberg and Robertson (1972) have pointed out, cannabis use, like recreational drinking, may be but a minor matter. To the outsider, however, information that a person uses cannabis may be sufficient to invoke a full image of the cannabis user—as delinquent, hippie, lazy, and therefore deserving of restraint by law. Heroin users are probably more likely to be stereotyped and uniformly classed, even though within the heroin-using community there are many variations in forms of use, commitments to legality, behavior in association with the drug, other drugs used, and receptiveness to treatment or rehabilitation proposals. Thus, the classifications of their world employed by heroin users are likely to be more complex than as well as different from those used by those of the "straight" world viewing the heroin scene. The straight-world judgments and descriptions that are incorporated into public action programs may diverge widely from either the actuality of conduct or the need within the heroin community; therefore, there may well be marked discrepancy between the receptiveness to programs by heroin users and the responses expected from them by legislators, physicians, police officers, and others. On the other hand, if the way the straight world orders its data about heroin users should be compatible with how those users live and how they see things and further if the straight-world classification leads to action proposals that somehow fit the beliefs, interests, or needs of heroin users, there might be greater concordance between the legislative expectation and its impact. The foregoing constitutes, not a requirement for classification, but a proposal for evaluating the classification of drugs and persons or the impact of controls by availing oneself of the additional information derived from knowledge of the drug-using world and how those in it live and what they believe.

Involvement

There are other sociological or anthropological approaches to classification. Some, for example, are keyed to an existing drug that is socially employed and order the people who use it according to their activities. A central concept that allows the prediction of activities—and of reported subjective effects—is that of involvement. Involvement is akin to Jaffe's (1970) notion of dominance or addiction; however, those investigators who have a social orientation tend to discount the psychiatric evaluation of compulsive ingestion and the implication that the drug dominates the user's life. *Immersion* is an equivalent social term.

Goode (1970) shows that it is possible quite accurately to predict drug-related activities (for example, engaging in illicit drug traffic), if one knows how often a person uses marijuana, to what extent his friends use it, and whether or not other illicit drugs are also regularly used. Johnson (1971) adds a further qualification that allows even greater predictive accuracy: those who traffic in marijuana are also more likely to have heroin-using acquaintances. Such findings tell us nothing about marijuana classification, but they do illustrate how users can be classified so as to allow very accurate estimates of one kind of drug-related activity. Such ordering of variables associated with marijuana dealing also make it clear that marijuana is not, of and by itself, predisposing to criminal trafficking conduct. Likewise, marijuana does not "lead" pharmacologically to other drugs; that is, no biological deficit is created that requires another drug. Yet involvement with marijuana—or other illicit substances—is associated with the risk of increasing interest in and experimentation with other drugs. If heroin is available, it can become one of the drugs tried by the involved user.

Knowledge of the determining action of social and behavioral variables can prevent the error of assuming that ingestion of the drug would by itself lead to a particular criminality or to other drug use. Although the work has yet to be done, one could readily assume that a similar set of behavioral variables, preferably supplemented by information about family background and personality, knowledge of genetics, biochemical idiosyncracies, and social setting would allow one to say which persons who try heroin would be likely to become dependent or involved in the heroin life. Not all users of heroin are addicted (Sackman, 1971). There is evidence for familial (Blum and Associates, 1972a), personality and neighborhood (Chein, Gerard, and others, 1964), and lifestyle (Preble and Casey, 1969) factors as influential—plus the inference of biochemical idiosyncrasy (Beecher, 1959). Therefore, present classification systems that attribute "high abuse potential" to heroin (or other drugs) could be made more accurate if such general statements of possible but by no means inevitable effects were made specific, that is, conditional upon variables acting in addition to the drug to produce a particular form of conduct—or subjective response—of interest.

Another illustration of the prediction of involvement is found in Aberle's (1966) work with Navajo peyote users. This hallucinogenic drug is used by some North American Indians in religious rites. The opposition of most Navajo Indians to the use of peyote can be shown to be due to its symbolic aspects. The cult of users is felt to threaten conventional Navajo ways and is incompatible with goals of most Indians for tribal development. Opposition is, however, directed toward the drug itself and to presumed drug effects: unbridled sexuality and loss of self-control. Investigation by outside observers has shown that both of these effects are nonexistent. Those Indians who do become peyote-involved find a variety of satisfactions; indeed, the more varied the satisfactions expressed by an individual, the greater his involvement in the cult. Early use is best predicted by simple opportunity for access to it. Within groups having equivalent opportunities, people who have suffered economic loss are more likely to begin using peyote. Such losses are measured by livestock ownership losses in particular; a correlate is anxiety as measured by frightening dreams. Involvement is also associated with greater contact with individuals within the cult and a reduction of associations with Indians who are not in the cult. As in the case of marijuana, one-time use of the peyote itself is but a crude predictor of later heavy involvement. Greater accuracy in predicting who will become involved depends on data about availability, the presence of cult members, the economic status of a region, and anxiety suffered by individuals.

Whether that involvement is good or indifferent or bad depends upon the values of the observer. If the observer is a non-Navajo scholar (typically an anthropologist), peyote use is not considered bad in itself or in its effects. Within the Navajo tribe, however, non-users tend to consider use of peyote as drug "abuse." A generalization may be derived here to the effect that "insider" and "outsider" (H. S. Becker, 1963) group judgments of one another can be harsh and can center on drug use as a central discriminating basis for such judgments. "Objective" outsiders may see the significance of drug use quite differently. Values and emotions of this sort can obviously contribute to the place a drug is given in a classification scheme that incorporates notions of abuse.

Impact of Regulation

When governments intervene to alter drug availability or to educate, punish, or treat users, the programs used are likely to alter the environments in which people live. It is theoretically possible and practically desirable to order, that is, to classify, such programs themselves according to the persons they affect, what environments they alter, and under what conditions they are effective.

People and places, as well as substances, are affected by regulations. Better understanding of regulatory rationale, as well as consequences, may result from the social analysis of regulations. For example, Zacune and Hensman (1971), using historical evidence, credit reduction of alcoholism prevalence to English pub laws that set up controls on the time and place of drinking in two eras. David Musto (oral communication, 1972), citing M. Cameron (1931), credits stringent repressive measures employed by the Chinese government from 1898 to 1912 with the control of opium use there. In contrast, the Iranian government reported at meetings of the United Nations Narcotics Commission that as of 1970 the result of its opium control measures was to increase heroin use.

Blum and his associates (1972b), in studying the impact of arrest on drug dealers, discriminated within the dealer group various subgroups differentially affected by arrest or its threat. For example, one group of middle-class casual dealers appeared deterred over time by illegality and threat of arrest, although they suffered low actual risk of arrest. Successful middle-class dealers, also at low actual risk of arrest, were not deterred. A group of lower-class dealers who were heavily involved in drug use but were economically unsuccessful in dealing appeared deterred; they were at high risk of arrest. Another group of lower-class dealers, also heavily involved in drugs and in other crime, were successful economically and socially through dealing; although often arrested, they were not deterred. McGlothlin (1973) finds the overall risk of arrest for marijuana traffickers between Mexico and the United States to be high. Blum and his associates (1973), in studying local police departments, could show how risk varied with enforcement activities by locale in association with functional (not public) police policies for priority targeting.

The foregoing do not illustrate a classification scheme. They do suggest that one might order kinds of regulation through law enforcement by kind of drug use by kind of population by place and time to create a scale showing high to low impact measured by drug behavior change. The same kind of ordering could be applied to educational preventive endeavors and, as is often recommended (Tinklenberg and Woodrow, 1974), to treatment impact.

Integrating Information

Thinking about the elements in Feldman's (1972) system, recalling those of Isbell and Chrusciel (1970), and noting the various components found by factor analysis to distinguish styles of drug use, as in those sociopsychopharmacological studies that simultaneously examine types of drugs and types of people, it is apparent that information from various levels of observation is usefully employed in constructing classification schemes. Although such an integration of data is implied in most systems beyond those of medicinal chemistry, the need for systematic integration becomes the more striking as one has reviewed the range of systems through that of social observation. Just as pharmacological schemes have implicit evaluations of drug users, the social schemes—such as Feldman's—have implicit information on drugs.

What is required if one assumes that classification schemes for control will combine diverse kinds of data explicitly? That explicitness is the first requirement. It is followed by procedural needs that are essentially of a logical and statistical nature. One must be sure that methods adequate to each level of data are employed in the investigations, that probability statements appropriate to each kind of data characterize statements of a predictive or descriptive nature, and that before combining the information, some transformations are made that serve to scale, normalize, weight, factor, and/or otherwise make it possible to deal with one quantified system whose diverse elements can be handled equivalently. The consistency of such schemes is defined by the adequacy of logic and procedures.

Criminal Law

The criminal law expresses the classification schemes of the common man insofar as these are shared or adopted by his legislators. In that sense, it symbolizes public views. The law also usually includes some kind of scientific classification system adapted by legislators for their purposes. In doing this, the law also attempts to describe the ways by which the conclusions entailed in a classification system can be put into action to influence society. Current classification systems and laws are usually identified as drug-control measures. Yet a person who accepts that description rather than analyzing the legislation may be misled. The U.S. Controlled Dangerous Substances Act is an example of an ostensible drug-control measure, which inspection reveals is a classification by the criminal law of several elements of which drugs are only the smaller part. Examination of that law shows, for example, that following the specifications of heroin, cannabis, and barbiturates, there is a three-part matrix: (1) substances (cannabis, heroin and the like), (2) types of behavior associated with a drug (for example, simple possession, possession with intent to sell, or selling), and (3) type of person (for example, an offender with less than three previous convictions and one with three or more previous convictions). A range of controls (penalties) is affixed to these features and varies as they do. The penalties range from a minimum of probation for a period of months—no imprisonment occurring—to imprisonment for life. If the components in the matrix are found by the courts to be cannabis, simple possession, and no previous convictions, the range of penalties allowed is from probation to up to one year in jail. If the components are heroin, selling, and three or more convictions (such that the person is classified as a habitual offender), the law provides for life imprisonment.

Sanctions set forth by the law demonstrate the objectives of law makers—or of those government figures, organs or interest groups who frame laws in the absence of legislative power or interest. The law also reflects their assumptions about the desirability of various sanctions. Kaplan in Chapter Fifteen considers the merit of various assumptions made and, elsewhere (1973), analyzes operations of the law in detail. The criminal law itself is a classification scheme of criminal sanctions, ordering them in relationship to drugs, conduct, and sanctions. Its objectives may be open or hidden, single or multiple. In drug legislation they have included the following objectives: deterring others from prohibited action; correcting or rehabilitating offenders; requiring penance of the offender; exacting vengeance upon the offender; expressing public morality or educating others to a moral goal; isolating offenders and thus protecting others from either the "contagion" of drug proselytizing, the trespass of their visibility, or the non-drug crimes they might otherwise commit; appearing to accommodate to national or international pressures or conventions; advancing the interests of bureaucrats or others as beneficiaries of power and wealth distributed to administrative components within the police-court-correctional enterprise; raising prices for producers or sellers or providing income by means of corruption through maintaining the illicit marketplace monopolies; or simply acting responsively without clear intentions as to impact. Although some of the foregoing may be unexpected consequences rather than latent intentions of lawmakers, the international arena is diverse enough to sustain the conclusion that at least sometimes drug laws achieve what was intended in drafting them.

Insofar as a drug control law or legislation precedent or judicial procedures linked to it specify the alternatives open to the courts, then the drug law also becomes a classification system about the beliefs and experience of a social system as to how people involved in drug use are to be classified (malevolent, greedy, mentally ill, physically ill, socially maladjusted, victims of their environment, and so forth) and, following such a diagnosis as to the nature of their failings, how they are best handled. Typical sentences include probation, work, imprisonment with or without rehabilitative services, mandatory treatment, or death. Less common are requirements that the offender be placed in another family (if a child), be exiled, change schools or work settings, undergo courses of religious or school instruction, or make restitution. It is beyond our scope to analyze these and other means for implementing control objectives insofar as the objects of control are humans and not drugs. Yet it is of the very greatest importance that policy-makers realize that the criminal law and its classifications express assumptions about how those human beings involved with drugs are best described and influenced. Any classification system that implies a given approach to description and influence but whose assumptions are not frankly determined and tested by evidence offers great risk of disappointment.

Acknowledging Alternatives

Harold and Oriana Kalant (personal communication, 1973) believe that there are a number of alternatives, which international collaborators ought to acknowledge and from which selections should be made. They suggest that the essence of present international legislation is the control of human behavior rather than of substances. Much of the scientific material as to drug properties serves only to rationalize these objectives. The discrepancies of logic and the limitations on the efficacy of control measures arise, at least in part, from the multiplicity of forces and events that intervene between substances and behavior. If this be so, then at least the following choices suggest themselves:

1. Recognize that substance-oriented controls do not represent the actual intentions and functions of international endeavors and drop them entirely.

2. Should controls be deemed desirable, direct them overtly and frankly at behavior itself, just as occurs in the case of the laws and regulations of some countries stipulating acts to be controlled in association with alcohol use.

3. Maintain substance-oriented controls, but with the admission that the intention is, nevertheless, to control humans and not chemicals. Conduct evaluation and research to learn how this is best done by learning what relationships exist among forms of drug production, sales and use, and those target behaviors that are disavowed or held dangerous.

4. Cease efforts to control drug-related behavior, accepting whatever individual or social costs are incurred.

5. Reexamine the control objectives, identifying those that best express international intentions. Identify those objectives that are most likely to be achieved through international collaboration. Consider the mechanisms necessary for the achievement of these limited objectives and implement them fully (Spong, 1972).

For far-reaching suggestions as to alternatives for international action that go well beyond issues of drug classification to consider the whole range of actions which need to be taken, including the presentation of important concepts as to what international collaboration requires, the reader is strongly advised to review the Report by the Committee on Crime Prevention and Control of the United Nations Economic and Social Council (1972, 1973). The scope of that report is beyond our specific concerns here; however, its relevance is such that it should be considered required reading.

International Classification

Richard H. Blum

III

For those who are concerned with controls, the classificatory work of national and international agencies is of interest. We limit ourselves here to international work.

WORLD HEALTH ORGANIZATION

The World Health Organization (WHO) of the United Nations has probably done or commissioned more psychoactive drug classificatory work than any other body, national or international. It has utilized scientists and clinicians from many countries, emphasizing in their selection knowledge of chemistry, pharmacology, and, to a lesser extent, psychiatry. We have earlier illustrated that work by reference to Isbell and Chrusciel (1970). The procedures employed in classification entail the work of committees of experts who avail themselves of the scientific literature and report their findings in publications.

It is evident that an interest in developing a uniform international system of drug classification underlies the work of WHO. This may be seen in a 1965 document which reviews existing national legislation that governs the classification of pharmaceuticals in general (Eddy, Halbach, Isbell, Seevers, 1965). Particular attention was paid to toxic or dangerous substances; the listing of national controls was limited to those applying to medical use (as opposed, for example, to poisons employed agriculturally or industrially). The report observed that criteria governing pharmaceutical classifications vary widely from country to country. Further, within national laws, it is common that "there is no uniformity in the classification laid down in the regulations." In the field of psychoactive drugs, apparently the same condition still exists. The Vienna Protocol on Psychotropic Substances may be considered the first international effort to produce uniformity internationally with regard to a broad range of psychoactive substances (as opposed to opiates, cannabis, and coca products enumerated in the Single Convention of 1961), classifications, certain criteria for these, and the levels of control and public action deemed appropriate by the drafters of the Protocol for each class of drugs.

In 1964, a WHO scientific group produced the report (World Health Organization Technical Report #287, 1964) in which they considered specific therapeutic effects of drugs, the liability for the production of dependence, and the evaluation of risk to public health either under medical use or when abused. The presentation centered on the biological foundation of drug dependence which, it was held, "serves as the basis for the evaluation of the sociological and epidemiological implications of drug abuse." A classification system was presented in which the drugs were grouped as "generic types," that is, morphine, barbiturate/alcohol, cocaine, amphetamine, hallucinogens, and cannabis type. Dependence on morphine, which was taken as an illustrative model, is described in terms of psychic dependence, tolerance, and early physical dependence with a subsequent abstinence syndrome. It was noted that the degree of dependence liability varied by drugs in this (opioid) class. However, all were held likely to produce physical dependence when given in sufficient doses, though, for some of them, for example, codeine (placed in the same class), psychic dependence resulting in compulsive use is infrequent.[*]

Some problems in the WHO scheme have been considered by Hakansson (1966) in a detailed paper on definitions. He observes on semantic grounds that WHO distinguished in its criteria for drug effects (and thus its classification of "types" of dependency) between nonempirical and empirical relationships, thus generating tautologies and untestable statements. He also observes the tendency to attach abuse definitions within the limited frame of reference of pharmacology and psychopathology, giving these interpretive dominance unrelated to empirical data. A third problem is the implicit incorporation of sociopolitical values in WHO definitions. Hakansson also notes that preexisting classification systems led WHO in 1964 to include a "cannabis type" dependency even though both definitions and data were particularly weak. Bejerot's (1965) criticisms of the referents for "drugs" are noted; Bejerot observed that substances producing euphoria (gasoline, glue thinner) are excluded as are some that lead to physical dependency (tobacco) and, further, that the WHO concept of dependence excluded drugs on which people depended, for example, insulin for diabetes. Bejerot suggested that such definitional problems are related to temporal and cultural notions of what constitutes health.

---

[*] Other work by WHO authors concludes that codeine is most unlikely to produce either physical or psychic dependence unless heavily overadministered (World Health Organization, 1970).

Hakansson (1966), Smart (1973), Christie and Bruun (1969), and others have addressed themselves to the many specific questions that are raised by the use, in any classification system, of terms such as *abuse, dependency,* and the like. In this chapter, we will not go beyond Hakansson in considering issues of definition except to note that the shifting emphasis by WHO over the past twenty years does reflect the problem one has as one gains information on new kinds of use and effects.

Still strongly debatable is the WHO position that defines abuse in terms of nonmedical use. As its critics note, "abuse" is a determining classification of drug-associated behavior central to any control scheme. As Birdwood (1972) argues, the value components in that judgment must be as evident as its multiple referents semantically are clear.

Zacune (1972) is also critical of the WHO definitions. Citing work by Lewis and Oswald in Scotland showing that withdrawal symptoms without compulsion to use occurred with fenfluramine, leading to arguments that "current definitions of dependence are confused and unworkable," Zacune writes (p. 29):

> This—the current WHO definition—is probably more useful albeit just as unworkable as past ones. Although it recognizes that physical dependence is an accidental feature . . . its insistence on specific types of dependence makes it difficult to define the distinctive characteristics of polydrug users and users of new substances. Polydrug users do not use one specific type of drug, but a combination of any that happen to be around.

Zacune, like Hakansson, finds the definition of dependence tautological. Further (p. 29):

> The authors of drug dependence definitions stand in danger of being accused of an excessively narrow concept of society which does not take into account the values of the (drug using) subgroups within that society; instead they may impose their own values and with them the implicit paternalistic notion of "social harm."

Hakansson, Zacune, Birdwood (1972), and Halbach (1971) have each commented on the frequent changes in WHO definitions from 1952 through 1965. Birdwood is critical of the narrowness of reliance on dependence as the major problem and speaks of "a dream-world peopled by pharmacological bureaucrats; an in-game for experts." His criticism is that such classifications have led to public action systems that exclude people in need of treatment. He mentions as excluded from drug clinics British barbiturate users. He also discusses modern polydrug use: "Young drug takers have turned the pharmacologists' dream into a nightmare. . . . Their dependence . . . is not on a particular drug, but on drugs in general, on being stoned out of their minds, on injecting."

Birdwood goes on; "If the cynic had his way, a drug is a substance which when injected into a rat gives rise to a learned paper"; and, like Hakansson, he proposes improved definitions.

Pharmacological criteria for evaluating morphine-type dependence liability that were presented in the World Health Organization Technical Report #287 (1964) were based mostly on animal tests and observations in "addict" patients. The value of research on monkeys to enable prediction of dependency liability in man was noted.[*] Note was made of the current procedures for evaluation of a new drug in the United States. These procedures utilize blind trials on monkeys, supplemental studies on hospitalized addicts if monkey outcomes were not unequivocal, and simultaneous pharmacological evaluation and clinical trials by the manufacturer, followed by review of the data by the Committee on Problems of Drug Dependence of the National Academy of Sciences–National Research Council. In the case of drugs judged therapeutically useful but found to have dependence liability, the Committee recommends controls to the Bureau of Narcotics and Dangerous Drugs, which initiates a notification by the government to WHO through the United Nations.

There can be no question that the research procedures outlined in the WHO evaluation recommendations are themselves valuable. Knowledge of the capability of a drug to produce dependency in monkeys or its subjective evaluation by addicts as a euphoriant with demonstrations of tolerance and physical dependence, plus normal pharmacological and clinical testing, are necessary. It allows decisions on the release of a substance for use and recommendations to physicians as to how it should be administered. The scheme will be recognized as helpful and careful.

The problems inherent in it are twofold. The addict population at the U.S. Public Health Service Hospital, at Lexington, Kentucky, which is used (and like procedures are recommended by the WHO group to other nations), is an unusual group of drug-involved, mostly opiate-using lower-class deviants. Having themselves gravitated to very unusual drug use, they may resemble others like themselves still on the streets. However, the prediction from Lexington addicts to either normal patient populations or to different social and private user groups is not necessarily exact. One does not doubt that the procedures employed demonstrate a dependence potential, but these procedures cannot estimate the proportion of medical patients likely to develop psychic dependency or the appeal of a new drug, possibly subject to the whimsy of fashions in use, to the large number of persons (particularly youths) interested in trying out psychoactive substances. The informational and control mechanisms are nevertheless useful to the physician in guiding him in his prescribing the new drug, once it is approved. Recommendations for control follow automatically from this medical

---

[*] This is because much work with opiates and monkeys has been conducted. However, other drugs may act quite differently. For example, chimpanzees resist alcohol and dependency. To achieve it, one must force-feed them large amounts as infants; when older they resist (Bourne, 1972).

science classification, yet the control scheme itself goes far beyond recommendations to medical practitioners. Control schemes regulate manufacture, distribution, storage, sales, and the enforcement of criminal laws against users and traffickers.

The pharmacological classification system recommended by WHO in 1964 and practiced under the Single Convention dictates controls beyond the field of medical practice, where the Expert Committee expertise lies, and beyond the kind of data available to anyone with regard to the utility of either the commercial or criminal controlling statutes and actions. Thus, a classification scheme representing the best efforts of competent pharmacologists leads, because of the law and administrative practice, to a linked control system that has no scientific basis. This was clear at the time to WHO officers; for example, Halbach (1968, p. 336) wrote, "Dependence . . . does not indicate the degree of risk or the need of appropriate control pertinent to the drug described. . . . It is not possible to establish an automatic link between biologically determined data and administrative action." The pathway from the classifications of drugs and assumptions about drug effects to estimates as to the efficacy of controls is crucial to understanding how public action systems may be based on inappropriate premises. Essentially the same assumptions operate in the 1971 (Vienna) Convention on Psychotropic Substances, for it too is based on a pharmacological scheme and moves directly to controls on a great number of psychoactive drugs. Under both the Single Convention and the Psychotropic Convention, WHO is empowered to make recommendations for classification to the Commission on Narcotic Drugs, which has the decision-making power. Under the Single Convention, however, the Commission either accepts or rejects the WHO recommendations, whereas in the Psychotropic Convention, the Commission reserves to itself much broader powers, allowing itself to disregard the WHO and consider other factors (economic, social, administrative, legal, and so forth) in making decisions. This administrative difference, although important in terms of UN Narcotics Commission–WHO relationships, does not alter the logical and empirical problems encountered in classifying drugs for control using a pharmacologically based system.

Another World Health Organization Technical Report (#273, 1964) elaborated the new terminology to replace the old definitions of drug addiction and habituation by the description of dependence on distinct types of drugs. This scheme for categorizing effects was linked specifically to the model drug:

> Drug dependence of morphine type is described as a state arising from repeated administration of morphine, or an agent with morphine-like effects on a periodic or continuous basis. Its characteristics include (1) An overpowering desire or need to continue taking the drug and to obtain it by any means; the need can be satisfied by the drug taken initially or by another with morphine-like properties (2) A tendency to increase the dose owing to the development of tolerance (3) A psychic dependence on the effects of the drug related to a subjective and indivi-

dual appreciation of those effects; and (4) A physical dependence on the effects of the drug requiring its presence for maintenance of homeostasis and resulting in a definite, characteristic, and self-limited abstinence syndrome when the drug is withdrawn.

Discussing effects the report went on:

> With morphine, the harm to the individual is in the main indirect, arising from preoccupation with drug taking; personal neglect, malnutrition and infection are frequent consequences. For society also, the harm may be related to the preoccupation of the individual with drug taking, disruption of interpersonal relationships, economic loss, and crimes against property are frequent consequences.

In conclusion, the report stated:

> The risk to public health should be and usually is of paramount importance as a criterion for the establishment of control for a dependence producing drug of any of the types described (morphine type, barbiturate type, cocaine type, amphetamine type and cannabis type) and in deciding the degree of control. At the same time socio-economic factors and social harm associated with drug dependence and drug abuse must be taken into account and may determine appropriateness of control in a particular case. The socio-economic factors largely determine society's attitude towards the individuals involved in drug abuse, but they are not characteristics that need to be considered in medical and scientific differentiation of the types of drug dependence.

A 1965 supplemental paper offered further details (Eddy, Halbach, and others, 1965). It introduced two new types of dependency, the khat type and the hallucinogen (LSD) type. With reference to all the dependency-by-model-drug-types, the emphasis was on laboratory findings showing behavioral toxicity and on clinical psychiatric descriptions implying defective conduct. For cannabis, for example (p. 729):

> For the individual harm resulting from abuse of cannabis may include inertia, lethargy, self-neglect, feeling of increased capability, with corresponding failure and precipitation of psychotic episodes. Abuse of cannabis facilitates the association with social groups and sub-cultures involved with more dangerous drugs, such as opiates or barbiturates. Transition to the use of such drugs would be a consequence of this association rather than an inherent effect of cannabis. The harm to society derived from abuse of cannabis rests in the economic consequences of the

impairment of the individual's social functions and his enhanced proneness to asocial and antisocial behavior.

The attempt on the part of the Expert Committee is welcomed because of their progress in discriminating among the reactions to different drugs in their classification system and in discriminating within the reactions to a given drug the several features of craving, compulsive use, tolerance, and physical dependency. Serious problems are introduced by the failure to qualify their definitions with a full statement of the complexity of nonmedical drug use. With regard to opiates, one asks if the Committee meant that continued self-administration inevitably leads to dependence, craving, and compulsive use? With regard to cannabis, did the Committee mean to suggest that repeated use does in fact produce compulsive use and psychic dependence along with unavoidable asocial or antisocial behavior? It appears to have been their intention to provide a descriptive approach that would use the model drug illustratively, showing what they believed could happen. Their emphasis, however, was clearly on ill effects. That emphasis accounts for the inference a reader draws of inevitable addiction, psychopathology, or social harm following use of such substances.

A sociologist, Jock Young (1971, p. 45), calls attention to how the classificatory scheme may be incompletely based:

> The Expert Committee being composed of pharmacologists and medical doctors has been understandably myopic in its concentration on drugs as the basis of a suitable classification. To describe adequately a particular form of drug use, then, we must use what I term a socio-pharmacological classification. Thus, we will need to divide drug users up into categories which describe patterns of drug use involving similar social meanings and beliefs, on the one hand, and drugs with closely related pharmacological effects on the other . . . morphine, meperidine, pethidine, dependency by members of medical and allied professions which occurs in most advanced industrial countries, or marijuana dependency by bohemians which occurs chiefly in Britain, North America, France and Holland. Implicit in this revised terminology is the notion that it is invalid to generalize about drug use without reference to a specific culture context.

And further (p. 212):

> The campaign against psychotropic drugs carried out under the auspices of the United Nations is, despite the medical and scholarly language . . . typically underscored by distinctly political considerations.

Zinberg and Robertson (1972, pp. 40, 41, 81)—a psychiatrist and an attorney—are also critical:

The concept of dependency per se in the WHO categorization includes the psychological response to any extensive drug use and raises it to an equivalent position with the pharmacological effects. People who are dependency-prone, it implies, become dependent more readily than people who are not, and strong drugs spell quick trouble for the former, though weaker drugs are less dangerous. "Independent people" by implication, can withstand a mild drug for a long time and have a fighting chance even with a strong one. The WHO position, in which strength and weakness could be considered moral properties, has puritanical overtones. . . . The WHO classification in fact perpetuates the medical tradition of presuming that people caught up with drugs suffer, except in unusual circumstances, from personality defects. . . .

The WHO categorization pays little attention to setting. . . . The attitude of the WHO and the psychoanalytic and the sociological approach all emphasized susceptibility and took heavy use for granted. Little attention was paid to the occasional user. . . .

It is our intention to show that modern drug users, though they are held to be deviants, differ little from nonusers—except in their attitude toward drug use. Their drug use is only an auxiliary trait for them, but society perceives it as a master trait. . . .

There is a problem in drug research when it is pursued essentially from the point of view of pharmacological action. . . . In one way or another scientists are trying to derive a method of predicting individual response to a psychoactive drug from consideration of the drug. They accept intellectually the proposition that drug, set (user expectations), and setting (environment) are interdependent in shaping the drug response; but they proceed . . . as if the one factor, drug, is more determining than the others.

A WHO scientific group addressed itself directly to therapeutic problems in research and classification of psychopharmaceuticals (World Health Organization Technical Report #371, 1967). Difficulties in classification of psychoactives were acknowledged; the scientific group agreed to adopt a classification based on clinical efficacy and principle actions representing (p. 7) "a compromise between different schools of thought . . . based on available knowledge of pharmacological action and clinical uses of drugs. . . . This classification is not intended to be definitive."

The new classification was of neuroleptics, anxiolytic sedatives, antidepressants, psychostimulants, and psychodysleptics. Substances formerly termed major tranquilizers were included in the first, minor tranquilizers in the second, and hallucinogens in the last group. Various schemes that were set forth describe drugs according to their common application in the treatment of major psychiatric disorders and in effectiveness for specific symptoms in psychiatric states. Attention was given to adverse clinical effects, and dependency outcomes were noted. The 1967 report was cautious, speaking in terms of risks rather than inevitabilities, and a thoughtful discussion of the methodology of clinical drug evaluations occurred. Biochemical and neurophysiological modes of action were considered and human behavioral, including psychopharmacogenetic, research was considered. Recommendations were made for the kind and scope of research in psychopharmacology, for interdisciplinary and collaborative studies, and for the establishment of research, training, and reference centers. The need for environmental and cross-cultural research on the clinical application of psycho-actives was noted. This report is a broad and sophisticated document, which, in recognizing major methodological and semantic problems, does much to show how improvement in evaluative methods—and subsequent drug classifications and, by implication, proposals relative to control—might emerge.

The WHO Expert Committee on Drug Dependence addressed itself in World Health Organization Technical Report #407 (1969) to the need for data and criteria in order to determine "the degree of hazard and the need for control of drugs of abuse." In the definitions offered, it specified a "public health prob-lem" in broad ways, including the frequent presence of drug abuse (as before, defined as "persistent or excessive drug use inconsistent with or unrelated to medical practice"), of dependence, of the danger of spread of use, of effects from drugs involving others than the user including effects on interpersonal relations or production of adverse physical, social, or economic consequences to others. The Committee set itself the task of characterizing the principle and the kinds of data needed so that societies can determine whether or not given drugs should be controlled. Such decisions by a society were said to be imperative. Controls were stated to be necessary if abuse was prevalent, if drug reactions affected others than the users, if spread was between users and nonusers, if illicit traffic occurred, if psychic or physical dependence occurred, or if the drug was to be used in medicine on a commercial basis.

The Committee affirmed the need for reliable and comprehensive data, recommended multidisciplinary endeavors including sociological, psychological, and epidemiological efforts, and called for "material essential for the develop-ment of legislative, educational, and therapeutic strategies" (p. 12). Cross-sectional and longitudinal studies were proposed as were studies of the impact of control measures. Considering those drugs not under international control, the Com-mittee observed that classification can be by chemical structure or pharmacologi-cal effect but that these were for theoretical use or early warnings about potential abuse: "Chemical or pharmacological classifications cannot, however, be used as the basis for determining the need for control nor the type of control required because (1) small changes in chemical structure may cause great changes in dependence liability (2) drugs with different chemical structures may fall within the same pharmacological groups, and cause similar types of drug dependence, and (3) within any group there is wide variation in activity and degree of abuse liability."

A five-fold classification system from high to low risk and from no to high medical use was proposed: LSD was to be in the A group of high risk and no medical utility. Barbiturates and amphetamines were in the B group with high risk and high utility. In the C group were drugs (for example, tranquilizers) with high use but low risk of public health hazard. The D group included compounds containing low amounts of dependency-producing ingredients. The E group was composed of very low dependence-liability drugs, for example, antihistamines. Special note was made, separately, that "cannabis is a drug of dependence producing public health and social problems and that its control must be continued."

Evidence in this 1969 report of an interest in impact data on control measures and on social-epidemiological studies is progressive. However, these acknowledgements do not offset the immensity of the difficulty posed by the definition of a "public health hazard." This definition embraces almost all possible forms of behavior and social activity (adverse interpersonal, physical, social, or economic consequences). By terming these "public health" matters, the Committee moves to make physicians and related professionals the arbiters of economic and social behavior. Furthermore, their judgments are deemed compelling as the basis for decisions by whole societies as to whether or not to introduce controls, for the Committee believes that controls themselves are mandatory if the medical judgment is that any widespread adverse effect occurs.

Just as "risk to public health" is a judgment that at this time is not amenable to scientific consensus for many of the drugs in social or private use— and may be a limited domain of inquiry—so the second consideration of "usefulness of the drug in medical therapy" is also subject to debate. Medical utility may be difficult to ascertain. For instance, simply because a drug is used widely does not constitute evidence for its efficacy. Medical usefulness is sometimes simply a matter of physician or patient habit (Balint, Hunt, and others, 1970) or convenience, a matter of placebo effect, and not proof of therapeutic virtue.

In the United States, investigators commissioned by the National Academy of Sciences and the National Research Council evaluated drug efficacy. For drugs released before 1962, only 19.1 percent of a total of 16,573 claims for effectiveness were found supported by scientific evidence. Only 25 percent of the over-the-counter drugs were found effective. Although United States law since 1962 requires that ineffective drugs be withdrawn from the market, the U.S. Food and Drug Administration did not require their withdrawal until court action in 1972. The study shows that efficacy is the one way of classifying drugs and that it can be linked to public action, in this case the requirement that the consumer be protected from buying worthless products because of false advertising or poor scientific screening on the part of pharmaceutical manufacturers. The fact that a government agency, the Food and Drug Administration, did not enforce the law may be interpreted as a sign that, as with other public action (control) measures linked to classification schemes, political and economic interests as well as administrative competence affect the actual workings both of data-gathering for classification and the enforcement of the laws based on such classifications.

Were international classification and control linked to the strict measure of demonstrable efficacy, it would require a considerable shift in emphasis. It would require an international review of the therapeutic value of drugs relying on competent and extensive investigative resources to make such determinations. One can predict, based on such efficacy studies as have been done, that to move from controls based on the belief that certain drugs are dangerous to controls based on the knowledge that certain drugs are useless would make a giant dent indeed in conventional medical practice and in pharmaceutical manufacturing and sales. Home-remedy practices would also be strongly affected.

The Committee classification appears, perhaps without so intending, to endorse the status quo in medical practice, which allows the use of drugs on the basis of acceptance of what is done, rather than on the basis of demonstrable utility. The current and proposed classification schedules, by incorporating that operational definition, institutionalize in the law the use of substances that are habitually prescribed regardless of other considerations. Anyone arguing for better definitions—that is, scientifically supported ones that would put drugs under control based on standards of efficacy—would be inconsistent were he at the same time to resist controls on drugs with demonstrable danger. On the other hand, consistency is also required for those who might argue that the costs to governments of assessing and controlling weak or useless substances is not justifiable, that is, is greater than the gain to consumers through such controls that would prevent their wasting their money or health on hopeless remedies. Such advocates must then be willing to demonstrate that the cost of present or proposed controls over dangerous drugs is worth the cost to the public in administrative expense or to consumers in the denial to them of often pleasure-giving substances. These are but general considerations. Real appraisals must be specific to substance, persons, and settings.

In any event, it is evident that the WHO 1969 report, although calling for an enlarged data base from which to make judgments, implied that social behavior that occurs in association with drugs (including the presumed effect that users have on others by "adverse physical, social, or economic consequences") is a medical matter. The thrust was to seek to compel legal action by nations if medical scientists concluded that "a public health problem" exists.

The seventeenth report of the WHO Expert Committee (World Health Organization Technical Report #437, 1970), elaborated upon concepts found in earlier reports. A scheme for classifying drugs by level of control required was presented. (The Committee's work occurred in conjunction with the work of the UN Narcotics Commission that prepared the Protocol, now Convention, on Psychotropic Substances.) Criteria for determining the need for control again were identified as the degree of risk to public health and the usefulness of the drug in medical therapy. Classification systems were required to be flexible enough to accommodate new substances, to provide for access to drugs for research as the essence of the mandate. The incorporation of previously uncontrolled substances was the sole and whole purpose of the exercise. Five classifications were proposed (these differing from the 1969 group), based on degree of risk and medical usefulness. The drugs in the A group have high risk and low utility. Those of the two B groups have substantial public health risk but either some (B1) or great (B2) medical utility. Drugs in the C group involve a substantial risk but also have moderate or great therapeutic utility. The D group includes compounds containing only a little of chemicals in Groups A through C.

Tentatively, a precursor category was also established; that is, substances that have neither risk or benefit but are used in the manufacture of potent drugs or are capable of being synthesized and so used. Lysergic acid was used as an example. In itself, it is not psychoactive; but it is used as a basis for the manufacture of the hallucinogen LSD-25 and is therefore a precursor, the sales of which can be controlled so as to prevent its use in illicit manufacture.

An important concept was that of classification by analogy. This was a procedure to be employed when there was little or no information available about a drug whose "chemical structure, pharmacodynamic properties, therapeutic indication, or routes of administration" showed similarity to drugs already recommended for control. The analogy classification is based on theoretical assumptions only and provides for control of a substance in the absence of any evidence of its effects. This method is the essence of the classification of new but unused opiates (opioids) under the Single Convention. This procedure is not incorporated in the Psychotropic Convention, whose requirement for "sufficient evidence" may be taken as dissatisfaction, among those drafting it, with the earlier "laboratory classification" by analogy in the absence of evidence of effects.

The seventeenth report proposed a control schedule that listed kinds of controls over manufacturing distribution, record keeping, international commerce, and prescription. Although no mention was made of criminal controls, these were implied in a control procedure proposing that Single Convention obligations (relative to opioids, cannabis, cocaine, and the like) for reporting be applied to drugs in the new schedules. Since national enforcement provisions are set forth in the Single Convention, the effect perhaps would be to invoke similar sanctions.

WHO CLASSIFICATION

A diversity of scientific opinion and of proposed classification schemes appears within the WHO publication. They vary considerably in the criteria employed and the methodological aspects, in the sophistication evident, and in the extent to which medical authority is proposed as a basis for judging behavior outside the physician-patient relationship and for requiring societies to introduce commercial and criminal law as well as strictly prescription controls. It is apparent that conventional chemical-pharmacological orientations have been dominant, although with the expanded notion of "public health risk" the beginnings are seen for employing epidemiological and social research. Similarly, as the scope and impact of controls advocated expand, we can note an occasional recognition of the need to see the consequences of such controls. In many of the recommended schemes, there is too often a lack of recognition that drugs—given in ordinary doses—do not by themselves compel specific outcomes, particularly deviant life-styles, so that the origins of behavior are too narrowly attributed to chemicals without regard for other factors operating. Similarly, a false confidence may be transmitted to the reader who believes that the definitions are clearer and the criteria for scientific appraisal better supported by research capabilities than is the case. These problems are in no sense the fault of the dedicated and competent WHO experts and staff; they are built into the inadequacies in knowledge about drug effects or control methods. However, the level of information preferred by most WHO authorities excludes many recent data that do bear strongly on drug clasification and control recommendations. Wider acquaintance with these data and a broadening professional base in WHO work would lead to better bases for classification work.

UN NARCOTICS COMMISSION

Classification under the jurisdiction of the UN Narcotics Commission is at present limited to the Single Convention on Narcotic Drugs. We have seen that controlled drugs are opioids, coca leaf and cocaine, and cannabis. The opioids include natural products—the opium form from poppies, opium derivatives (heroin, morphine), and synthetics of similar chemical structure. These drugs, within or between classes, have widely varying degrees of dependence liability as measured either in laboratory studies with animals or men or in observations of natural populations. If and when the Psychotropic Convention comes into force, the Commission will have full responsibility for the classification of all psycho-active drugs under control or suggested for control.

Problems in the Single Convention classification system are well known by now. "Narcotic" is a legal label, which, by using an earlier pharmacological term, creates semantic confusion, for not all of these substances have soporific or analgesic effects nor are all of them capable of producing tolerance, physical dependency, and relapse. Among the drugs controlled, the range of effects is great; for example, morphine under certain conditions of dosage clearly leads to tolerance and physical dependency whereas cannabis leaf smoked under ordinary conditions does not. The high level of control now uniformly required under the Convention and accepted by most (but not all) countries is inappropriate if one assumes that control intensity should in any way be linked with pharmacological potency or with varying conditions and risks in actual use. Such assumptions are themselves questionable. Some persons (prohibitionists) might wish to disallow any psychoactive drug in social or private use; some laissez-faire persons might wish that no drugs be controlled by the criminal law or perhaps even by civil regulations governing production, purity, sales, and the like. Examination of the language of the Single Convention, with its emphasis on control by means of the criminal law and on suppression (of production, commerce, use), suggests that the philosophies of its architects tended in the direction of conservatism, emphasis on drug dangers, and faith in the criminal law and commercial controls as suitable instruments for influencing human drug-taking conduct.

Inconsistencies within the Single Convention classification (for example, in grouping drugs of different effects and use styles in the same category) and incongruities in its control provide an excellent example of the problems in developing over time classification and control schemes. Political and moral pressures, special interest groups, and scientific knowledge and ignorance all have contributed. Perhaps the Single Convention is best understood through awareness of the historical and political processes that influence international action. Scientific features play only a secondary role.

A review of legislative history and an evaluation of current classification schemes indicates that basic assumptions about drugs, behavior, classification, and controls should be examined. Information-search procedures must be improved. Means to convey information to policy-makers for its integration and application by them need facilitation and flexibility in classifications, and controls must be incorporated into schemes that are provisional rather than deemed permanent.

The Vienna Convention on Psychotropic Substances is not yet in force, and, consequently, its classification system will not be examined in detail. Were it to come into force, the UN Narcotics Commission would have final power in determining drug classifications, albeit WHO would advise and recommend, and information from unspecified "other sources" is admissible. The four-schedule classification scheme is much like that found in the U.S. Dangerous Substances Act of 1970 and does not avoid the problems of evidence, logic, procedure, and generalization that attend pharmacological schemes and abuse definitions occurring in that law or in the similar laws of other nations. The criteria bearing on classification in the Convention are suitably complex: they are the dependence liability of a substance; demonstrable psychoactive effects; abuse or ill effects similar to those of already classified substances; present or potential abuse so as to constitute a public health or social problem warranting international control; therapeutic usefulness; and such economic, social, legal, administrative, and other factors as may be relevant. Major questions are not addressed. These include adequacy of direct scientific and economic evidence bearing on the criteria that the Commission would require; the assessment of the practicability, cost, and impact of control measures required once a classification is made; and procedures for appeal to authorities beyond the Commission and its parent body, the UN Economic and Social Council, with regard to classificatory decisions.

There seems little doubt that, through the broadness of the criteria and relevant factors stipulated, the convention represents an increasing awareness of the complexity of classification and control in the international community. Given that awareness, one hopes that positive steps may be taken to improve the information utilized in international decision-making and program-planning.

Interest
Groups

Richard H. Blum

IV

The question of factors that operate in the decisions about drug classification linked to drug effects immediately leads to the arena of highly charged moral, social, and political issues that surround estimates of drug effects and recommendations for kinds of public action in response. Insofar as discussions of classification go beyond such effects as demonstrable tissue pathology or disturbed metabolic function to describe how drug use influences personal traits or how people act toward one another, at work, in learning, in having religious experiences, and the like, it is evident that considerations broader than those of health are involved. Even though many citizens rest content with allowing psychiatrists to be the experts in the description of some of these behaviors (those considered results of mental or emotional disturbance), the psychiatric authority is not generally accepted as the proper base from which to recommend public action. Some of the strongest challenges come from within psychiatry and psychopharmacology. Other strong challenges come from attorneys and law enforcement personnel. Some come from religious leaders, some from social scientists, and not a few from drug users themselves. The competing domains are medicine and its associated basic sciences, those in the administration of justice, moral and theological thinkers, social scientists and social philosophers, and drug consumers.

From within each of these groups come challenges to existing classifications of drugs, drug effects, and drug users. Especially charged are the debates (over what is good and bad and over the kinds of public action that are implicit in the descriptions of drug effects or associated conduct) and competitions for power and responsibility for influence over national and international programs that seek either to influence the manner of drug use or, contrariwise, to prevent specific governmental influences from being exercised. Special interests also strongly influence these debates, including commercial drug interests (manufacturers and sellers); professionals and bureaucrats working within a given social response system; and local, national, or international political interests. These latter are of course expressive of moral, economic, and cultural differences.

The medical and moral debate is illustrated by a statement of an unconventional psychiatrist, Thomas Szasz (1971, pp. 39–47):

> Many psychiatric problems are not medical but moral problems. . . . Judgments [about addiction or abuse] have nothing whatever to do with medicine, pharmacology or psychiatry. . . . Our present inclination . . . is either to ignore the moral perspective or to mistake the technical for the moral. . . . Drug abuse as we know it is one of the inevitable consequences of the medical monopoly over drugs. . . . We have allowed a moral problem to be disguised as a medical question and have then engaged in shadow-boxing with metaphoric diseases and medical attempts ranging from the absurd to the appalling to combat them.

With regard to the challenge to medicine from law enforcement Michael Sonnenreich, an attorney in the U.S. Department of Justice, describing the development of the U.S. Comprehensive Drug Abuse Control and Prevention Act of 1970, observed (1971, pp. 9–10):

> This classification for drugs is primarily a regulatory one. There was clearly a need to control the use of drugs for research and also their legitimate use in the commercial markets. This control has been accomplished by establishing five schedules which categorize the drugs in terms of their known dangers and their medical use, if any. A rational and cohesive approach to the entire concept of regulating dangerous drugs (now called controlled substances) has been effected. . . . The focal point of this entire bill is the penalties it provides for criminal violations. . . . What we have tried to do is to distinguish among the kinds of people who become involved in the drug culture. . . . For example there is . . . an experimenter . . . there is the chronic user. At the top is the trafficker . . . [there is] the person who gives marijuana to his friends . . . [there is] the actual seller.

The medical approach as opposed to the criminal law approach is argued by A. Freedman (1971, pp. 15–20):

> To write a bill that adjudicates about one third of the prescribed medicines in this country (potentially criminalizing an enormous popula-

tion of legitimately medicated patients)—to write a bill that is so scientifically unsound as this bill still is—to write a bill with three (drug classification) schedules . . . to have written the kind of a bill that would give the Attorney General initial and final authority to decide on legitimate medical practice, to define what is and what is not a dangerous drug, and who shall use it, and when he shall use it, as the bureau (U.S. Bureau of Narcotics and Dangerous Drugs) has done, is absolutely a throwback in history.

In matters of drug control we send the Commissioner of the Bureau of Narcotics and perhaps one co-opted member of the Establishment to negotiate at the United Nations or World Health Organization *in camera* and without advice or consultation from the medical profession or the general health community. . . . You are having your lives with respect to drugs regulated sans review.

And a nonenforcement attorney, arguing social as against criminal controls, considers the U.S. Comprehensive Drug Abuse Prevention and Control Act of 1970 (Robertson, 1971, pp. 21–31):

This bill claims to classify drugs according to harm and modifies penalties for users. . . . It really is just another incarnation of the police approach to drug control which since 1914 has dominated official action and caused so many of the problems we face today with drugs. . . . we will reap from this law what we have reaped from past laws: more drug use, more police power, and more controversy. . . . It is time to replace the formal restraints of the law with the informal controls naturally present in the everyday context in which drugs are used. . . . It is time to shift the public focus from blanket condemnation to the actual medical and social harms which some drugs produce. . . . One of the chief reasons that overcriminalization survives is that the moral content of the laws is usually masked as a health or safety measure. . . . It is not at all clear that many forms of drug use are mentally or physically harmful or, even if they are, that the state has the right to impose its conceptions of health on the individual.

Moving from that particular law to an analysis of United States drug laws generally, a lawyer challenging the statutory approach over the pharmacological reports (Levine, 1971):

I have recently completed a detailed study of the drug abuse laws of the fifty states and the federal government. This study indicated that the dangerous drug laws define and classify dangerous substances differently than pharmacological authorities. The study further indicated that the statutes vary drastically in defining and classifying controlled substances. The principles used by the legislatures in defining and classifying dangerous drugs are not ordinarily apparent.

And a husband and wife pharmacologist team with a historical and social perspective reviewing drug legislation in North America, write (Kalant and Kalant, 1971, pp. 115, 116):

> From this brief historical review, it can be seen that both the Canadian and American laws against opium and marijuana were initiated by groups which were concerned, on moral grounds, with the practices of foreign peoples or domestic minority groups. . . . Present day critics of the laws on marijuana have attacked bitterly the way in which these laws were passed. But it must be remembered that moral arguments on such topics were as valid and cogent to the society of fifty years ago as scientific and medical arguments are today. The change in the nature of what we accept as convincing arguments in the health field is simply one more evidence of the way in which society has changed. The international agreements have a similar history. . . . The point we wish to make is that some laws restricting use of certain drugs have been deliberate responses to specific problems, while others were originally proposed by small pressure groups and accepted by an indifferent majority. The legislation as a whole, therefore, *cannot* be regarded as a uniformly well reasoned group of acts based on sound scientific evidence and thoroughly discussed by the public before their enactment. There should be no need, therefore, to regard drug laws as sacred or unchangeable.

Those moral views which were and are incorporated into drug legislation constitute much of the unchallenged basis for other criminal laws—incest, homicide, and theft, for example. In all likelihood, a society does not need scientists to contribute at all to its lawmaking as long as a society is morally homogeneous. Perhaps it is only when moral diversity and conflict, as well as heterogeneity of behavior (pluralism) emerge that "objective" standards are called into play by which to shape and judge the laws. That secular scientific objectivity is itself, as the Kalants observe, a culture value and perhaps a culture phase. When scientific —including economic—values do come into play in drug lawmaking and law criticism, then their relativism and functionalism (pragmatism) introduce the concept of evaluation. Evaluation asks why does the drug law exist, what effect does it have, how much does it cost? The moral view is thereby challenged by evaluation which, for moralists, constitutes a threat to fundamental beliefs. Moralists or other absolutists (see Lipset and Dobson, 1972) in turn judge the scientific view—and the intellectuals who promulgate it—and are likely to conclude that some form of heresy exists ("radical," "revisionary," and the like). These conflicts are immediately apparent as one classifies drug classifiers and identifies interest groups in drug legislation. The question of who decides which viewpoint to adopt, let alone the criteria to be employed in judging the goodness of a classification and control scheme, depends, it would appear, not so much on the "facts" but on who have power and responsibility and what their beliefs and interests are.

WHO CLASSIFIES?

The description of interest groups in classification and control schemes is elucidated in studies of the history of recent drug legislation (see Eisenlohr, 1934; Lowes, 1966; Renborg, 1957; Samuels, 1969; Terry and Pellens, 1970; Little, 1971). In any one country one might wish to map the structures of power and interest promulgating, debating, and most influencing actions taken. These would differ according to the locale of action, for community programs are much more likely to represent the interests of local groups, whereas international programs represent those of governments and international bodies. Even so, such basic descriptive work at the community level is missing, for there is no anatomy of power and interests to tell us, for any country or locale, how various action programs represent the influence of, for example, drug users in need of help, the police advocating "cracking down," physicians seeking to establish treatment centers, merchants seeking to avoid any user service facilities in their areas, local government setting up services in response to crime rate rise, and the like. Nationally, it may be easier to designate classifiers on single issues, as Grinspoon (1971) or Musto (1973) have done in studies of United States marijuana legislation. When matters become complex, as is the case in the United Kingdom, Scandanavia, and North America today, such mapping would be a chore indeed.

The history of international legislation is also clearer for past than for present. Existing studies indicate that democratic developed countries of the West have had much influence in structuring international legislative systems, including basic classifications. To what extent the United States has, since the 1930s, as many claim, been the primary source of pressure for control and the major contributor of enacted legislative-classificatory schemes we are unable to say.

Not all classification schemes that come to bear on public action are derived solely by governments. Certainly the pharmaceutical industry and those medical scientists working in universities and nonindustrial laboratories have contributed strongly. Also, much of that work has not been intended for use in legislation or to guide public action. Consider, for example, the workaday systems employed by the pharmaceutical industry to record sales, to set priorities for research, to be used logistically in planning materials purchases, or to guide marketing efforts in one or another area. No one knows to what extent it would be possible to document the work in classification by the pharmaceutical industry or to describe segments of that industry along lines pertinent to drug regulation. As Bruun (1972a) points out, lack of research on the industry—as opposed to that by it—is itself noteworthy. It might be of interest, for example, to map the industry itself, showing which firms in which countries have been most involved in the production of drugs identified as sources of "abuse," to measure the carefulness of clinical trials used by various firms before their applications for permission for full marketing privileges, or to document the funds spent by firms to lobby governments or on scientific groups so as to emphasize or deemphasize one or another regulatory feature. Such data would certainly contribute to the better understanding of the role of the pharmaceutical industry both in the development of national and international policy and in contributing to premature release of psychoactive drugs.

Many classification schemes that are influential outside industry are unofficial; that is, they are not enacted legislatively or necessarily approved by professional bodies. Physicians employ a number of pharmacopoeias, as, for example, the *Extra Pharmacopeia, Physicians Desk Reference, British National Formulary, Monthly Index of Medical Specialties,* and the *American Medical Association Drug Evaluations.* Furthermore, many hospitals and medical schools have their own formularies, usually organized by disease entity or symptoms and showing drugs recommended for use.

CLASSIFYING CLASSIFIERS

Comparison of the evaluations of cannabis offered by Weil (1972), with those made by Isbell and Chrusciel (1970) reveals remarkable differences in the level and kinds of criteria used and in the resulting classification and control systems. Perhaps these differences could be better understood if we learn more about the classifiers—their training, experience, culture, moral stance, and the like. For example, recall Aberle's study of the Navajo (1966). He found those noncultists who called peyote cultists drug "abusers" were nonusing, less well-educated, more conventional persons. Better educated Navajos were—like outside anthropologists—more often neutral, not antagonistic to the cultists or using pejorative language in describing them or the effects of drugs on them. Other studies of drug use in small societies (Blum, 1969a) have shown how disparate the views of foreigners and natives can be.

Within larger and more diverse modern societies, such differences in evaluation of drug effects that depend upon the position of the evaluator are strikingly apparent. For example, with regard to alcohol, marijuana, and LSD (Blum, 1969a) politically liberal—defined by voting records assembled by political party advocates—legislators appear less concerned with control through criminal law and coercion and more likely to define ill effects, as with alcoholics, as a matter of illness rather than unacceptable moral deviancy. In another investigation (Blum, 1969a), narcotics officers were compared with academicians and professional people. The former had far more negative views of users and of drug dangers than the latter. Both the police and academicians in the United States tended to have negative views of each other.

Classification systems for those who evaluate drugs may be a useful device. Control over the operation of personal bias is normally built into well-run experiments and clinical trials by procedures that prevent evaluators from knowing which drug is being given to which patient. Failure to observe very careful controls over bias can have far-reaching effects on the findings (Rosnow, Rosenthal, and others, 1969). To better understand how classification and control systems are constructed, one might wish to add to procedural safeguards the study of events that influence the selection of evidence, its appraisal, the preference for control measures, and their appraisal. At the very least one expects the political positions, occupation, education, moral-religious position, residence locale, age, and personal drug preferences of people to affect their judgments. Some features are readily ascertained from interviews or surveys. For instance, it has been found that in the United States the better educated liberal young are more likely to deny that marijuana use is dangerous than are less well educated, more conservative, older persons (Blum and Associates, 1972a). It seems likely that the broader the category of drug effect (as, for example, "dependence" or "abuse") and the less objective the means and definitions of measurement employed, the more powerfully matters of personal opinion do influence the outcome judgment.

Personal opinions about drugs are themselves predictable on the basis of education, age, family background, economic status, and political stance (Blum and Associates, 1972a). It is not at all difficult to envision how these ordinarily hidden influences affect construction of drug classification systems that allow nonobjective standards for the assessment of effects.

Even objective standards can be employed to widely different ends in the choice of research designs. Compare, for example, two studies on cannabis effects. Zinberg and Weil (1970) in the United States had subjects smoke small amounts of ordinary marijuana and were able to report essentially no behavioral toxicity. Durandina and Romasenko (1971) in the Soviet Union injected massive doses of hashish into dogs and were able to report tissue pathology and death. Both are perfectly legitimate studies but one is tempted to speculate as to the existence of rather strong differences, between the two sets of authors, in the moral positions, personal experiences, and possibly the intentions to influence others' opinions.

One learns much about classifiers from a study of thousands of United States professors (Ladd and Lipset, 1972). Political positions were found correlated with professional discipline; liberalism was greatest among social scientists (64 percent) and law professors (51 percent); was low among biological and medical scientists (medical professors, 38 percent; biochemists, 38 percent; physiologists, 35 percent; and chemists, 35 percent); and was lowest among engineers (24 percent). Liberalism was greater among those who had achieved more academically, among those in elite universities, and among those most influential (government consultants and high achievers). Within elite schools, medical professors were more conservative than natural scientists. Social scientists were most critical of the police, a finding compatible with international study findings (Emmerson, 1968) cited by Ladd and Lipset (1972) that in nineteen underdeveloped countries, "students in the social sciences, law and humanities are more likely to be politicized and leftist than their colleagues in the natural and applied sciences." This is not the case in the U.S.S.R. (Lipset and Dobson, 1972), where natural science and medical students are more radical, that is, critical of the state. Just as political liberalism was found correlated with drug legislative views among (California) legislators, so are there correlations among professors between discipline and drug control opinions. Ladd and Lipset (1972) found that marijuana legalization was endorsed by 54 percent of the social scientists, 44 percent of the law faculty, 33 percent of those in medicine, 31 percent in biological sciences, and 30 percent of the chemistry faculties. The authors observe how professionals who are involved in "practical" work (for example, physicians in practice) are more likely to be conservative than those engaged in research, social criticism, or membership in Trilling's "adversary culture."

It is reasonable to conclude that values and opinions on politics, the police, and drug control affect the work and recommendations of those professionals who have interests in or responsibilities for drug classification for the purposes of public action. If so, then those classifications from chemical through medical through social might readily be transformed according to the expected correlated positions of those working at each level (discipline) who contribute data to classification and control recommendations. The most conservative control-oriented schemes would be chemical; pharmacological ones would be midway; clinical psychiatric schemes ought to be found less oriented toward law-enforcement control; those offered by academic law professors would be, like social science proposals, most liberal, that is, most likely to have the fewest drugs classified as so dangerous as to require uniform strong controls and most likely to recommend other than criminal laws as the means for drug control.

The reader can test this hypothesis against the descriptions of each system and, in his reading of this volume, can test the position of each of the authors to see if scholarly discipline by itself allows the prediction of what classification-and-control schemes are explicitly or implicitly endorsed. Whether or not that particular test for one source of bias is revealing, it would generally appear wise for any nonscientist who relies on a classification scheme to know the background, bias, and moral/political interests of those who have prepared that scheme.

CULTURAL RELATIVISM AND POLITICAL REALITY

The relativistic feature of social classification schemes sets them off from conventional pharmacological and chemical ones. The data from the Navajo illustrate the broad and important phenomenon that the meaning associated with a drug varies from one culture or group to another, as does the significance of how people use the drug and the various effects—including correlated behavior —that are experienced or observed. One sees this readily in Western countries where strong debate can be generated as to whether alcohol is a beverage (liquid food), a medicine, or a drug. Some temperance people call alcohol a poison.

Similarly a person's drunken behavior may variously be considered "good fellowship" by his also inebriated friends; "foolishness" by a more sober friend; "criminal" by a policeman called in to quell the associated noise and fighting; "disgusting and debasing" by a temperance-worker neighbor; "psychopathological alcoholism" by the psychiatrist called in by the drinker's wife; and, by the drinker himself, "good fun," "confusion," "awful sickness," or "terrible remorse," depending on which stage of the weekend binge he is in when one talks to him.

Some of these same features of differing standards and differing behavior samples can be found in group conflicts as to drug categories. For example, there are throughout the Western world many young people who enjoy using cannabis and believe it both good and safe. Opposed to them are nonusers who believe it immoral and unsafe. Those of the younger group press for legalization and are joined by many older persons who, though they do not use the drug, concur in the moral and objective standards and the evidence. Those who believe it immoral and unsafe resist legalization and may press for continued high penalties for possession and sales. If compromises are proposed, for example, the Advisory Committee on Drug Dependence (Wooton Report) in the United Kingdom (1968), the National Commission on Marijuana and Drug Abuse in the United States (1972), or the Le Dain Commission in Canada (1970) or, unofficially, in Egypt (Soueif, 1972), they are likely to be sociopolitical in nature, combining at the very least judgments of present use and risks coupled with estimates about the future and response to political factors.

Across cultures the definitions of drug use and drug abuse, or of particular features such as "dependency" or "health benefit" vary as much or more. Cannabis use is accepted in some countries and is subject to high criminal penalties in others. Opiate use has likewise been accepted in many places and indeed has only recently, in this century, come to be viewed as either dangerous or criminal. Likewise, alcohol use is accepted in Christian lands but is rejected in Moslem countries, notwithstanding that within Christian lands there are rejectors and in Moslem lands acceptors. The same differences in the acceptance and rejection of use may be found with regard to many other psychoactive substances.

One can readily conceive of a classification of countries according to their stance on drug control to demonstrate cultural relativism. It has not been done to date, but would incorporate measures such as the number of drugs controlled, the number of persons coming under control, the intensity and variety of sanctions applied, the funds and personnel mobilized in public action programs, and the like. As a separate index, drug interest might be measured by determining advertising expenditures, drug sales (content analysis), references to drug issues in the press and by politicians, proportion of drug scientists at work, and the like. Interesting political and social-change correlates to such indices might be evident, as, for instance: Are technologically advanced countries with heterogenous populations (United States, U.S.S.R.) more likely to be enforcement-oriented in their stance? Are underdeveloped countries with decentralized governments, that is, tribal controls, likely to be least controlling and least interested? Are countries of equivalent size and technological status likely to differ as their suicide and homicide rates differ, suggesting a relationship between drug control stance/interest and these measures of personal/interpersonal harm? Such research would be interesting and ought to shed light on now hidden variables that contribute to pressures to or not to classify and control psychoactive drugs.

Clearly, drug classification systems that estimate risk or benefit and that call for any form of social control or public action will not meet the same degree of acceptance either within or among countries where there is a range of practice and opinion respecting any of the classified drugs. Whether classification and control schemes arise at all must be attributed to matters of cultural and social values, whether these be linked to definitions of morals or crime or health or politics. The cross-cultural evidence offers some evidence as to when definitions of a drug problem are likely to arise, for example, when more powerful new drugs are introduced into a society; when a society is undergoing rapid and difficult social change; when existing institutions (medical, religious, festive) for integrating (controlling) drug use are breaking down; when large numbers of young people in high socioeconomic categories are removed, by virtue of their family values, from a felt obligation to adhere to conventional moral/drug conduct; when drugs or their styles of use are perceived to symbolize a feared or hated or despised "out group." A more thorough review of factors associated with the origins of drug use and of drug problems will be found in the report, *Origins of Drug Use and Drug Problems,* prepared for the National Strategy Council of the United States (Blum, 1972a).

To the extent that drug use is perceived as a "problem" by any vocal group, they are likely to become an interest group pressing for action. In nation states, action implies some classification scheme under law, be it a classification of drug users (for example, which drinkers of alcohol are to be treated or arrested), of settings of use (which circumstances are legal and which are illegal for the use of peyote), of producers (who may legally grow and/or manufacture and who may not), of sellers (licit and illicit) and of the drugs themselves (dangerous or not, beneficial or not, approved or not). These classifications can be culture specific and will reflect the beliefs of the classifiers and the operation of interest groups. These features in turn become part of the context in which drug classifications for public action emerge.

If one considers these practical pressures, it is evident that such classification-and-control schemes reflect many influences, not just the findings of one discipline of scholars or practitioners (for example, pharmacologists, psychiatrists), but a variety of information, beliefs, interests, pressures, and the like. It would be arrogant and ignorant for a scientist to insist that his discipline should be the one to determine everything about the drugs of interest and what public action should be taken. It would be foolish for scientists representing all disciplines to insist that research data alone should determine public action, for ordinarily public action will take place when other interest groups are aroused; when legislators respond; when laws are drafted; when public discussion takes place; when additional interests are determined; and, finally, when through one set of compromises after another, a public action program is endorsed. How much compromise there will be depends on how beliefs, interests, and power are distributed within a nation or in the international community. For minor matters where little is invested, little compromise may be required. For major matters where there is homogeneity of belief, interest, and power, little compromise is necessary. But for major matters when there is much invested by way of belief, emotion, interest, money, and power—which is the case of psychoactive drugs in much of the world today—then classification schemes and their resulting administrative apparatus and linked public action programs will very likely reflect multiple forces and their temporary resolution through compromise.

Examples of practical forces at work can be found in studies of the history of legislation. These are beyond the scope of this section. For the reader who is interested in the development of international legislation, the following references are recommended: Eisenlohr (1934), Lowes (1966), Renborg (1957), Samuels, (1969), Terry and Pellens (1970), and Little (1971). A history of and commentary on the work of the UN in drug control by Bruun, Pan, and Rexed will be published in 1974. A project of the Consortium, it is tentatively entitled *The Gentleman's Club: International Control of Drugs and Alcohol.*

For the reader who is interested in the much narrower area of the World Health Organization and its work since the 1950s in the drug abuse area, refer to Hakansson (1966) and Zacune (1971). For those who are interested in national comparisons, Shirley Cook (1970) offers insights to the reasons for differing national responses to illegal drug use. William Lanouette (1972) compares the development of the U.S. Dangerous Substances Act of 1970 and the United Kingdom Misuse of Drugs Act of 1971. Legislative histories of individual countries exist, but these will not be cited here.

RANGE OF PURPOSE AND LAWS

Differences in values and interests lead to differences in purpose. Therefore, different kinds of classifications schemes emerge nationally and internationally. Some are broad and seek to deal with that most popular issue of "drug abuse" (that is, disapproved, unhealthy, or illicit use), which forms the basis for our work here. Drug laws themselves may be classified according to their intention as the following taxonomy shows. From that one sees that the control of "abuse" is but one category of action among many, for taxation, regulation, and a variety of other purposes are also served by legal classificatory schemes. There are other schemes as well, some subsumed not under the law but under institutional practice. A good example is that of the pharmacopoeias which are used to classify pharmaceuticals as such for medical and manufacturing reference purposes. Administrative classifications also exist, as, for instance, those governing the stages in the trial of new drugs under drug safety and quality control laws and those determining tax rates, shipping requirements, manufacturers and dispenser's licensing, and other such features.

Our collaborator Jonathan Wolfe has constructed a taxonomy of laws governing drugs. Wolfe's taxonomy restricts itself to the stated objectives of laws not to the latent functions, the actual or unexpected consequences, which result. Religious and tribal codes, while of great importance where operative, are excluded.

I EXPLICIT DRUG LAW OBJECTIVES

Revenue Supply
>taxation
>licensing
>monopolies
>records

Consumer Health and Protection
>licensing requirements for production and sales
>drug purity
>advertising controls
>prescription requirements
>monopoly control
>proofs of drug efficacy
>proofs of drug safety
>warnings as to toxicity
>protection of special religious (drug) practices
>price controls
>labeling as to contents and dosage
>provision for low cost distribution as part of public medical care
>>delivery
>support for research and development

Prevention of Abuse
>elimination of drug supply
>>prohibitions on possession and use
>>prohibitions on sales
>>prohibitions on associations or places of association
>>penalties to deter abuse
>>crop substitution
>>precursors
>>religious law (sanctions by or in support of)
>restriction on drug supply
>>licensing of sellers
>>limitations on supply
>>(state) monopolies
>>record keeping
>>licensing of distributors (physicians, scientists, etc.)
>>licensing of research workers and establishments
>>prescriptions
>>religious law (sanctions by or in support of)
>>quotas
>education
>support for research

Rehabilitation
    civil commitment
    criminal commitment
    compulsory reporting of addicted persons
    education and advertising
    obligation to undergo treatment
    obligation to provide treatment
    provision of social welfare or other support
Organization and Administration
    authorizing and defining the functions (structures of administrative
       bodies)
    funding administrative organs

II FOCUS OF CONTROL
Raw Materials
    agricultural controls
      prohibition laws
      licensing laws
      government monopolies
      taxation laws
      crop substitution
Chemical Precursors
    chemicals/materials used in manufacture
Manufacture
    prohibition of manufacture
    licensing
    monopolies
    labeling
    drug purity laws
    inventories
    taxation
    quotas
Distribution
    sales
      prohibition
      licensing
        consumer
        physicians
        pharmacists
        wholesale distributors
        other suppliers of psychoactive substances
        researchers
        dentists, veterinarians, midwives, etc.
      monopolies
      record keeping
        physicians
        pharmacists
        wholesale distributors

> retail dealers of psychoactive substances (other than
>> pharmacists)
>
> researchers, dentists, veterinarians, etc.

taxation

limitations

> limitation on time of sale
> limitation on age of buyer
> limitation on place of sale
> limitation on amount of sale

advertising

> prohibition
> review and limitations
> warnings

import/export laws

prohibition

licenses

records

monopolies

taxation

limitations to certain ports

quotas

consumer controls

prohibition of use

registration of user

age limitations

time limitations

place of use limitations

limitations of amount used

activity limitations

research and development controls

> defining research activities, research workers, and establishments
> stipulating research substances and their uses
> stipulating research subjects and safeguarding procedures

III TREATMENT LAWS

Compulsory Reporting to Government of Addicted Persons

civil commitment

criminal commitment

> treatment enabling legislation (establishing programs, facilities, and
>> funding)
>
> legislation restricting treatment to particular physicians, clinics, or
>> other especially licensed entities
>
> legislation defining eligibility for treatment
> legislation requiring mandatory tests to detect users

IV PREVENTION: EDUCATION

Education in the Schools

> optional drug education
> compulsory drug education

Drug Education of Professionals
Media
Warnings
Compulsory Education of the Citizenry

With that taxonomy we conclude this section. The listing serves to remind that there are diverse objectives for drug control laws and many alternatives for their form and implementation. We have earlier suggested that classification systems serving control objectives can be improved by being based on a broader range of information and more explicit and systematic procedures for their construction and revision. In the same way, the objectives of legislation can benefit from an awareness of alternatives and improved information—and improved utilization of that information—assessing the appropriateness of an objective in a given situation. There are many alternative mechanisms that can be put to work in the international implementation of control schemes. As one may infer from Woodcock's Chapter Sixteen, these alternatives may be additive and complementary and might well capitalize upon international resources beyond those ordinarily conceived as part of formal multilateral endeavors. Almost certainly, such resources already exist—or can readily be generated—and can be applied in the revision of classification schemes as well as in the development of legislation and administrative and other implementation. The first step is for the policy-maker to become aware of the information and methods that exist. The second is to join together those willing to put these into service to create collaborating resources.

What Do
Drugs Do?

Keith F. Killam

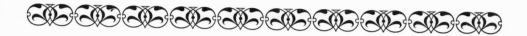

V

That question, "What do drugs do?" is basic to any classification scheme that is used to plan public action. In this chapter we shall speak to the contribution of the basic scientist in gathering information about the action of drugs. In delineating this specific area of basic science pharmacology, we imply the investigation of fundamental processes rather than studies of evaluations of specific therapeutic regimens. The basic scientist uses living tissue as a model for both normal and pathological states found in man. These studies usually involve animal experimentation in its broadest sense; and, in some instances, the investigator manipulates the organism in such a way that the signs derived from that manipulation mimic specific disease states in man. Obviously, caution is needed in the intepretation of material so gathered, but there are many basic problems that can be worked out, at the onset, only with animal experimentation. Another strategy open to the basic scientist is the observation of genetic mutations of animal populations that produce pathologies which mimic those in man. In order to evaluate the contributions that one can make at this level of discourse, it is important to have a basic understanding of what is meant by pharmacology or the interaction of chemical agents with biological preparations.

If we begin at the cellular level, drugs or chemicals ultimately interact with other chemicals. The chemicals within the body comprise the structural units, the fluids bathing the structural units, and the particulate matter suspended in the bathing fluids. Thus, the interaction between chemicals from the outside may occur in the body at many places. If one considers the sites of interactions as targets, then some type of specificity can be deduced by analysis of the precise chemical structure of both the target site and the exciting chemical. At the target site, the usual response of the chemical union is the formation of a drug-target site chemical complex. The affinity or tightness of binding between the chemical and the target site will determine both the quality and the duration of the consequences of that union. If the complex is tightly bound, structural changes may result with secondary or tertiary consequences. With looser binding of a drug-target site complex, the drug may compete with a natural chemical. The result may be a slight modification of function. This leads, in turn, to the concept that the relationship between the chemical and the target site and the binding is in fact a statistical event. The amount of chemical will increase the probability of hits at the target sites; and the degree of tightness of binding at the site will determine whether the site has access to other molecules of the same type or of natural substances. If a particular change in function is infrequently observed with a drug, it may be possible to enhance the probability of the change occurring by simply increasing the amount of drug present.

The consequence of a probabilistic approach or a statistical approach is a method of describing or accounting for threshold effects. By slowly increasing the level of a drug, one should be able to detect the amount needed to produce an observable effect. As the amount of drug is increased further, there should be a dose range over which there is a linear response to linear units of increase in the amount of drug. Finally, there should appear a dose range, wherein no further effect may be observed, even with excess of the drug. These general observations are taken as evidence for drug-target site interactions, target site occupancy, and the probability of formation and dissolution of the complexes.

In the process of forming and dissolution of the complex, the drug molecule may undergo change, the target site may undergo cleavage, or fragments of each may form new complexes. This is called biotransformation. The subsequent products of biotransformation may be less effective than the parent drug, more effective, or have completely different target site specificity. The observable change expressed to the outside world depends upon the role of the target site and its original function. As a corollary, a multitude of targets and their modifications will express the algebraic sum of alterations taking place at all the sites in the body.

If one moves from the cellular concepts to the whole organism, it is obvious that for a drug to have an effect, it must gain access to the delivery system, the circulatory system. The natural way for drugs to gain access to the circulatory system is to be absorbed across biological membranes. The most obvious absorbing surface is the skin. However, because the skin has a very dense exterior to prevent water loss and the conservation of heat, undamaged skin does not absorb chemicals very well. The gastrointestinal and the pulmonary systems represent absorbing surfaces where most chemical transfers take place between the outside world and the circulatory system. Facilitating transfer, these membranes secrete fluid media that dissolve a drug and alter its characteristics, maximizing the exchange. Both systems are bidirectional in that both absorption and excretion go on simultaneously. The two systems are specialized in that the pulmonary system handles gaseous exchanges whereas the gastrointestinal tract specializes in the processing of solids and semisolids. However, neither is exclusive. The gastrointestinal system has an additional factor to be considered in drug action, in that materials absorbed from the system usually are conducted first to the liver, where some degree of biotransformation occurs before the material is then passed out to the general circulation. This accounts for the need to increase the amount of drug when taken orally as compared with that which might be insufflated into the lungs.

With the introduction of the hypodermic needle into medical practice, other routes of entry into the circulatory system and the body in general became available. The intravenous route of applying drugs gains access to the circulatory system directly. Intramuscular or subcutaneous injections provide reservoirs of drugs locally in the particular tissue. The access of the drugs from these reservoirs to the general circulation is dependent upon the specific resorption processes of that particular substructure, muscle or skin.

Once the chemical has passed the absorbing membrane, it is taken up in the circulatory system. Thus, blood containing the drug will bathe every part of the body. Any selectivity of drug effect on a particular organ is simply a case of a better match between the drug and the target sites of that organ. As the amount of drug circulating increases by increased intake, threshold amounts may be present to alter the functions of another organ. Thus, specificity or selectivity of effects can only be ascribed to discrete dose levels. Both qualitative and quantitative changes in the observed effects are related specifically to the amount of drug available in the body. When so-called toxic side reactions are described, the non-selectivity of the drug actions is being demonstrated.

As is the case at the cellular level, biotransformation of the drug-target site complex is a major contributing factor in the duration of a drug-induced change. Another factor to be considered at the organ level is the avenue of excretion of the chemical products. The transport system carries material to and from all organs. As indicated above, the absorbing surfaces of the gastrointestinal tract and the lungs perform excretory functions as well as absorbing functions. In addition, there are three other excretory processes. The first is the kidney. It performs as a selective filtering system, handling particular drugs and chemicals. The second specialized excretory system is the sweat glands. The sweat glands handle many of materials processed by the kidneys. Finally, the liver, in addition to its other biotransformation functions, has a special excretory process as channeled by the bile duct and the gallbladder. Drugs in the circulation may be combined in the liver with bile salts and stored in the gallbladder. These complexes will pass into the gastrointestinal tract, where they may be resorbed or passed through the intestinal system as waste products.

A final consideration at the organ level for the duration of action is the number and kind of storage sites or reservoirs of drugs. This represents a special kind of drug-target site complex. The most common reservoir is the body fat. Repeated administration of lipid-soluble drugs may in time saturate fat deposits, resulting in a prolonged action of the drug after the intake has stopped.

At the whole body level, the effects of drugs must be translated into the algebraic sum of the effects on all systems. At the outset, to describe the spectrum of activity of a particular drug one needs to evaluate the basal or intrinsic patterns of activity in contrast to those as a result of the internal or external adaptations. Basic scientists continue to investigate at the cellular, organ, and whole-body levels the interaction between changes in the internal and external environment that occur spontaneously and day by day. Armed with these data, one may then begin to describe primary and low-order changes induced by drugs. With repeated exposure to a particular chemical, a number of kinds of adaptations occur within the body to reduce its effectiveness. This is termed tolerance.

Tolerance may result from speeding up or making more effective the mechanisms of biotransformation that reduce the effective concentration of drug available in the circulation. This comes about as a response primarily of the liver to the demands upon it. The chief response is to make more sites available for biotransformation. This is called enzyme induction. The subsequent specificity of the new sites for biotransformation is related to the structure of the inducing chemical and whatever other substances may be present in the body at the time. In some instances, the newly induced sites of biotransformation will outlast the presence of the inducer in the body. This becomes of prime importance when we think of environmental pollutants, which may in subtle ways change the bio-transforming machinery of the liver. A reduction in the responsiveness associated with an absolute reduction in the amount of circulating material may be also achieved by having the excretory processes themselves become more efficient.

A second form of tolerance is the loss of sensitivity to the drug at the site where it acts. Tolerance to the drug may extend to other drugs with similar action. This phenomenon is known as cross-tolerance. This has been postulated for drugs such as the opiates. The specific mechanism and change that goes on at the particular site is not well understood.

A final class of adaptations is related to the adaptability of the organism itself. Mammals have extremely complex and redundant pathways to maintain their normal functions. Simply by adapting to the intoxicated state, the organism may generate alternate ways of exhibiting the primary function knocked out by the drug. Some of the implications underlying what is known as state-dependent learning may be examples. By state-dependent learning, we mean that the presence of a particular chemical will govern the kind of response a subject exhibits to a conditioning stimulus. Without the chemical being present, the subject generates a totally different set of responses, achieving the same behavioral endpoint.

With this brief description of the number of areas and concepts in pharmacology that must be borne in mind when we discuss how do drugs act, we shall now comment briefly on the strategies and tactics taken by the various basic scientists in examining the mechanism and site of action of particular drugs. Those trained in chemistry may, on one hand, design new molecules that will compete for specific substances found in the body, or they may design new molecules based upon information already gathered about older drugs that have perhaps multiple effects. The attempt is to reduce the so-called side effects and enhance the primary effect. As we have pointed out above, this is simply a trade-off (governed by the amount of drug available for the most part and only secondarily related to site specificity). Other chemists may study the way in which a particular drug may be biotransformed, as for example with one exposure to the drug, with multiple exposure to the drug, and with the exposure to multiple drugs. The establishment or recognition of the biotransforming pathways and the particular end products may also come from such research. When sufficient quantities of the particular end products can be isolated, these then can be tested as drugs or chemicals in and of themselves. Other chemists continue to delve into the inner workings of the cells and particular organ systems. We know that specific organ systems have differing functions, and thereby the cells must have different machinery to handle the different chemical problems asked of the organ system. As the technology provided by biophysics progresses, the analytical methods are more refined to detect trace quantities of particular substances. In addition, the attempt may be to relate changes from the cellular level back to the whole organism.

The investigator primarily trained in physiology will examine drug effects as they affect either isolated systems or the integration of the body as a whole. He may focus specifically on a particular system and use the other parts of the adapting organism as the controlling factors. A typical question would be "Does a particular drug change the function of the heart as the primary event, or through the control usually exerted on the heart from the brain?" More and more, physiologists are using animals equipped with sensors that monitor a body function in such a manner that the animals will be able to go about their daily lives, but still be observed for the subtle changes occurring as state or drug changes.

The continuing emphasis upon looking at organisms in their natural state and assessing drug effects thereon, emphasizes the role of the investigator trained in psychological techniques. Within these frameworks, the particular subject may be described in terms of his normal adaptive response to his environment or he may be subjected to particular tasks governed by the investigator. In the latter case, the subject may either adapt specifically to the stimulus or he may generate other kinds of behavior in response to the priming stimulus. We see that the particular response elicited by the drug may be described in terms of the behavioral consequences, perhaps in terms of neurophysiological changes, perhaps in terms of other physiological events, or in terms of events that occur at the cellular level.

Across this wide spectrum of investigators as basic scientists who look at how drugs act, there are obvious limitations imposed by the approaches they use and the technologies available for them to quantify the changes. The chemist may be able to tell very precisely what chemical changes can occur, but he may not be able to describe the events that are occurring in a particular neuron when abnormal behavior is being generated. The physiological psychologist may be able to define the part of the brain that is altered at the particular time, when a behavioral change is occurring, but he may not be able to define precisely the chemical event that is going on. The research of the future obviously will employ the wedding of as many of these disciplines as is feasible, commensurate with the development of technologies.

Following this brief consideration of how drugs may act, and describing the general investigatory role of one or another basic discipline, we would like to now examine what we know in general about how drugs do act. The fundamental difference between what will be presented here and what is conventional thought in pharmacology is that we prefer not to be organ-focused. For example, as noted earlier, one may have a drug that works primarily on the heart, but it is also obviously affecting the liver and the kidney. Thus, when somebody says, "I'm taking a heart drug," this is shorthand for saying "I'm taking a drug that has some selective targeting on the heart." We present, here, a different concept of these processes. As we see it, there are four general categories of drugs: First, there are *drugs that effect cures*. These are primarily limited to chemotherapeutic agents. Secondly, there are *drugs that are replacements* for either genetic errors or wear and tear on the body itself. The third category are *drugs that modify or accentuate specific kinds of nervous activity*. The fourth and final category are *drugs that induce other symptoms*. They do not cure the disease process, they simply control it.

In the category of drugs that effect cures, or those useful against invading organisms, we include prophylactic drugs as well as drugs useful in direct therapy. As prophylactic drugs, we include topical disinfectants. The drugs useful in direct therapy are governed by the identification of the invading organism and its sensitivity. Then one poisons selectively the intruder, hoping not to destroy the host at the same time. As we indicated above, the processes of tolerance can develop by having the invader change his responsiveness to the drug. This is why constant research in use of chemotherapeutic agents is necessary.

The category of drugs used in replacement are, as we indicated, of two general classes. The one includes drugs that bypass genetic mutations of the particular subject; the other class simply makes up for the wear and tear on the organism. Aging takes its toll on the endocrine systems, as does traumatic injury. In these instances, replacement drugs are given for the rest of the subject's life, in contrast to those drugs that effect cures. In the latter instance, the drug is present only during the time when the invading organism is there. The responsiveness of the subject to replacement therapy obviously will fluctuate as the stress upon the subject fluctuates from day to day.

The third category of drugs, those that modify or modulate nervous activity, are those that specifically change or alter the transmitter systems in the nervous system. The communication between nerve cells is amplified and modulated normally by a number of chemical substances. These substances are produced in the nerve terminals and bound into prepackaged forms, ready for the next impulse to come down the nerve. When the nerve cell fires, the packaged material is ejected and attaches to the target site on the next neuron. The termination of these events can be by biotransformation of the transmitter substance or the repackaging of the substance back into the original neuron. There are specific chemicals that interfere with the production, the storage, the release, the binding at the target site, and the mechanisms by which the nervous event is terminated. Thus, one might be able to accentuate or nullify the action of one type of transmitter system versus the others. Depending upon the therapeutic event or therapeutic endpoint desired, this may either be a chronic or an acute administration regimen.

The final class of drugs, those that in fact are only symptomatic treatment, accounts for better than half of all the drugs used in therapy. These drugs, and they can vary with respect to the target site, may simply change the adaptive process without specifically changing the disease entity in and of itself. For example, anticonvulsant drugs do not cure epilepsy, they simply control the convulsive disorder. The antischizophrenic drugs, such as chlorpromazine, do not cure schizophrenia, they control the subject's symptoms so that he may be more amenable to other kinds of therapy. A subject who may have a headache, instead of assessing whether or not his eye glasses—or something else—is the source of his trouble, may reach for aspirin automatically to alter the symptom, the headache.

The foregoing, a thumbnail sketch of pharmacology, the discussion of what various kinds of scientists do, and the different approach to the question of "What do drugs do?" is presented not to make the reader more cognizant of the effect of any particular drug, but to change the point of view about the interface between chemistry and biology in general. There is no chemical substance that cannot be used for a different purpose than that accepted for medical therapy. Tomorrow's drug of abuse may be already on our shelves used today for another reason. If the mythologies about drugs and their effects can be altered by a basic understanding of the interface between chemistry and biology, then, part of the mystique will be gone, more rational areas of therapeutics may evolve, and more effective control procedures may be designed.

It should be recognized that the philosophy underlying the above scheme of classification keeps in perspective the totality of the characteristics of each drug. It keeps apart clinical assumptions and intent from the diversified effects. At the same time, as information about a drug accumulates, the full spectrum of activity becomes an ordered mosaic rather than a disjointed collage. More realistic decisions about use and control should be governed by priorities weighing the total cost-benefit rather than targeted classifications.

In this framework, the contributions of all research and therapeutic efforts would contribute to the decision making about usefulness and control. In essence the strengths and limitations of each viewpoint become assets rather than liabilities. There are no protections for inequities save for informed bases for advice allowing the legal base to adapt to the ebb and flow of information, accommodation and adaptation.

The basic scientific approach to the study of drugs—pharmacology—seeks to explain the changes induced by chemical or biological systems from the cellular levels to the interaction of individuals. Each investigator (and thus his data) is the product of his training and capabilities. Placing the information so derived in perspective should focus, not upon expectations of drug selectivity, but on the compromise of the composite of all of the effects from a single drug. The resultant philosophical approach to drug classification should yield maximum freedom for therapy, positive rationale for controls, but at the same time should defuse mysticism related to expectation of drug effects.

Medical Science and
Drug Classification

Daniel Bovet

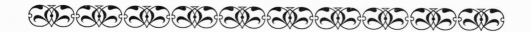

VI

From the standpoint of medicine, the beneficial uses of drugs far outweigh their damaging uses. In consequence, the emphasis in existing classification systems is on drugs with desired effects, what these effects are likely to be, how they are brought about, and what substances are employed to achieve the treatment goal. Pharmaceutical history may be viewed as genuine progress, for not only is the rate of discovery, production, and use of drugs increasing rapidly, but also, even with adverse effects fully acknowledged, the medical gains to this time, measured as relief of pain or improvement in illness or malfunction, have outweighed the costs. Certainly, drug discovery, production, and use should not in themselves be taken as proof of virtue; sometimes the contrary holds. Nevertheless, given today's world, where the unforeseen consequences of technology and what had been thought to be progress are often ugly surprises, the pharmacologist may still take an optimistic view of his field and its future, just as the average man enjoying the benefits either of medicaments or social drugs such as wine and beer will also appreciate the good without denying the occasional bad.

What tomorrow will bring is always uncertain. In pharmacology we can expect it to bring many more drugs serving many more medical purposes (see Evans and Kline, 1972). We can expect more sophisticated methods that yield more understanding of how drugs act and thereby how the body—including the brain and mind—function. With these developments, we can also expect the expansion and greater complexity of drug classifying systems, both those used in science and those applied to public action. Scientific sophistication as well as social wisdom will be required for those lawmakers who plan tomorrow's drug legislation and related social programs.

TERMINOLOGY

The term *drug* is quite widely used, often in the absence of any definition. As noted in earlier chapters, the decision as to whether or not a substance is to be classed as a drug at all is a critical one. Sociologists will say (Goode, 1972) that the decision is really a social process, perhaps not a real decision at all—just a matter of what happens over time in the use of plants and chemicals and the language that grows up around evolving practice. Perhaps that is why pharmacologists have been so broad in their own language when trying to develop a definition that fits all substances, circumstances, and effects. On the other hand, the pharmacologist is aware that so many substances do affect bodily processes that for purely scientific reasons the definition must be embracing. Modell (1967), for example, says that a "drug is . . . any substance that by its chemical nature alters structure or function in the living organism." Goodman and Gilman (1965–1968) state, "A drug is . . . any chemical agent that affects living protoplasm." Hence, "pharmacology . . . embraces the knowledge of the history, source, physical and chemical properties, compounding, biochemical and physiological effects, mechanisms of action, absorption, distribution, biotransformation and excretion, and therapeutic and other uses of drugs," whereas the study of the biochemical physiological effects of drugs is itself pharmacodynamics (see Killam, Chapter Five). For ourselves, we offer a more limited definition: Drugs are substances—either chemically pure and well-defined, impure, or a mixture of vegetable, animal, or mineral products—capable of altering one or several functions in the living organism by altering its constituents by means of chemical, physical, and/or physicochemical properties. *Medication* implies a much more restricted term, one related to the purposes for which a drug is used. A medicament is understood to comprise (Public Health Code of France) "all substances or compositions which are represented to be curative or as possessing preventive properties with respect to human illnesses . . . as well as all products which can be administered to man in order to establish a medical diagnosis, or to restore, correct or modify organic functions."

Central to classification schemes are a number of other terms, the definitions of which are not by any means always clear in practice, terms that embrace much more than conventional medical thinking or practice. Fundamental to the process of classifying and legislating medicaments for social control is the recognition that the concept of a drug "problem" is itself often ill defined.

The Canadian (Le Dain) Commission of Enquiry in 1970 approached drug classification and control with a broad perspective, distinguishing among medical, nonmedical, and illicit use. For the Commission, *medical use* occurs when drugs are given or taken for generally accepted medical reasons, whether under medical supervision or not; all drug use that is not indicated on generally accepted medical grounds is considered to be *nonmedical use*.

The definition of *nonmedical drug use* embraces the following areas:

Illicit drug use corresponds in principle to drugs or practices—the drugs that are nominally forbidden by law. The Canadian report is precise on this point: "Clearly nonmedical use is not to be equated with illegal use. The use of alcohol by adults is generally nonmedical but is—except in Moslem lands—legal, whereas the use of marijuana in most countries is both nonmedical and illegal" (p. 3).

Illicit use, in turn, is to be distinguished from a particular style or outcome of use. For example, *drug addiction* or *drug habituation,* as defined by the WHO Expert Committee on Addiction Producing Drugs (World Health Organization Technical Report #142, 1957), attend primarily to substances, styles, and outcomes, mostly involving opiates (heroin, morphine, and the like) but embracing barbiturates, alcohol, and other drugs linked to these uses and responses.

Drug addiction, or the French equivalent, *toxicomanie,* is yet another distinction. Abandonment of the English word *addiction* was recommended by WHO, yet one finds it widely employed. For example, Jaffe (1970), Preble and Casey (1969), and others find it useful in describing the intense involvement in the drug life that accompanies "drug dependence" especially with opiates but that is not a necessary consequence of opiate administration. It implies the centering of all interests on drugs and on drug-using comrades, a way of finding meaning in life and of keeping active, and perhaps a symbolic rejection of straight-world values.

The foregoing are to be distinguished from *drug dependence*. This term is recommended by the WHO Expert Committee of Addiction Producing Drugs (World Health Organization Technical Report #273, 1964) and by the WHO Scientific Group on Evaluation of Dependence-Producing Drugs in order to seek greater precision in descriptions encompassing particular forms of use for many drugs. The WHO definition reads: "Drug dependence" is a state of psychic or physical dependence, or both, on a drug arising in a person following administration of that drug on a periodic or continuous basis. The characteristics of such a state will vary with the agent involved, and these characteristics must always be made clear by designating the particular type of drug dependence in each specific case; for example, drug dependence of morphine type, or barbiturate type, or amphetamine type, etc.

Within the concept *dependency,* WHO distinguishes between *physical dependency,* a relatively precise description of a syndrome involving tolerance, craving, and, according to some, relapse in which the role of the drug itself can be specified (even if not fully understood biochemically) and psychological or *psychic dependency*. The latter term implies a requirement for "compulsive" or otherwise uncontrolled drug use due not to the interaction of chemicals in the drug with metabolic processes as is presumed with physical dependency, but rather a state of need or interest in the user that, for many possible reasons, comes to be focused on a drug and its repetitive use. Yet it will be seen that these two forms of dependency are not as clear as might be hoped. For example, psychological factors (for example, learning) may well play a strong role in the development of physical dependency, certainly relapse is otherwise difficult to explain. Psychic dependency is a restatement of the mind-body dichotomy that is so treacherous philosophically. It deemphasizes the physiological processes underlying "mind" and may obscure metabolic idiosyncrasies, or even learned autonomic functions, which—as, for example, in psychogenetics—can account on biological grounds for differences among animals in their reactions to psychoactive substances.

One further distinguishes *drug abuse*. Eddy, Halbach, and others (1965) in the WHO document ask that "drug dependence" be equated with "all kinds of drug abuse." Yet, in spite of the WHO plea for such synonomous usage, one must recognize that other writers employ *drug abuse* to describe, not specific drug dependencies, but a wide variety of forms of drug use, even that conduct of drug users that may not be an outcome of use, of which the observer disapproves.

PERSPECTIVES

The examination of terminology and usage shows that there is considerable variation in how people speak of drug effects and drug users. Underlying the differences, which introduce notable confusion and unnecessary debate of the sort that semanticists deplore, one may identify quite different perspectives and criteria. The *legal* position speaks of "illicit" and sometimes that is synonomous with "abuse." The *moral* view underlies "abuse" as disapproval but may be found if "addiction" is believed by the speaker to be a state of depravity or weakness. The *psychiatric* view implies a kind of personality that is "dependent" or medical diagnoses related to "dependency" or "toxicomanie" and may presume special relationships for kinds of personalities to kinds of drugs as, for example, "heroin addicts" most often being "psychopaths" (Pichot and Buchsenschutz, 1972). The *biological* view may presume biochemical-metabolic processes entirely as accounting for "dependency" and "addiction." One may also identify a *social* view, which focuses on the beliefs of the user or the observer, that is, "abuse" as disapproved behavior, "addiction" as centering on interests or meaningful activity, or "nonmedical use" as descriptive of social activities (drinking) or religious rituals (wine in the Mass).

It is evident that diverse criteria are brought to bear even when the same term is employed. Consequently, the language of description in drug classification easily suffers confusion and leads to misunderstanding. That misunderstanding can be superimposed on the substantive issues of data, that is, what do drugs do, how do people react, how are risks defined, and what relationships are there among various control measures and the reduction either of risks or of benefits?

CONTROL FOCUSED ON MEDICAMENTS

Most drugs that are the subject of laws aiming to control social or private use are also—or have been purported to be—medicaments. Such a statement requires that folk medications, for example, those employed in Ayurmedic medicine, be considered medical practice. A notable exception to the overlap are the hallucinogens, rarely used in Western or Old World folk medicine. These are used religiously and sometimes socially. The correlation between substances employed as medicaments and those self-administered for social, private, or religious reasons (or at least in such settings) means, at the outset, that medical scientists and practitioners have a great interest in the development of classification systems that set the limits of acceptable medical practice. Usually these limits are set in collaboration between medical (or other biological) scientists and lawmakers, but quite often their views and data base are disparate enough to create areas of dispute—if not outright conflict—between the two groups. Among all possible drugs (poisons, industrial chemicals, pollutants, plants, and the like), those that are medicaments are most subject to legal sanctions extending to medical practice. Because drugs that have diagnostic or healing functions also appear in greatest demand for nonmedical reasons and to the extent that overlap exists among drugs that produce desired medical effects and those with actual or presumed important social and private effects, then biological scientists have additional interests in classification systems, for their knowledge of drug effects ought to be of some assistance in understanding or predicting the nonmedical use of drugs. Note that we say only "some assistance," for one must not presume a similarity of effects under medical and nonmedical administration. The interest of the biological scientist in classificaton schemes embracing drugs used socially or privately (in some instances termed *abuse* or *misuse*) is also aroused because of the possibility of learning more about medical uses, that is, clinical effects, by observing nonmedical practices. This point is made by Tinklenberg in Chapter Twelve.

One observes that among the medicaments most subject simultaneously to legal controls for medical, research, and social/private use, there are but few, in contrast to the immense number of drugs in existence. Although it is inexact to speak of a common characteristic, one may say that this group of drugs, which are attracting most legal and public attention today, are for the most part linked by either an actual or a presumed ability to affect the mind and behavior in ways that both patients or users and observers are likely to say are primarily good, that is, widely desired, but also bad, that is, in some way toxic or undesirable. In this volume, we agree to use the word *psychoactive* to embrace these substances, although others may call them psychotropic, narcotic, drugs of abuse, or the like. Within the special class of medicaments that are psychoactive one finds the efforts at classification for public action and, in consequence, an awareness of the problems of method, fact, and viewpoint that occur as one attempts to set up criteria for establishing the good and the bad, the acceptable circumstances for medical and nonmedical use, and the kinds of effects that ought to be known in order to make public and private decisions as to what uses are warranted.

We see immediately that there are disagreements, not only about classification particulars but also as to what drugs belong within the general class of substances defined as psychoactive and subject to public control. A definition of *psychoactive* that seeks to encompass these present and future drugs is that found in the (Vienna) Convention on Psychotropic Substances: A psychoactive substance "has the capacity to produce central nervous system stimulation or depression or hallucinations or disturbances in perception, thinking, mood or behavior."

The emphasis of this definition is on effects—generally speaking, effects on the mind and behavior. In consequence, basic to all initial decisions is the question: Is the drug psychoactive or not? If it is, the allocation to a subcategory rests on being able to determine the effects on the mind, on behavior, of a given substance. Pharmacodynamics, because it treats with these effects, albeit at biochemical and physiological levels, necessarily becomes a means for producing information for making nonmedical decisions, that is, decisions about laws and regulations. Problems are built into this procedure, not only because of the scientific limitations of pharmacodynamics but because of the difficulty in translating biochemical and physiological findings into the language of lawmakers, in extrapolating laboratory data to the actual conditions of drug administration, and in the differing assumptions of scientists and lawmakers (and, of course, among scientists and lawmakers and other citizens) as to what the data mean, what the laws mean, and what the desirable and undesirable effects of those laws —as well as the drugs themselves—are or will be.

DRUG DEVELOPMENT

Throughout such discussions, persons with a medical orientation will have an interest in facilitating the discovery, production, and use of demonstrably beneficial medicaments, for they will be aware that this is an age of great pharmacological activity, the benefits of which they will not wish to see blocked. For example, a physician cannot happily see an incident of some misuse of opiates lead to the creation of laws that so control medical practice that patients in great pain cannot be relieved thereof. The cost of such control of a relatively rare misuse would be the prevalence of great pain and anguish. The physician will, on the other hand, be aware that because adverse effects do occur, including those related to toxicity, the proper conditions for the medical administration of drugs must be stated so as to secure in practice rational, safe pharmacotherapeutics.

The unexpected effects of drugs, that is, side effects, can be capitalized upon to lead to new uses and new classes of compounds. Indeed, psychopharmacology began in this way. On the other hand, interest in side effects may be the essence of nonmedical use as people enjoy drugs for pleasure, relaxation, mystical experiences, and the like. Here the achievement of the side effects (viewed from the physician's professional standpoint) become the presumed motives for use. Among these motives it must be emphasized that sensory experiences as well as organic changes are sought; motives as well as drug effects can appear to be nonspecific as humans "play" with drugs in the expression of curiosity and the pleasure of discovery. Yet, other than playfulness is also found as the adverse effects of drugs are put to use for exploitative, aggressive, or lethal purposes. These are seen in chemical warfare, in crowd control with "nerve gases," in the manipulation of drug-dependent persons, and in suicide and homicide by drugs. These are also part of the discovery process.

The rate of pharmaceutical development may best be understood by looking backward. One of our most ancient documents in the history of medicaments is an Egyptian papyrus. The Ebers papyrus, which probably originated around 1550 B.C., contains prescriptions for cathartics (castor oil), antiparasitics (root of pomegranate), and emetics. Their use has reached us after surviving for thirty-five centuries. The therapeutic domain has been progressively enriched by the opium poppy and the mandragora—introduced by Dioscorides in the first century; by gold and mercury—introduced into the medical armamentarium by Avicenna (980–1037); by the use of sulfur and the discovery of the effects of mercury in the treatment of syphilis (Holmsted and Liljestrand, 1963) as practiced by Paracelsus in the sixteenth century. We owe to the seventeenth century the discovery of the properties of cinchona bark (quinine) and to the eighteenth century the introduction of digitalis. However, the real development of drugs occurred in the nineteenth and twentieth centuries as a consequence of chemical progress and particularly in the wake of developments in organic chemistry.

In 1827, E. Merck announced the production of morphine, which had been isolated for the first time by Sertuner in 1806, and of emetine and of strychnine (Tempkin, 1964). The introduction of anesthesia by means of gas occurred in the nineteenth century: nitrous oxide (1842); ether (1844); chloroform (1847); later the bromides were introduced (1864) and chloral (1869); then the local anesthetics (cocaine, 1864; stovaine, 1903; procaine, 1905). All these represented significant stages in the battle against pain.

At the beginning of the twentieth century, Dreser introduced acetylsalicylic acid (1899); Takamine produced epinephrine, the first synthetic hormone (1901); Fisher and von Mering synthesized barbituric acid derivatives (1903); while the systematic studies of Cattell in 1910 resulted in "606," the "magic bullet" against syphilis, the first term of the arsenobenzol series, which were to be followed by an explosive development in medical chemistry. The studies of the alkaloids, the vitamins, the steroids and polypetide hormones, the antibacterials, and the antibiotics—all derived from the most varied fields of synthetic and organic chemistry—have allowed improvement of known medications and the development of new types of therapeutic agents: the androgens, estrogens, progesterones, analgesics, anti-inflammatories, antiallergics, antidiabetics, diuretics, antibacterials, and antiparasitics. More products were discovered in the twenty-five years between 1930 and 1955 than during the preceding 3,500 years. It is estimated that approximately 75 percent of the medications prescribed after 1960 were discovered only within the last twenty-five years.

Two concrete examples will illustrate the ways and the rapidity with which progress has been made possible in medical chemistry. Penicillin is the first example. It was discovered by Fleming in 1928 and isolated by Chain and Florey in 1940. The first penicillin compounds, although they appeared at that time as miraculous products, have nevertheless been improved remarkably since then. Successive studies have, first of all, permitted the development of retarded-action penicillin, then long-term-acting pencillins, penicillins that are acid-resistant, pencillinase-resistant, oral penicillin, penicillins that are effective against resistant strains, penicillin analogues, derivatives less likely to produce allergic reactions, and, finally, the broad spectrum penicillins that by their polyvalent activity combat infections against which we were helpless up to that point.

A second example demonstrates the progressive increment in pharmacological activity that can be achieved through research. Consider the diuretics in carbonic anhydrose inhibitor series that began with sulfanilamide; in only a few years their efficacy, as measured by the effective dose, has increased 100- to 1,000-fold.

The introduction of more effective medications has had positive effects on public health. Witness decreased mortality from infectious diseases, decreases in infant mortality, increase in population growth as a function of longer life expectancies, and the enhancement of human lives as individual pain and disability is reduced. One must not contend that these public health developments are due solely to pharmacological progress, for simultaneously one has witnessed improved technology and delivery of medical services, better nutrition, remarkable advances in sanitation, and other health-advancing achievements.

For example, if one examines the Statistical Annuals of the French Government covering all French territories, one finds that infant mortality dropped regularly (except during World War II) from 28.4 deaths per thousand in 1870 to 11.1 deaths per thousand in 1965. The number of deaths of children under one year old dropped from 201 per thousand in 1870 to 21.9 in 1965. In the United States, taking another example, influenza and pneumonia deaths were reduced from 155.9 per one hundred thousand in 1910 to 31.6 per one hundred thousand in 1965. The deadliness of tubercular meningitis in France before the introduction of antibiotics was 100 percent, but it is now estimated to be about 7 percent. Bronchiopneumonia killed about one-third or those suffering from it before antibiotics and only about 6 percent now. As a corollary, life expectancy has increased. In France, for example, in 1805 life expectancy was about thirty-three years; in 1970 it was about seventy years. Given such developments, human beings will be grateful for public health advances and to pharmaceuticals insofar as they have played a role.

Beginning very early, human beings have learned the value of drugs. They have sought them out, in folk medical explorations, in pharmacognosy, in university or institute laboratories, in clinical research, or, combined with an economic interest, by means of the pharmaceutical industry. The growth of the latter has itself been rapid during the past fifty years. Today it is estimated that 80 percent of all drug research is financed by industry. If there is a close relationship between investment and discovery, one must expect that the industry will be the major source of new medicaments.

The trend is for new medicaments to replace, not supplement, old ones.

The short period during which a product is likely to be used widely (estimate, perhaps fifteen years) should be considered in the light of product protection by means of increasingly widespread international patent agreements that affect pharmaceutical inventions. This means increasing pressure on pharmaceutical industries to produce new drugs and a marketplace that, thanks to patent protection, is also encouraging.

CONSUMPTION

Simultaneously, we see a number of broader economic features that increase the consumption of drugs, and some of these same features may lower relative drug cost to individuals. These factors include rising rates of personal income, increased advertising to physicians (and indirectly to patients and non-medical users), growth in the relative numbers of physicians and paramedical personnel dispensing drugs, the increased role of the nation-state as provider to or insurer of individuals so that drug purchase costs are shared by taxpayers, increased competition within the pharmaceutical industry (with decreasing trade barriers, as in the European Economic Community and its associate countries), and in some places competition between legitimate and illegitimate producers and sellers as well (these latter may be simply smugglers who avoid taxes or illicit dealers who can undersell drug dispensers because their markup is less[*]). All of these factors provide a large market, while the natural wish to feel well and to avoid pain, coupled with the increased availability of substances warranted to achieve these ends, provides the motives for medical consumption.

Traditional medical practice (Balint, Hunt, and others, 1970; Blum, 1960) contains strong elements conducive to prescribing even in the absence of certain medical need, as, for example, the use of the medicament to symbolize the doctor's "giving" something to the "wanting" patient, the reliance on the repeat prescription as a way of maintaining the doctor-patient relationship in cases where psychological defenses mitigate against the better communication that might identify and treat functional complaints, and the speed with which prescriptions can be written when a busy practitioner does not want to take time out for a thorough examination and more rational treatment regime. No doubt there are other features that also are conducive to prescribing—or, as in the foregoing cases, to overprescribing. For example, Lennard, Epstein, and others (1971) propose that under the pressure of wishing to increase sales, pharmaceutical companies in their advertising tend to define previously normal states as abnormal and thus deserving of therapeutic—in particular drug-therapeutic—intervention. The advertised definition of a mother's crying as her little girl goes off to school for the first time as "depression" in need of "treatment" by an

[*] Blum (personal communication) reports that in his study of drug dealers he found California housewives who had prescriptions for barbiturates buying them from illicit dealers at one-half the druggist's price. Some of the same dealers who were selling the son marijuana were selling the mother her sleeping pills.

antidepressant drug, is an illustration. A further facilitator of prescribing may be the fact that the patient—or the insurance company or government—pays for the drugs, not the doctor. There is no penalty to the physician for overprescribing even though we see, in Italy and the United Kingdom, for example, a great waste of drugs prescribed but not used.

Above and beyond these facilitating features are those that are part of technological society in general. They may be summarized as an increasing trust in increasingly available technological products by which to control nature, including illness and disability or, for the psychoactive specifically, human nature. The trust seems well founded, given the recent history of medicine. It is not, however, without its side effects—as students of ecology, with increasing pessimism —have pointed out.

At this point we may say that, short of catastrophic change, the trend is for more drugs, more medicaments, and more people using medicaments. There will be greater diversity and specificity in drug functions and effects, greater consumer pressures for use, more physician readiness to prescribe, and such competitiveness in industry—accompanied by large sales and, we presume, profits—as further to encourage research and yet more development. Inevitably, the pharmaceuticals produced will have undesirable side effects, for one cannot expect completely to avoid toxicity. There will be expanding social and private as well as medical use. And one anticipates—insofar as there is public anxiety over either the novelty or ill effects of such new uses—counterpressures for legislation and control. If Tinklenberg and Woodrow (1974) are correct in stating that the cross-cultural evidence reveals rates of "abuse" of from 3 percent to 7 percent in adequately studied society, with higher rates being unusual—such as the Mexican village alcoholism rate of 50 percent among males aged forty and over, as reported by Maccoby (1972)—then one expects that the counterpressures for control will not ordinarily be based on evidence of widespread prevalence of ill effects or of real "epidemics" as some have contended. The log normal distribution described by Tinklenberg and Woodrow (1974) and found in Canada to characterize the incidence of use of many drugs (Smart, 1973) does, however, link the definition of extreme or abusive use to the average level of use of a given drug in a given society.

Musto (1973) argues that for the United States at least historical data indicate that pressures for the most stringent control of new kinds of drug use arise when a disapproved (feared, hated) minority is identified with the use of a substance. If this is so, then it would appear that the pressures for control are partly directed toward controlling people (the minority) not drugs, or preventing the spread of the minority's perceived characteristics to the majority, probably especially to the children of the majority. In a way, one may view the process as resistance to the "democratization of delinquency" that the empirical evidence (see Blum and Associates, 1972b) does show occurring in the spread of drug use through drug dealing.

REGULATION AND REACTIONS

One of the easiest sectors to control by law is that of research, especially academic and clinical research on drugs, since scientists are notoriously law-abiding, às Blum's comparison of students and faculty on the same college campus showed (1972b). Pressures for control on research are likely to handicap studies on drug effects, including those pharmacodynamic investigations that are fundamental to comprehending the range of drug actions and outcomes on which any law containing drug classifications based on effects must rest. It is possible then to foresee an unstable—or if you will, unsatisfactory—scientific-legal system in which the response to change contains elements that negate the very feedback and information flow that is required for the rational guiding of change, that is, informed social policy based on accurate data derived from research (see Lind, Chapter Fourteen).

If regulations become so stringent that drug research is impeded and drug production no longer pays because the market is restricted, one would then anticipate reduction in pharmaceutical industry research activity and subsequent reliance on a more limited medical armamentarium. That could mean some potentially treatable illnesses will go untreated, and some diminishable pain will not be diminished. The history of human inquiry and the strong urge to combat illness and pain are such as to suggest that such controls also constitute an unstable system* (not considering the economic or intellectual incentives to produce and the powerful reasons for nonmedical use) for, to date, human beings have been reluctant to accept controls on "progress," especially the relief of suffering, for the sake of forestalling or suppressing undesirable effects.

Resistance to controls also arises as part of a philosophy of life—and of government—that puts its emphasis on the cultivation of individual freedom and resistance of intrusion on that freedom. Leake (1961), when considering "the scientific status of pharmacology" as retiring president of the American Association for the Advancement of Science, resisted further controls saying, "We have altogether too much bureaucracy as it is, and if we are to preserve our standards of individual freedom and responsibility in our social unity, we must do all we can to reduce government control and regulation."

---

* In the United States where legislation (the Kefaufer-Harris Amendments of 1962) requires manufacturers to prove drug effectiveness, there is an on-going debate between those who argue that such laws protect the public and those who claim that they work to slow development and release of beneficial compounds. Economists Friedman and Peltzman, arguing the latter, show that since the law there has been a decline in new drugs introduced. United States government health authorities and spokesmen for the pharmaceutical manufacturers disagree, contending that the rate of introduction of important new agents has been stable for two decades. They also suggest that fewer drugs introduced can denote progress insofar as new drugs now introduced are more efficacious and less dangerous and contribute less to a market already so crowded with drugs that physicians are dangerously confused. (*Washington Post,* Feb. 8, 1973, U.S. Senate hearing report.)

If the history of medicaments—and economics—suggests strain built into stringent control efforts, does that suggest the annihilation of social regulation of medicine? We are neither historians nor futurologists, yet we would venture to state that is not the case. It appears that the more regularized the social situation in which drugs are administered, the greater the predictability of the emergent behavior—including drug effects. The parallel to laboratory conditions is readily seen. If we see that predictability of effects (and thus diminished anxiety or undesirable side effects) is achieved through social regulation, just as it is through medical supervision (medical supervision is an excellent illustration of social regulation or a kind of control on settings of use), it is hard to imagine any but the hardiest anarchist opting for greater chance rather than greater certainty. Experience of modern societies with situations in which there is no control—including, for example, those in which there is insufficient control over the pharmaceutical industry by means of testing and licensing of new drugs before they are put on the market (for example, thalidomide in West Germany or the United Kingdom)—does not allow one to conclude that laissez-faire is the optimal rule for the marketing of medicaments.* Medical scientists will be the first to argue against laissez-faire in drug research, production, or sales. One must therefore anticipate that social controls over drugs will continue to be used and elaborated, and that whatever disequalibria exist by virtue of controls will be the cost of controls. The problem, of course, is to optimize the system. That will require improved classificatory schemes and improved research as well as maximal, mutually respectful communication among citizens, lawmakers, the drug industry, and scientists.

PSYCHOACTIVE DRUGS

Psychoactive drugs represent one of the most ancient domains of pharmacology. Because their effects on mind and behavior are easily visible, early man seems to have been quick to identify psychoactive plants and to put such substances to use in religious, healing, social, and personal ways. There is evidence of very early use of beer and wine among neolithic agricultural populations, and among nonliterate hunting and gathering peoples—such as the American Indians —there are knowledge and use of a variety of plants productive of hallucinogenic effects. The data suggest that the present importance of psychoactive drugs is an expression of mankind's continuing pharmacotropic history.

In the civilized world, one finds a history of at least several thousand years of use of cannabis and opium, as well as the more recent introduction of

---

* In the same U.S. Senate hearings in which pro and con arguments were heard about the requirements for demonstrable efficacy before release, data were introduced showing that a heart drug (propranolol), banned in the United States but allowed on the market in countries with less stringent testing requirements, was associated with producing heart failure in patients receiving it (at a rate of 9.2 percent in one group and 13 percent in another). (*Washington Post,* Feb. 8, 1973, U.S. Senate hearing report.)

distilled alcoholic spirits. Yet the discovery of surgical anesthesia marks a technological turning point, the introduction into modern medicine in the nineteenth century of manufactured psychoactive compounds. This has been followed by the discovery and introduction into medical practice of other very important psychoactive drugs, the barbiturates (used as hypnotics, sedatives, and anticonvulsants), the synthetic analgesics, and, also in the first half of the twentieth century, the amphetamine stimulants. Of special importance to modern psychopharmacology was the introduction during 1953 and 1954, of three medicaments—chlorpromazine, reserpine, and meprobamate. Anticipated by the studies of Lewin (1924), Kraepelin (1892), and Moreau (1845), the 1950s marked the beginning of chemotherapy in psychiatric illness. Three groups of medicaments emerged following these initial discoveries. Classified by their applications in clinical psychiatry, the classes are the antipsychotics (also called neuroleptics and tranquilizers), the antianxiety drugs (for example anxiolytics), and the antidepressants. The results of their use have been so impressive as to be called by Kline the third psychiatric revolution. One should note that drugs in these classes are of value in treating minor as well as major psychiatric disorders, and they also have extensive applications in geriatrics, family medicine, terminal care, and the like.

The direct benefits resulting from the psychopharmacological revolution have been most impressively seen in the reduction in most nations in the number of patients in mental hospitals. In the United States during a decade of 20 percent population growth, there was, for instance, a 10 percent reduction in psychiatric bed patients. In France, Delay (1956) reports that following the introduction of antipsychotic drugs, the average period of mental hospitalization has gone down from 122 to 59 days. That these reductions in number of hospitalized patients and duration of hospitalization have simultaneously been associated with other innovations in psychiatry, especially community psychiatry with its emphasis on outpatient care and on milieu therapy (that is, open-door or other more effective ward-management procedures). Greenblat, Solomon, and others (1965) state that drugs have by far the greater effect when compared with milieu therapies. The effect of the two developments together may well be additive. The advent of psychopharmacology has supported innovation in concepts of care and those innovations have in turn facilitated chemotherapy aimed at reducing the number of persons in the hospital.

The very importance of psychoactive drugs, first in psychiatry and then in all of medical research and practice, has been one of the problem sources for classification schemes. Schema have grown up emphasizing one or another outstanding feature of one drug (or a subgroup) yet combining these inconsistent features into one overall scheme. What emerges may sometimes be useful in teaching and in research and has, perhaps for those reasons, become a matter of habit in medical thinking. These habits, however, are not usually helpful in advising on law or social policy governing nonmedical drug use.

In Table 1 we offer a classification scheme of the sort used by medical

Table 1. MEDICAL DRUG CLASSIFICATION ADAPTED
FOR LEGISLATIVE SCHEMES

General class of drug or therapeutic use	Specific drugs in that class: illustrative examples
A. General anesthetics	
1. Gases	Nitrous oxide, ethylene, cyclopropane
2. Volatile[a] substances	The ethers, chloroform (obsolete), halothane, methoxyflurane
3. Nonvolatile substances (intravenous) (see Barbiturates)	Ultrashort-acting barbiturates (sodium thiopental, hexobarbital)
B. Alcohol	Ethyl alcohol
C. Hypnotics and sedatives	
1. The barbiturates	Amobarbital, secobarbital, phenobarbital, pentobarbital, thiopental
2. Nonbarbiturate sedative-hypnotics	Bromides, paraldehyde, chloral hydrate, ethchlorvynol, ethinamate, glutethimide, methaqualone, methyprylon
D. Anticonvulsants and antiepileptics	
1. Barbituric-acid derivatives	Phenobarbital, mephobarbital, primidone
2. Glutarimides	Amino-glutethimide
3. Hydantoins	Diphenylhydantoin, ethotoin, mephenytoin
4. Acetylureas	Phenacemide, pheneturide
5. Oxazolidines	Trimethadione, paramethadione
6. Succinimides	Phensuximide, methsuximide, ethosuximide
7. Carbonic anhydrase inhibitors	Acetazolamide
E. Drugs for Parkinson's disease	
1. Centrally acting muscle relaxants	Mephenesin, methocarbamol (Robaxin®), chlorsoxazone, carisoprodol
2. Centrally acting anticholinergics	Trihexyphenidyl
a. Atropine derivatives	Benztropine mesylate, orphenadrine and chlorphenoxamine, caramiphen hydrochloride
3. Centrally acting catecholamines	L-dopa
F. Analgesics	
1. Narcotic analgesics	
a. Opium alkaloids	Morphine, codeine, thebaine, heroin, apomorphine
b. Synthetic narcotic analgesics	Meperidine, methadone, pentazocine, alphaprodine, anileridine
2. Non-narcotic analgesics and antipyretics and anti-inflammatories	
a. Salicylates	Sodium salicylate, acetylsalicylic acid (aspirin)

General class of drug or therapeutic use	Specific drugs in that class: illustrative examples
b. Para-aminophenol derivatives	Phenacetin, acetaminophen, acetanilid
c. Pyrazolon derivatives	Antipyrine, aminopyrine
G. Neuroleptics and antipsychotics	
1. Phenothiazine derivatives	Chlorpromazine, promazine, triflupromazine, fluphenazine, perphenazine, prochlorperazine, trifluoperazine, thioridazine
2. Rauwolfia alkaloids	Reserpine, rescinnamine, deserpidine, syrosingopine
3. Butyrophenones derivatives	Haloperidol
4. Thioxanthenes	Chlorprothixene
H. Antianxiety drugs (minor tranquilizers) (See C. Hypnotics and sedatives)	
1. Antihistamines	Hydroxyzine
2. Benzodiazepine compounds	Chlordiazepoxide (Librium®), diazepam (Valium®)
3. Anticholinergic	Benactyzine
4. Miscellaneous	Meprobamate (Miltown®, Equinal®)
I. Antidepressants	
1. Tricyclic antidepressants	Imipramine, amitriptyline
2. Monoamine oxidase inhibitors	Tranylcypromine (Parnate®), Isocarboxazid (Marplan®), Nialamide (Niamid®), Phenelzine sulfate (Nardil®)
J. Psychic stimulants	
1. Phenylalkylamines	Amphetamine
2. Others (not derived from phenylalkylamines)	Methylphenidate, pipradrol
3. Xanthines	Caffeine, theophylline, theobromine
4. Miscellaneous	Cocaine
K. Hallucinogens (or psychotomimetics or psychotogenics)	Mescaline, lysergic acid diethylamide (LSD), dimethoxymetamphetamine (STP), psilocybine, phencyclidine (PCP), cannabis (marijuana, hashish, ganja, bhang)
L. Analeptics (central nervous system stimulants of the convulsant type)	
1. Cortical analeptics	Pentylenetetrazol
2. Mixed analeptics	Nikethamide Picrotoxin Ethamivan Bemegride
3. Spinal convulsants	Strychnine

[a] Volatile solvents for nontherapeutic use (glue-sniffing): toluene, acetone, benzene, etc.

texts and adapted for legislative schemes. It is illustrative only and does not seek
to present all drugs conventionally grouped in any of the categories. The table
was constructed by reviewing texts—Soviet (Zakusov, 1966), French (Hazard,
Cheymol, and others, 1969), English (Paton and Payne, 1968), English-Cana-
dian-United States (Goodman and Gilman, 1965–1968; DiPalma, 1964), and
United States (Cutting, 1964; Usdin, 1970)—supplemented by McGeer (1971),
and then constructing a composite.

Observe that in some cases—Groups A, C, E, and L (general anesthetics,
hypnotics, anti-Parkinsonism agents, convulsants and the like)—the clinical
classification base coincides well with experimental data based on studies of
behavioral effects, on cerebral metabolism, and on electrophysiology. When a
neurologist or a pharmacologist speaks of anticonvulsants (antiepileptic, anti-
Parkinsonism) drugs, the former as clinician and the latter as laboratory investigator will be able to use the same terms, for at several levels of effects the drugs
are consistent and correlated and thus constitute a well-defined nosological entity.
Insofar as these consistent observations are used to create a classification category
—that is, of anticonvulsant psychoactive substances—the classification scheme is
accepted by and useful both to the practicing physician and the research scientist.
If, however, one were to note that anesthetics such as nitrous oxide, ether, and
also phencyclidine (Sernyl, see K) are used socially for pleasure, as is the case,
then the scheme breaks down, for the effects noted by the street-scene observer
are no longer at the neurological level. The scheme then ceases to be consistent.

We see in Table 1 that another subgroup rests, not on neurological
descriptions of effects, but on clinical psychiatric observations. In Groups G, H,
and I in the table, the classification criteria rest on the capability of the drug to
relieve the symptoms of a given type of psychiatric disorder, that is, anxiety,
depression, or psychoses. This group differs from the classification by effects on
such entities as convulsions and sleep only because psychiatric symptoms have
less well-defined animal or laboratory counterparts. Yet other groups are constituted as subgroups among the foregoing, with the criterion being the mechanism of action. For example, among the antidepressants there is a distinction
between those that increase biogenic amines by blocking the enzyme mono-
aminoxydase (tranylcypromine) and those that presumably act by interfering
with the re-uptake of released transmitters. Still another group, subgroups J and
K in Table 1, are classified, not by the symptoms they relieve, but by some of the
symptoms they (may) produce. Thus LSD is classified as a hallucinogen because
it is commonly reported by those ingesting it to produce changes in sensation,
changes that are summarized (sometimes inaccurately, in fact) under the term
"hallucination." Nicotine is stimulating but smokers also report they are calmed
and, when given to someone undergoing nicotine withdrawal, the drugs seem to
relieve distress, even pain. Thus we see that for groups classified according to
symptom production (or relief), the term used as the classification key—that is,
hallucination, stimulation—is but one of many effects possible, yet the name
of the group rests on an essentially psychiatric judgment as to a major effect,

a judgment more or less corroborated by laboratory studies depending on the level of observation made. One notes too that for cannabis, the key-word conventional classification as an hallucinogen is rarely descriptive of reported subjective effects. Yet those who would class cannabis as a euphoriant introduce a classification—pleasure-producing—that is based on subjective effects reported across almost all groups by nonmedical users.

We see in Table 1 that Group I has subgroups based on chemical names, for instance, tricyclic derivatives. Sometimes groups are built up on the basis of chemical typologies, for instance, a pharmacologist may describe the action of a new drug (or a new observation in a known one) as being like the action of a known chemical compound—for example, he may say that drug X is chlorpromazine-like or drug Y appears to be of the morphine type. The examples in Group F show that the foregoing analogous subgroup procedure, based on classifying a new substance because it is a type like another chemical, is not restricted to any one major category; that is, in Table 1 subgroups are readily formed by pharmacologists whenever they use one drug (chemical) as the type or model by which to judge other drugs. We see that in Table 1 neurological, symptom-treating, key-symptom-producing, mode-of-action summaries, and chemical-name structure commingle as category-constructing criteria and that subgroups within one category may be constructed on the basis of secondary (and tertiary) criteria (for example, the chemical or mode-of-action subgroup within a clinical-treatment-effect major group).

Consider "sedatives" are listed in Table 1 under C, although some textbooks exclude that term. Such exclusions may be based on the fact that "sedative" effects may be observed in chemically unrelated substances and may appear in most of the principal groups that we have considered. Within the general anesthetics, (B) alcohol, (C) hypnotics, (D) anticonvulsants, and (E) anti-Parkinsonism groups have sedative effects. For instance, a sedative effect may follow the administration of weak doses of hypnotics—barbiturates or nonbarbiturates—during treatment with antiepileptic drugs or anti-Parkinsonism drugs, or following the consumption of alcohol. Within the analgesic group (F), the sedative effect is produced by opium derivatives (laudanum) and by some antipyretics (acetylsalicylic acid). Within the drugs utilized in the treatment of psychiatric disorders, the sedative effect is characteristic both of the antipsychotic drugs (G) and the antianxiety drugs (H). They may also appear with antidepressants (I). Within the hallucinogens (K), sedative action is often associated with cannabis. Also, different types of drugs, in which the pharmacological effect on the central nervous system appears but secondarily, have a direct or indirect sedative effect, for example, as it occurs with spasmolytics and the antihistamines.

The foregoing inconsistencies may not trouble the medical scientist if the basis of his system is not intended to be an external logical or aesthetic standard. Ordinarily, he simply wishes to display a great variety of psychoactive substances, ordering them in some way; that the order is created by different levels of observation or semantic processing is not serious as long as the classification scheme, for example, Table 1, is used only for display purposes. When, however, reductionism takes place and the action of a drug is simplified so that its effects are conceived as only (or even primarily) those ascribed to it by the key-word of classification nomenclature, then one gets into trouble.

RESEARCH AND SPECIFICATION OF DRUG EFFECTS

One of the areas in which the most systematic research has been done is the elaboration of adequate techniques to screen synthetic products with a view to their therapeutic application. Generally speaking, the results have allowed us to recognize, within the chemical series that have been most studied, satisfactory and sometimes surprising correspondence between the experimental data obtained from man and from animals. In many cases, the experimental studies of psychotropic agents in animal behavior permit one to elucidate the precise mechanisms of action and to answer certain questions regarding their utilization; for example, the effects of prolonged administration, synergy with associated medicaments, dependency phenomena, and the like. From a general point of view, the effects of psychotropic medications, that is to say, the action that they exert on behavior and upon states of consciousness, reveal directly—or indirectly—the functions of the central nervous system. Spectacular results have been achieved in the domain of molecular pharmacology with regard to the knowledge of intimate mechanisms of the activity of the principle types of psychoactive drugs. Moreover, in many cases, pharmacological investigations have allowed us to expand our knowledge of the structural and functional bases of central nervous system activity.

Without entering into a discussion that would exceed the scope of this chapter, we shall limit ourselves to outlining—according to the conceptions suggested by Berger (1960)—the two types of possible psychotropic mechanisms of action. One group of products—volatile general anesthetics—for example, ethyl alcohol—owe their activity essentially to the physical properties of their molecule and in particular to their ability to be diffused in the organism and their lipid solubility. The analysis of their effects reveals that on the cellular level their general action is related to parallel alterations of cell membrane permeability and of the respiratory metabolism of the cell. The second group of products owe their activity to the structural analogy that their molecules have with certain neurohormones or chemical transmitters. In the case of the psychostimulants, for example, in the case of the amphetamines, the synthetic product substitutes itself in some way for the natural hormone, the effects of which it stimulates, modulates, or opposes. The pharmacological properties of numerous psychotropic drugs have a similar mechanism of action which may be interpreted in terms of imitative and competitive effects with regard to the neurohormones such as the catecholamines, the serotonins, or the acetylcholines.

To move from the molecular or cellular level—that is, from concern with cell membranes, receptors, and the like—to considering what happens to the whole organism, as, for example, what the clinician observes when he gives a drug or what the subject reports when he takes one, requires a great leap. One hopes it is a great leap forward. Two things must be introduced: one an awareness of increased complexity, that is, of more factors influencing what is observed at the one-person than at the one-cell level; and second, the use of broader concepts (often termed intervening variables) to try to account for what is happening. If one is engaged in research, one seeks to control as many of the possible factors influencing the drug outcome as one can, as, for example, the dose, the form (tablet, solution, or the like), the manner of introduction (for example, by mouth, by injection, by inhalation, or surgically), the number of and time between administrations, and so forth. Even so, the experimenter cannot control many factors important in human subjects, as, for example, what the human thinks will happen to him, how he responds to the doctor and to the perceived sensations attributed to the drug.

If the drug is given by a clinician as part of treatment, then there are some factors that are expected to play a role which the physician takes into account but for which he cannot make exact estimations. Typically these include the patient's age, weight, and sex; the patient's physiological state according to the time of day, time elapsed since the last meal, menstrual cycle, and the like; the patient's particular resistance or susceptibility to related medications (antagonists or synergists); the social setting in which treatment is given—whether the patient is ambulatory, hospitalized, in a home (asilaire)—the positive or negative elements within the setting, the relations between physician, patient, and drug administrator—psychotherapy, placebo effect, presence of others; the patient's pathological state (patient's presenting complaint); and, finally, the individual's characteristics with regard to the patient's particular genetic makeup.

Because of the complexity of controlling for all likely influences in humans, the limited number of safe and ethical research procedures one can employ with humans, and the need to screen drugs before their employment with humans, much of the work on drugs is done first in animals. Of particular importance in evaluating those drugs effects that are fundamental to classification schemes for public action are efforts to assess effective and lethal doses. Killam in Chapter Five and Halbach in Chapter Eight attend to much that bears on this discussion. Here we simply note that a basic description of a drug requires that one know how much of it, given in what form, manner, and so forth, produces a given behavioral result (for psychoactive agents) and what dose kills the animals receiving it. Ordinarily the effective dose (ED) is defined as that yielding the X result in 50 percent of the animals given it and the lethal dose (LD) is that killing 50 percent of the animals. These are average values only. One finds that the range of results varies quite considerably on animals of the same species. Genetic studies have shown that much of this variability is inherited and that one can either increase or reduce the intensity of the effects—for a given dose (that is, alter ED_{50} and LD_{50})—by breeding different strains of animals (Bovet, Bovet-Nilti, Oliverio, 1969). Humans, too, differ in their reactions and drug susceptibilities depending upon genetic factors. The pharmacology of the future is likely to be pharmacogenetics, for through such research a much greater predictability of drug responses can be expected to be obtained.

By now it is clear that one cannot make the simple statement that a drug does X or causes Y or produces Z. Consider the lethal dose procedure above: the very existence of a standard called LD_{50} demonstrates that the same dose has different effects, killing half of the laboratory animals and not killing the others. The actual effects are not that simple either—for example, death may be quick for some and slow for others; among those who live will be those (depending on the drug) suffering permanent impairment, while others may appear to recover completely. As one considers this variety of outcomes, varying with many conditions, one finds it useful to think in terms of probabilities, not certainties. Indeed, Killam, in Chapter Five, introduces us to thinking of pharmacodynamics per se in probabilistic terms, from target sites to organ systems to behavioral outcomes. Probabilistic thinking means that we accept uncertainty; we realize we are estimating, as we know more about a phenomenon and the forces determining it, the accuracy of estimating increases; and we use statistical methods of description and inference, as Joyce describes in Chapter Nine, to present the array of data representing the phenomenon and to create standards for judging whether or not the outcomes observed are due to understood factors (those experimentally manipulated) or to events that we do not comprehend.

It may be helpful to realize the importance of the conditions of drug administration as determining outcomes, including effectiveness and toxicity. A classical experiment in pharmacology demonstrates that the same dose of strychnine that is likely to initiate convulsions in a few seconds when it is injected intravenously, acts only after a certain latency period when introduced subcutaneously, and remains apparently ineffective when administered orally. Parenteral administration of morphine presents high risk of acute intoxication, whereas inhaling opium smoke does not. The high degree of toxicity of nicotine when it is ingested, as a base, or in contact with mucous membranes, contrasts with its absence of symptoms of true intoxication resulting from tobacco smoke. The weak concentration of the alkaloids in smoke and their rapid elimination assures the short-term (!) innocuousness of smoking.* We know the advantages that anesthesiology has obtained from administering volatile anaesthetics by inhalation and the advantages of such a mode of administration in terms of the ability to control the depth of anesthesia at different moments of the operation; the same example allows us to illustrate the contrast between the reactions of a subject to different doses of the same products. A phase of mental overexcitation and overagitation—which results from blockage of cortical inhibitors—regularly precedes the analgesic phase of loss of spontaneous mobility and of muscular relaxation that characterizes the anaesthetic phase proper. The picture of alcoholic

---

* Again depending on the criteria, one can show that cigarette smoke does kill individual cells—the membranes lining the mouth.

intoxication—with its very different behavior over the time sequence of a drinking bout—has made such observations all too familiar.

TOXICITY AND RISK

Therapeutic research has a double objective: the increase of the effectiveness of drugs and the decrease of their toxicity. The attempts to increase the therapeutic coefficient of psychotropic drugs and the control of toxicity aim to increase their safety margin, that is, the difference between an effective and a toxic dose. In spite of the technical progress along these lines, we are far from resolution of the problem of drug toxicity. A certain number of spectacular accidents have been due to insufficient control measures. Examples include elixir of sulfanilamide in the United States in 1938, stalinon in France in 1955, thalidomide in Germany in 1961. Daily medical practice also reveals the toxic effects in drugs that can be overlooked. For example, one study (Cluff, Thornton, Seidl, Smith, 1965) compared an active surveillance of patients for adverse reactions to routine in-hospital reporting. They found that 5 percent of *all* admissions were caused directly by drug reactions, while an additional 15 percent of admitted patients had an adverse reaction while in the hospital. These rates were four times higher than routine reporting had revealed. Noting that the average patient had received nine different medications before his bad reaction, they found that the more different medication given the greater the chance for a bad reaction. Psychoactive drugs were low on the list of those leading to adverse reactions. Wade (1973) writes that 3 to 5 percent of all hospital admissions in the United States are for drug reactions. Once in general medical hospitals, 18 to 30 percent of all patients experience an adverse drug reaction. Such reactions are estimated to double the length of stay for these patients.

In addition to specific effects, toxic outcomes can be related to use by patients of several compounds simultaneously and to insufficient education about drug safety, both of the medical profession and of the public. Concern about adverse reactions should, of course, be in the perspective of the consequences of nonuse of a drug. If for example, the cost of avoiding adverse reactions is failure to cure an illness, then obviously one will elect the lesser disadvantage.

Each "therapeutic act"—and the consumption of all medicines constitutes such a therapeutic act—also carries with it a "therapeutic risk." From the ethical point of view, it is natural to consider that the risk which the physician has a right to take varies in relationship to the seriousness of the patient's prognosis. With respect to this, much emotional illness entails but a limited immediate risk to the life of the patient. However, if one considers suicides related to depression of alcoholics and suicides of schizophrenics as a measure of risk, then these mental illnesses do pose high risk to life. The decision to use psychoactive drugs should be based, in part, on such risk estimates. When life risks are low, one may wish to argue to reduce drug risks by limiting drug prescribing. If it is granted that any psychoactive drug use carries some hazard, then one can see a basic argument for reduction in the nonmedical use of psychoactive substances.

WIDENING MEDICAL INTEREST

In medical research as well as in classification, one must recognize a tendency on the part of some workers to be disinterested in the nonmedical uses of psychoactive substances. Indeed, historically, there has been little pharmacological interest until recent years in some drugs that have been used almost exclusively nonmedically as, for example, the hallucinogens (cannabis, and the like). Lewin (1924) was an exception, as was Moreau (1845)—yet today one still finds classifications stressing medicaments as defined by physicians (not by self-administering users). Hazard, Cheymol, Lévy, Boissier, and Lechat (1969) define psychotropic drugs, as does Usdin (1970), in the restricted sense of drugs used in the treatment of psychiatric disorders. Yet, as we consider the balance of risks in relationship to decision-making as to when and whether drugs ought to be employed, we must realize that nonmedical as well as medical uses strongly require simultaneous consideration. It may be that, for example, the same drug and the same people may be involved in the two different settings (for example, physicians or patients self-administering morphine or amphetamines illicitly).

Since the last century, the introduction from Asia and the rapid extension of opiates in the Western world have revealed the multiple effects of that group of alkaloids, the use of which presumably expanded rapidly because of their analgesic properties and their euphoriant effects. In consequence, medical scientists as well as churchmen and international lawmakers first focused their attention on the "phantastica" of natural origin (curiously ignoring the West's own natural drug, alcohol). The beginning of the studies of synthetically derived psychoactive substances began mainly after the introduction of amphetamine into the treatment of the narcolepsies (Prinzmetal and Bloomberg, 1935) and the interest aroused by the effects of this product on animal and human behavior. Beginning in 1943, the self-observations made by Hofman on the hallucinogenic activity of LSD-25 spurred immense interest in nonmedical uses of synthetics by users, researchers, lawmakers, and the public.

Rapid evolution, increasing production, more prevalent utilization, and diversity of associated outcomes help account for current concerns about the nonmedical use of drugs. Yet these interests must not obscure the need for research and guidelines related to risk decision-making as, for example, more precise ways of estimating the risks to a patient if he is or is not given a drug or placed on a drug regime as a therapeutic act.

UBIQUITY OF DRUG USE

As a framework for understanding methods and problems in classification, we must realize that in drug use we are dealing with nearly universal behavior. As Talalay (1964) observed, taking drugs is as ordinary as dressing oneself or combing one's hair. It is often so habitual as to be unnoticed by the doer. Ray (1972) estimates that of 1,000 persons, 750 will have some symptom of what they considered illness during a month, that 500 of these people will treat themselves with an over-the-counter (OTC) drug, and 250 will see a physician. For these self-diagnosing and self-treating Americans, there were more than 4,000 OTC preparations available from which to select. Their buying yields annual profits for cold remedies alone of $500 million and for vitamins and laxatives of $200 million.

Is self-diagnosis and self-treatment a medical or nonmedical use? Certainly a physician has not been seen, so one may say "nonmedical." Yet the drugs are advertised and approved governmentally and a doctor may once have recommended it to the consumer. Indeed, physicians often recommend OTC preparations (Blum and Associates, 1972b)—the frequency of such recommendations being related to their own use of them. Further, the repeat prescription (see Balint and others, 1970) creates a situation in which the patient does take drugs without seeing the physician over long periods of time. But if self-medication is medical use, then what of the illicit user who self-diagnoses and prescribes for his depression by taking amphetamines or treats his anxiety with heroin?

The point is that there are many people who need professional assistance and, perhaps, prescribing. One distinguishes between presumed medical diagnosis and need and the actual illicit social behavior. Yet even such presumptions become awkward when, as in methadone treatment in the United States or heroin clinics in the United Kingdom, one finds the physician essentially following the patient's own initial "prescription," that is, the illicit opiate user changes to the status of a medical patient, but the nature of his drug use (opiates) does not change. The setting is altered—and perhaps the behavior—but not the class of drug.

An analogous illustration of the complexity of affairs is found in weight control. In terms of etiology, those who are overweight may suffer from basic disturbances in their internal signaling systems (Schachter, 1971), from differing hunger set points autonomically or ventral medial hypothalamic disorders (Nisbett, 1972), from deviation from cultural standards (after all, in some societies thin women are disparaged), or from a self-critical standard or stereotype symptomatic of other self-rejection or conflict leading to diet even though they are of normal weight or even underweight. In the case of the obese, they may be said to be dependent on or addicted to food. Such persons, with quite different possible etiologies, may self-prescribe illicitly (amphetamines) or nonmedically (OTC substances); they may be treated medically yet improperly—"fat doctors" giving amphetamines on an assembly line (Lewis in Blum and Associates, 1972b); they may be treated medically and ethically but without improvement (staying fat); or they may be treated medically with success—or nonmedically with success. Since we know that obesity is widespread and is a health hazard (associated, for example, with diabetes or heart disease), why is society not as worried about food addicts as about drug addicts? Indeed, there may be overlap, at least if there is "iatrogenic disease" as the fat patient becomes amphetamine dependent in the "fat doctor's" hands. Interestingly, children with eating behavior problems seem to be at greater risk of using drugs in dangerous ways as adolescents (Blum and Associates, 1969b and 1972a).

We see that it is not only with "drug abusers" that one must face the problems of etiology, diverse standards for judgment, various settings for "abuse" and drug employment, and various outcomes as an interaction effect. Overall, one asks what are the reasons that make one problem (drug addiction) of more political and social interest than the other (food addiction)?

MEDICAL RESPONSIBILITY

It is, however, only in the case of drugs that physicians—and pharmacists —find themselves gatekeepers charged with controlling levels and situations of use and using clinical observations to set therapeutic levels. This responsibility, although socially acknowledged and legally endorsed, is subject to debate as to its limits, as lawmakers make inroads on the physician's freedom to act (whether that be control of morphine, amphetamines, or heroin) and as physicians, in turn, respond irritably to such interference (see Brown and Savage, 1971). Implicit in the physician's right to administer a substance is the promise of the substance—or the doctor—of probable efficacy and known risk. This assumption of responsibility separates medical use from other drug or substance uses, for in the case of nonmedical use, illicit use, or simply the availability of other utilized substances (be these foods or household poisons), a professional does not undertake personal decisions on another's behalf to seek both efficacy and minimal risk. The difficulty, of course, is that the range of probable outcomes is so great and the decision-capability of physicians so varied that lawmakers have come to feel that society, not the individual physician, must set the limits for acceptable medical practice. Since it is probable that the range of adverse drug outcomes is even greater when medical responsibility is not assumed, society through its lawmakers also assumes it must intervene with formal rules to minimize risk to those self-administering drugs in social or private situations. Since the risks of under-control of drugs are evident (opium-use epidemics, thalidomide, teratogenesis) and the risks of overcontrol less visible (that is, the presence of a bad reaction is more dramatic than the uncertainty as to what would have happened had a forbidden drug been employed), one may anticipate that pressures for control will be increased as bad outcomes are made visible. Thus, whatever the system of classification or the medical assumptions of pharmaceutical potency and benevolence ascribable to therapeutic acts, the physician must expect to be subordinated to social controls over his prerogatives and practice.

The foregoing may appear removed from the pressing concerns of policymakers seeking to devise public action programs and the classificatory schemes on which they depend. Yet the features that influence estimates of drug effectiveness must be familiar to the policy-maker, as they are to the pharmacologist and the clinician.

The policy-maker, like the scientist, must think in terms of probabilities and methods to increase the accuracy of estimate, not only for drug effects, but for the impact of control systems themselves. The lawmaker needs to think of risks and benefits, not as simple and absolute concepts, but as a range of outcomes that need to be jointly evaluated by some formal decision model. This cannot be done, of course, if there is semantic confusion, and we have seen in the review of common terminology just how much uncertainty can be introduced by the language of "drug abuse" and by the differing perspectives that common terms may either represent or conceal. Finally, any approach to drug policy must be seen to begin with the near-universality of drug use and, generally, the optimism of users or physicians as to pharmaceutical utility. There are, of course, therapeutic and pharmacological nihilists, but even many of these drink wine or take aspirin. In any event, although it is important to distinguish who is responsible for drug giving and to acknowledge the much better control over outcomes (that is, uncertainty is reduced, probability statements become more accurate) when settings are controlled—which is one goal of medical practice—we cannot be so certain of the functional distinctions between medical and nonmedical drug uses. There, as in all other aspects of scientific observation and terminology, we are dealing with somewhat arbitrary concepts and with uncertainty. This general statement applies to classification systems for social control, however they are elucidated.

SUMMARY

From the standpoint of the pharmacologist and medical practitioner, drugs are primarily benign; their capabilities for relieving pain and curing illness are more often seen than are their powers to produce ill effects. This experience has guided mankind in its long search for and use of drugs as medicaments. These same urges will continue to expand chemical therapies. The history of pharmaceutical medicine shows very rapid expansion in the recent past and allows the prediction that many more drugs with much more diversity and specificity of effects will soon be developed. The challenge to classification schemes linked to public action, as, for example, laws governing drug production and use, will be to handle these new substances in a sophisticated way. By that is meant the development of data from many levels of investigation unified conceptually and so structured as to indicate key communalities among such classificatory subgroups as are developed.

Existing classification schemes can be useful in some areas of science and medicine, but a problem occurs when nonspecialists relying on existing medical classifications fail to appreciate the inconsistent criteria for the scheme overall. Insofar as classificatory schemes are used simply to display the range of psychoactive drugs highlighted by one or another key feature—such features implying a family of chemical, neurophysiological, and clinical correlates—they may be instructive. On the other hand, if one simplifies concepts, believing key-word descriptions to be the sole qualities of drugs, then misunderstanding and misapplication are likely.

Those classification schemes that order psychoactive drugs have the most bearing on contemporary international law. Yet, among the vast numbers of substances that are drugs by definition, only some are medicaments and of these only a very few are psychoactive. The correspondence between those psychoactive drugs used medically and those employed nonmedically, that is, for pleasure escape or religious reasons or whatever, is considerable. The immediate consequences are that the medical scientist must take a great interest in classification schemes and in legal control measures for several reasons. (1) His research on drug structure, action, and effects constitutes data used in constructing classification criteria. (2) Public concern about drug use politicizes drug-handling policies that affect medical practice. (3) Legal control measures may inhibit research. (4) Legal control measures may interfere with medical practice and, hence, with the ease and welfare of patients. (5) New drugs or new data about drugs may be gleaned from observations on nonmedical drug practices. (6) The medical scientist or practitioner will be concerned with those nonmedical uses of drugs associated with adverse effects on health.

The role of the pharmaceutical industry and the characteristics of modern societies deserve special mention, especially when one has the future in mind. Both the industry and people at large, that is, drug consumers, have an interest in expanding the range and capabilities of psychoactive substances. Pressures for greater research investment and for the intensive marketing of new drugs are great. These, coupled with the rapid diffusion of newly marketed drugs (and sometimes not yet marketed ones) into illicit use, the tendency to define ever greater forms of "normal" moods, feelings, or goals as appropriate for chemical manipulation, and other forces create great demands on existing screening methods and on the criteria employed to judge efficacy, benefit, and risk. Pharmacodynamic, clinical, and epidemiological methods will require increasing sophistication to meet this challenge. It is probable that legislative controls that would aim to reverse mankind's pharmacotropic tendencies and modern production catering to these would, at best, introduce strain and quite likely would prevent the production and medical use of new drugs that could be therapeutic. On the other hand, laissez-faire in drug production and marketing has been shown to lead to serious infringements on the public health. In consequence, the medical scientist, like the lawmaker, will most likely seek to establish a balance, a balance based at least in part on solid research data as to the kind and extensiveness of drug effects on differing population groups under differing conditions of administration. The use of research for the specification of effects and the clarification of definitions of benefit and risk, as well as the assessment of control measure impact on research and medical practice is of paramount importance. This interest in the specification of action and effects, as, for instance, of effectiveness and toxicity by dose, manner and frequency of administration, and population characteristics, joins the research scientist, medical practitioner, and policy-maker in a common goal. Its pursuit requires that these groups also can accommodate uncertainty, accept complexity, utilize a broad range of explanatory constructs, use care in their definition of terms, apply rigorous standards for evidence and proceed with flexibility and respect for one another.

Nature and Limitations
of Drug Screening

Harold Kalant, A. Eugene LeBlanc

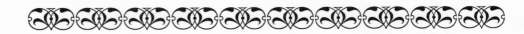

VII

Over the centuries in which new drugs were introduced to the practice of medicine on a chance basis, at infrequent intervals, the testing of drugs was largely a matter of experience gained during the practice of medicine. New agents appeared so infrequently that their acceptance or rejection could scarcely have been considered a serious concern for anyone but the physicians and the occasional unhappy patient who suffered an undesired effect of the new drugs. With the development of the modern pharmaceutical industry, however, new drugs have developed at an astonishingly high rate (see Chapter Six), their potencies are very great compared to the drugs formerly in use, and they are disseminated so rapidly throughout the medical world that the risk of serious undesired effects is now a major concern to many different people. Accordingly, governments have been forced to become involved in the development or regulation of drug screening methods for the protection of the public.

Drugs are screened essentially for two different purposes: to determine their efficacy as therapeutic agents for specific purposes and to assure their safety with respect to possible toxic or undesired effects. Efficacy is primarily the concern of the individuals or companies that develop the new drugs. A drug that does not do what it is claimed to do or does not do it as well as agents that are already available will in principle not be accepted by the medical profession. Intensive advertising may lead to temporary acceptance of an inferior product, but medical experience is likely to lead to its rejection in due course. A case in point is the fate of some ill-starred combinations of antibiotics that are less effective than the separate ingredients (Jawetz, 1968). Over-the-counter drugs may survive considerably longer, even if scarcely more efficacious than placebos, because the general public is not in a position to make objective comparisons of competing drugs. This suggests the need for a critical examination of the role of advertising in the promotion of drugs, particularly those affecting mood, but the subject is beyond the scope of this review.

In the field of efficacy testing, governments tend to limit their attention to what we may call quality control. An example is the introduction of specifications for purity, potency, and bioavailability—that is, the readiness with which the stated amount of drug in a given preparation can enter the body and exert its intended effect (*A.M.A. Drug Evaluations,* 1971). The function of government agencies in this connection is basically no different than that of any consumer protection service.

The main concern of governments with respect to drug screening is the question of safety. Most governments now have a rather elaborate set of requirements for early screening, before a drug is permitted to be used either in clinical trials in man or in routine medical practice. The purpose of those tests is primarily to ensure that the drug, in the doses and modes of administration in which it will be employed clinically, has a sufficiently low likelihood of producing toxic or undesired effects. Among the latter, there has recently been particular concern with individual and social ill effects arising from what has been variously called drug abuse, addiction, or drug dependence.

Every drug has potential toxicity. Any agent that in any way modifies a function of the body can, in sufficiently high doses, modify that function to a degree that will prove harmful rather than beneficial. The purpose of screening is therefore not only to identify but to quantify the risk, that is, to determine the relationship between beneficial or therapeutic effects and harmful effects at any given level of dosage. Fundamentally, the screening leads to a cost-benefit analysis in which the potential hazards must be weighed against the potential therapeutic value.

One can never anticipate either all the potential therapeutic actions or all the possible hazards that may arise in the use of any new drug. In general, the screening methods employed to detect drug hazards are therefore empirically based. In other words, as experience reveals a new type of harmful effect that had not previously been known, the screening methods incorporate new procedures designed to test for the new hazard in future drugs. Therefore, screening is never finished, because new types of toxicity may be identified after the drug has been in use for some time. This means that screening, properly defined, must include not only the tests that are used in advance of the release of a drug to the market, but also a continuing monitoring of possible ill effects that can be detected only after the drug has been in use for some time.

The purpose of this review is to outline briefly the logic and methods of drug screening, the limitations and values of the procedures employed, and some suggestions of possible future lines of development.

OBJECTIVES AND METHODS OF DRUG SCREENING

New drugs arise from a number of different sources. At the risk of some oversimplification, we can identify four categories:

1. *Folk lore and folk medicine.* Some of the most valuable drugs in current clinical practice have been adopted, in improved form, on the basis of previously known therapeutic roles in folk medicine. New drugs which come via this route are relatively easy to screen, because there is already a clear indication of the intended use and probable action. One of the classic examples is digitalis, which Withering explored in the treatment of heart failure because of its use by a local folk healer in the treatment of "dropsy" (Holmstedt and Liljestrand, 1963). The European explorers who brought curare to Europe knew that it was used as an arrow-tip poison by Indians of the upper Amazon jungle and that it paralyzed the animals struck by their arrows. This naturally directed the attention of Claude Bernard and later pharmacologists to explore its use as a muscle-paralyzing agent, and it was subsequently employed as a muscle relaxant during anaesthesia. Cinchona bark was used by Peruvian Indians for the treatment of fevers, and this fact directed the attention of later investigators to examine its specificity in the treatment of malarial fever; this in turn led to the exploration of its use for killing the malaria parasites.

2. *Chance observation.* One of the most striking of this manner of discovery of new drugs is that of penicillin. Alexander Fleming observed, and recorded, the fact that chance contamination of bacterial cultures by a species of common mold caused inhibition of growth of the bacteria in a zone immediately surrounding the clumps of mold. Howard W. Florey and Ernst Chain exploited this observation to isolate from the growing mold the substance that was directly responsible for the antibacterial action (Holmstedt and Liljestrand, 1963).

3. *Systematic chemical manipulation of existing drugs*—This is probably the main route of development of new drugs today. A large number of derivatives of a known chemical are prepared by systematic stepwise modification of the chemical structure, and the derivatives are then screened to see how the spectrum of actions of the original drug is modified by the successive chemical changes. This may lead to specialization of the effect in a particular direction that makes one of the new derivatives better than the starting substance for a particular therapeutic purpose. For example, when sulfanilamide was first introduced for its antibacterial action, it had a number of side effects, including a tendency to cause acidosis by inhibiting the enzyme carbonic anhydrase. Selective chemical modification of sulfanilamide led to a new series of substances known as the benzo-thiadiazines, which, in addition to varying degrees of carbonic anhydrase inhibitory action, also have other actions on the kidney that have made them the most widely used diuretics and antihypertensive agents in contemporary medical practice. Another side effect of sulfanilamide was a tendency to lower the blood sugar. A different series of systematic chemical modifications of the molecule led to the

development of the oral antidiabetic agents in use today (Mudge, 1970; Travis and Sayer, 1970).

4. *Rational synthesis of specific drugs for biochemical actions.* As the level of sophistication of knowledge concerning various biochemical processes increases, a point may be reached at which it is possible to synthesize deliberately a compound that will affect a given enzymatic process in a desired way. Such syntheses depend upon a previously acquired knowledge concerning the structure-activity relationships of natural substrates for the enzymes involved. In this sense, therefore, the deliberate rational synthesis of drugs may be considered an extension of the previous approach.

For example, the understanding of the mechanism by which sodium and bicarbonate are transferred across the wall of the tubules in the kidney indicated that the enzyme carbonic anhydrase played an essential role in the reabsorption of sodium. Acetazolamide was known to be a carbonic anhydrase inhibitor, and it was therefore predicted that it should act effectively as a diuretic by impairing the renal reabsorption of sodium ion. Pharmacological tests confirmed this prediction. A more elegant example is that of allopurinal, used for the treatment of gout. The biochemical investigations of the conversion of purines to uric acid had established the structural requirements of the purine molecules with respect to their ability to bind to the enzyme involved in uric acid synthesis, as well as to be effectively converted to uric acid. It was then possible to make a substitution on the purine molecule that would permit it to bind but not to be converted to uric acid. Such examples are still relatively scarce in the development of new drugs.

5. *Systematic screening for specific therapeutic purposes.* Occasionally, a particular treatment requirement is considered so important that a mass screening program will be undertaken to discover suitable new drugs. An example is the screening program that has been operated for some years by the National Cancer Institute in the United States, for the testing of potential chemotherapeutic agents for cancer. Any agent that is proposed, regardless of the presence or absence of a pharmacological rationale and regardless of the source of the material, will be tested on a routine basis.

Given such a diversity of sources of new drugs, and such a wide range of materials to be tested, we should not be surprised that screening must cast a very wide net indeed. *No drug has only one action.* Therefore screening for both therapeutic and toxic effects has to cover as wide a range as possible of potential actions.

Therapeutic screening usually includes a series of steps designed to examine a whole range of possible pharmacological effects. In practice, the new drug will be given over a range of doses to rats or mice, and the animals will be observed in relation to a checklist of different effects: Do they go to sleep, or have convulsions, or become hyperactive? What happens to their breathing? Does the fur bristle, or the tail stiffen? Does the pupil dilate or constrict? Is the heart rate or blood pressure affected? Is food intake altered, or response to painful stimuli reduced?

From these and similar observations made according to the checklist, the investigator obtains some indication of the most promising leads to explore in more complex types of study. For example, a drug that appears to affect the heart or circulation will be studied for its effects on the contractility of the isolated heart or strips of heart muscle. Effects on blood pressure will lead to an examination of drug actions on the sympathetic and parasympathetic nervous systems, and the biochemistry of norepinephrine and its receptor interaction, or on the response of the brain to incoming stimuli from blood pressure receptors in the walls of blood vessels. If a new drug shows a clear effect on the behavior of the animal, suggestive of a major action of the central nervous system, the investigator may go to more complex tests such as the Bovet-Gatti profile of drug effects on various forms of spontaneous and conditioned behavior (Smythies, Johnston, and Bradley, 1969).

Such screening may indicate that the new drug has a relatively high degree of selectivity for one specific type of therapeutic indication, or it may reveal a variety of new uses for a drug that was previously considered promising for one purpose only. An example of the latter situation is provided by chlorpromazine. This drug was originally introduced as preoperative medication intended to improve relaxation of the patient under anesthesia. It was found to lower the body temperature, and this led to its employment in surgical hypothermia such as that used in cardiac operations. Its relaxant effect led to its exploration as a major tranquilizer in the treatment of schizophrenics. Laboratory testing revealed that it was also a potent local anesthetic, antihistaminic, and an antiemetic. This latter action led to its use for the treatment of motion sickness and nausea and vomiting, and stimulated the development of a whole line of derivatives of chlorpromazine with a greater ratio of this effect to other actions. Chlorpromazine was also found to be a moderately effective blocker of noradrenaline, and consequently to have a blood-pressure-lowering effect similar to that of reserpine. Its local anesthetic actions suggested that it would also have a membrane-stabilizing effect, like that of quinidine, which could be used in the treatment of cardiac fibrillation. This example makes clear the need to have as wide as possible a range of screening procedures, in order not to miss potential beneficial effects of drugs in addition to the action that was originally being investigated.

Obviously, such a process cannot be called looking for a needle in a haystack, because the investigator does not even know it is a needle that he is looking for. A screening procedure is really an attempt to find whatever there may be in the haystack, needles or otherwise. Its value is determined by the suitability of the tests used, and by the economic cost of the screening relative to the potential values that may be found. The area of behavioral effects is perhaps one of the best illustrations of the limitations of available methods. Screening procedures such as the Bovet-Gatti profiles, though they may be the most sophisticated search devices available to date, are relatively crude methods of differentiating drugs that may have selective actions in psychiatric abnormalities. Since there is not yet a suitable animal model for schizophrenia or for manic depressive psychosis, new drugs have to be tested for behavioral effects on normal animals; results of such tests may have relatively little predictive value with respect to their actions in disease states.

It is equally true that the toxic effects can be extremely variable and unpredictable. Some toxic effects are simply the quantitative exaggeration of the same action that is employed therapeutically. Digitalis in large doses may produce heart block or ventricular fibrillation by a mechanism that is fundamentally the same as that which underlies its beneficial effect in heart failure or atrial fibrillation. In the same way, amphetamine psychosis is probably a manifestation of the same process of central nervous system arousal that underlies its beneficial effects in preventing fatigue or relieving depression. In contrast, other toxic effects may be apparently unrelated to the therapeutic actions of the drug. For example, elevation of body temperature by large doses of amphetamine is probably not directly related to the arousal effect, although both may be connected with the actions on release of noradrenaline in different parts of the central nervous system. A recently reported toxic effect in amphetamine users is necrotizing angiitis, a condition characterized by scattered foci of inflammation and destruction of tissue in the walls of blood vessels, which some investigators believe to be an allergic reaction quite unrelated to the primary effects on the central nervous system. Systematic chemical manipulation of the drug molecule may alter the ratio of one effect to another, so that in addition to increasing a specific desired therapeutic effect, it may greatly enhance the severity or probability of an unrelated toxic effect. For example, the conversion of amphetamine to paramethoxyamphetamine (PMA), in addition to enhancing the hallucinogenic effect in a mescaline-like fashion, also greatly increases the hyperthermic effect of amphetamine, and a number of deaths have recently occurred in Ontario among illicit users because of the intense fever.

Most of the foregoing description relates to a search for qualitative information concerning the kinds of effects that a new drug may produce. But screening also deals very importantly with quantitative assessment, that is, with defining the frequency and intensity of effects, both therapeutic and toxic. When initial screening has shown a new agent to have enough promise of clinical usefulness, the screening must be extended to include quantitative studies not only in individuals but within populations. Studies within the individual aim at establishing the difference in dose-effect relationship for the desired therapeutic actions and the toxic actions. Progressively larger doses are given, and one observes the threshold doses at which the various effects appear. The objective is to determine how large a margin of safety there is between the doses necessary to produce the desired and the undesired effects.

For example, low doses of amphetamine tend to produce primarily arousal, increased heart rate, pupillary dilatation and other effects similar to those of sympathetic nervous activity. With much higher doses there commonly appear sensory illusions which, at least in some patients, may become structured and give rise to hallucinations and delusions of persecution (Kalant, 1973). Mescaline is known primarily as a hallucinogenic drug, which produces characteristic patterns of colors, light flashes, and geometrical illusions. At lower doses, however, it also produces amphetamine-like effects on the heart rate, the pupil, and other organs innervated by the sympathetic nervous system. This similarity is not very surprising, since mescaline is closely related chemically to amphetamine and is in fact a trimethoxy-amphetamine. They differ in the degree of separation between the doses required for the sympathetic nervous system effects and the effects upon higher sensory and interpretive functions. As the doses of both compounds are raised, the overlap in their properties becomes more and more marked and specificity tends to disappear.

When the screening is extended to a whole population, variability between individual members of that population is encountered with respect to the sensitivities to any given effect of a drug. A simple analogy is the common experience of the spoiled egg salad at a large picnic. The whole group attending may be exposed to the same degree of staphylococcal food contamination, yet some are completely unaffected, some suffer only mild cramps, and others may have to be hospitalized for severe food poisoning. The screening of a new drug should ideally include large-scale testing on whole population groups, but this is seldom done because of expense and also because the drug is usually intended for some therapeutic purpose that is unlikely to be applicable to a large, healthy, and essentially normal population. One striking example of such a large-scale test was that conducted by Jacobsen and his colleagues on amphetamine when this was first introduced into clinical use in Denmark (Jacobsen, 1939). More than a thousand healthy normal people were given the drug to take on a regular daily basis and were asked to record their symptoms daily. The majority of these subjects experienced mainly the stimulating and fatigue-postponing effects, which most of them found to be quite pleasant. For them, the only untoward effects were a certain tendency to sleeplessness at night and some reduction of appetite. In contrast, a significant minority detected mainly the autonomic nervous effects such as the rapid pulse rate and palpitation of the heart. Most of these subjects found the sensation quite unpleasant and indicated that they would not ordinarily wish to use the drug. A comparable result was obtained by Beecher (1959) in his early studies of the subjective effects of morphine. Only about 10 percent of the normal subjects who received this drug for the first time found the effect pleasant; the rest found it unpleasant, primarily because of nausea.

There is, however, one important difference between screening for therapeutic and for toxic effects. The therapeutic effects are in general confined to the same individual who is receiving the drug and to the period of drug administration. In contrast, the toxic effects may outlast the period of drug administration and may also be exerted upon the later generations born of the subjects receiving the drug. Therefore the strategy of toxicity testing, as opposed to therapeutic efficacy testing, must include at least four different types of assessment:

1. Acute toxicity testing involves the determination of dose-response curves for noxious effects and the definition from these of a standard measure of toxicity or lethality such as the LD_{50} (lethal dose for 50 percent).

2. Chronic studies involve the administration of the drug in doses and over periods of time related to the expected patterns of clinical use. Structural and functional disturbances are monitored by a variety of physiological, chemical, and anatomical examinations. This would include such examples as the production of obstructive liver disease, suppression of blood-cell formation in the bone marrow, precipitation of diabetes, impairment of learning or memory, and so forth.

3. Delayed manifestation of toxicity refers to toxic effects found long after the administration of the drug has been discontinued. A well-known example is the onset of lung cancer, which may occur years after the person has stopped smoking. The stimulus to cancer formation is presumably the accumulation of carcinogenic tars from the smoke that has condensed in the lungs. However, a lengthy period of local tissue effect is required for the production of cancer, so that the onset of the demonstrable disease may be considerably delayed.

A less well known but equally dramatic instance is the production of permanent brain damage by mercury intoxication. Neurobiologists have established that there is a slow gradual decline in the number of functioning cells in the brain once the point of full maturity has passed. There is a sufficiently large reserve of brain cells that the functional effects of this steady loss do not become evident until the onset of what is recognized as senility. Chronic mercury intoxication is believed to accelerate the rate of brain-cell destruction, so that the same aging process occurs with greater rapidity, and impairment of learning ability and memory become evident in the form of a premature senile mental change (Weiss and Simon, 1973). It has been suggested recently that chronic heavy intake of alcohol, or of cannabis, may produce the same type of effect.

4. Damage to subsequent generations can occur for several different reasons (Joffe, 1969). Perhaps the commonest cause of teratogenesis is interference with the biochemical development of the fetus *in utero* at certain critical stages of formation of various organs and tissues. Thalidomide is a good example; infants have been born limbless because of an effect of the drug at a critical stage of the development and differentiation of the limb buds.

Chromosomal damage, affecting the reproductive cells of one or both parents before conception, is another possible mechanism of damage to the offspring. On the whole, there is considerably less evidence to support this type of effect in relation to most drugs. It has been claimed, for example, that LSD, cannabis, caffeine, and many other drugs produce such damage but the studies that have been carried out to date are upon the chromosomes of peripheral white blood cells rather than reproductive cells. There is insufficient evidence to permit any conclusion as to whether this type of damage is reversible or irreversible, and whether it can be specifically implicated in any abnormalities in the offspring.

A third mechanism by which a drug may affect the progeny is interference with the normal rearing behavior of the mothers. Animal studies, for example, have shown some drugs to interfere with milk production or with the normal patterns of maternal care for the babies. While this has not been specifically invoked to explain any such effects in humans, it seems quite reasonable that drugs that severely alter consciousness or motivation could produce such effects if taken by the mothers of recently born infants.

Most European and Western countries have now made mandatory the preclinical testing of new drugs in all these different ways. There is no difficulty thinking of still more tests of safety whose inclusion would be desirable, but each such addition increases the cost, duration, and difficulty of the testing period. Any program of testing therefore represents a compromise between the maximum amount of information that would be desirable and the maximum cost or difficulty that is acceptable for reasonable commercial operation of the pharmaceutical industry. This point is highly relevant to the following discussion of the limitations of screening.

LIMITATIONS OF DRUG SCREENING PROGRAMS

Selection of Subjects

Perhaps the most common and widely recognized problem associated with the choice of subjects in drug screening is the difficulty of extrapolation of results from one species to another. Most drug testing is initially done in rodents, that is, in laboratory rats, mice, guinea pigs, and rabbits. This is easily explained because of the relative cheapness of large numbers of these animals, and the availability of standard-bred subjects that give reasonably predictable and reproducible results. There is now an abundance of evidence, however, indicating major differences among rodents, dogs, cats, sheep, various species of monkey and ape, and man.

These differences apply not only to the sensitivities to a particular effect, but also to the balance of the various effects produced by any given drug. A classical example is that of morphine, which in dogs, apes, and man is primarily a sedative or behavioral depressant. In mice, it produces marked stimulation of the sympathetic nervous system, giving rise to the characteristic erection of the tail ("Straub tail"), hyperexcitability, and running. In the cat, it produces similar sympathomimetic signs and may provoke furious rage and attack behavior.

This species difference also applies to toxic effects. For example, one recent drug test gave evidence of visual impairment in the experimental animals being used, which almost led to rejection of the drug for trials in man. However, it turned out that the visual impairment was due to a bleaching of the macula alba in the eye of the rat. Man does not have a macula alba but a macula lutea, which is evidently unaffected by the same drug. This species difference might have led to the unjustifiable rejection of a therapeutically useful drug.

In other instances, the error could be in the opposite direction. There are many instances of species differences with respect to the predominant pathway of elimination of the drug. Cannabinoids, for example, are eliminated mainly in the feces in the rat and in the urine of the rabbit. If a drug were initially tested in a species that eliminated it chiefly in the feces, while man excreted it principally in the urine, it would be very readily possible to fail to anticipate toxic effects when the drug was administered to patients with kidney disease. It has been remarked justifiably that man is "the ultimate experimental animal." In view of the numerous species differences, it is essential that clinical tests of new drugs in man be regarded as a continuation of the experimental assessment.

Differences in age and sex of the experimental subjects may also influence the results of drug trials (Vessell, 1971). Many biochemical systems are either absent or incompletely developed in the infant at the time of birth. The exact identities and severity of such deficiencies vary according to the species, as does the rate at which the systems in question attain their maximum activity in post-natal life. The drug-metabolizing systems, for instance, are incompletely developed at birth. The newborn infant has an incompletely developed system for clearance of drugs and bile pigments from the liver, and for several weeks after birth has a slight degree of jaundice due to the excess bile pigments that are carried in the plasma bound to protein. Sulfonamides or aspirin, given during this stage, may displace the bile pigment from the plasma, causing it to pass into the brain where it may seriously damage certain brain centers, giving rise to the picture known as kernicterus. The same doses are devoid of such toxicity in the older child or adult.

In rats and some other species of experimental animals, there is also a difference between males and females with respect to the rate at which they can metabolize and eliminate many drugs. The quantitative study of toxicity must therefore be carried out in both sexes. This difference does not appear to be present in human beings, although there is evidence that women may be more sensitive than men to the actions of some drugs, such as phenolphthalein cathartics (Munch and Calesnick, 1960) and phenothiazines (Goldberg, Schooler, and others, 1966), independently of the possible sex difference in the rate at which the drugs themselves are metabolized.

One source of unpredictability of drug results which has received increasing attention in recent years is genetic variation (Vessell, 1973). Within a given population, hereditary anomalies in certain families have been recognized to cause relatively rare but dramatic examples of drug toxicity. For example, a genetically determined variation in the activity of an enzyme (cholinesterase) in the blood renders some subjects extraordinarily sensitive to the paralyzing effect of succinylcholine. This drug, used to produce muscular relaxation during surgery, is ordinarily broken down extremely rapidly by the cholinesterase once the infusion of the drug is stopped. Patients with the congenital variant of the enzyme break it down with extreme slowness and may remain paralyzed for an hour after the end of the injection. Another anomaly consists of a severe disturbance of energy metabolism in some subjects who are anesthetized with halothane for surgical purposes. They respond to this drug by a sudden severe loss of control over the production of heat by metabolic reactions, and may actually die of severe fever (Gordon, Britt, and Kalow, 1973).

In other instances whole populations differ from each other with respect to genetically determined sensitivity to certain drugs. A classic example is Primaquin sensitivity among black and Mediterranean races. These groups have a congenital difference in the structure of hemoglobin in their red blood cells, which renders them extremely sensitive to the destruction of red blood cells by an effect of the antimalarial drug Primaquin. If toxicity testing were carried out only on white European or American subject populations, a comparable effect of a new drug could not be recognized in advance.

Change in Circumstances

Most of the drug screening procedure, particularly in the preclinical stage, is carried out on normal healthy subjects. In some instances there are no animal models or equivalents of the specific disease for which the therapeutic effect is desired. Therefore a drug that might be clinically useful could be overlooked. The tricyclic antidepressants such as amitriptyline and imipramine act simply as sedatives in normal subjects. In other instances, the situation may be the opposite in that the effect of the drug in the normal animal may parallel that in the human patient, but the effect may be markedly altered by the occurrence of certain diseases in patients for which no model existed in the animal. For example, the failure of metabolic breakdown of female sex hormones in the liver of the patient with cirrhosis may cause excessive hormonal activity, with uterine hemorrhage, in doses which would otherwise be considered clinically reasonable.

In other instances, changes in toxicity could, at least in theory, result from an alteration in the environment of the users. Abnormally high levels of mercury were recently found in the blood of residents living downstream from an Ontario river into which a paper mill poured large volumes of effluent contaminated with mercury. This might well be predicted to increase the sensitivity to toxic effects of other drugs on the brain or bone marrow. Numerous recent studies have drawn attention to the hepatotoxicity of organic solvent vapors inhaled by the workers in many industrial plants. This might in the same way enhance the sensitivity to the hepatotoxic effects of a variety of drugs in ordinary clinical use. One may recall the manner in which disulfiram (Antabuse) was discovered as an antialcohol agent. Workers in a rubber factory, who employed the chemical for curing rubber tires, experienced severe flushing and fall in blood pressure when they drank even a small amount of alcohol (Hald, Jacobsen, and Larsen, 1948). In this instance, the coincidence led to the discovery of a clinical use for disulfiram. But it is not difficult to imagine numerous circumstances in which unexpected toxicities of clinically employed drugs might be due to such changed circumstances.

Uncertainty of Target

Toxicity screening is always made difficult by the fact that one is testing for unknown future complications that may arise during the clinical use of the drug. As a result, one is forced to set up methods of detection without being sure of what one wishes to detect. A classic example is that of iproniazid, which was initially introduced for the treatment of tuberculosis. It was found that some of the patients receiving this treatment became euphoric, and some with clinical depressions were symptomatically improved to a marked degree. This action was shown to be correlated with an inhibitory effect on an enzyme known as mono-amine oxidase. A number of similar drugs, also inhibiting the same enzyme, were developed for treating depressions in other patients, some of whom were also receiving other antidepressant medication. In a number of cases, the other medication included amphetamine, and the combination of amphetamine with the monoamine oxidase inhibitors gave rise to severe toxicity including hypertensive crisis and cerebral hemorrhage. When the drugs were initially being screened for the purpose of clinical use as chemotherapeutic agents for tuberculosis, it would have taken extraordinary luck or genius to think of testing them for their effects on monoamine oxidase.

The implication is that screening is never definitive and must be treated always as an ongoing process. The evolution of the clinical uses of the drug may lead to toxicities that could not have been anticipated during the initial development. One outcome of this fact has been the establishment of extensive toxicity reporting programs. Various governments have set up procedures by which individual practicing physicians can report to central data gathering offices (see Chapter Ten) the occurrence of unexpected toxic reactions to drugs used clinically. Perhaps the most sophisticated development of that type is the Boston Hospital Survey (1973) involving the establishment of a computer data bank in which complete details of the drug history of all patients experiencing toxic reactions are entered. This permits the recognition of relatively infrequent or rare patterns of toxicity arising from drug interaction that might not otherwise be detected by the individual physician.

It follows from the foregoing that the detection of toxicity is essentially a function of time, numbers of subject-dose exposures, and prominence. We have already referred to the significance of time as a factor in the detection of brain cell damage by mercury. Another example is the occurrence of abnormal pigmentation in the skin and viscera of psychotic patients receiving large doses of phenothiazines over long periods of time. This type of toxicity would not be detected in the ordinary type of screening program. The numbers of subject-dose exposures are important with respect to the possibility of detection of relatively rare events. For example, aminopyrine is capable of producing a severe and possibly fatal depression of white blood cell formation, probably by a type of allergic reaction. This event, though catastrophic, occurs in fewer than 1 in 10,000 subjects treated with the drug. Therefore, it would be extremely improbable that any ordinary clinical trial would be capable of detecting this type of toxicity. As a result it was not detected until the drug went into wide clinical use. A similar development occurred in relation to bone marrow depression by chloramphenicol. The diabetogenic effect of the benzothiadiazine antihypertensive agents and the production of liver disease by the oral antidiabetic drug chlorpropamide were similarly detected after these drugs had entered routine clinical use.

The significance of prominence, defined as a factor in the detection of toxicity, is well illustrated by the studies of Schmidt and de Lint (1972) on mortality statistics among alcoholics. In the present context, prominence is meant to refer to the degree of obviousness of the connection between the ingestion of the drug and the observed toxic effects. For example, cirrhosis of the liver has long been known as a complication of alcoholism, because it occurs with very low frequency among nonalcoholics. In contrast, heart disease, various types of cancer, and peptic ulcer all occur with great frequency even among nondrinkers. Therefore the excess mortality due to these causes among alcoholic populations was not identified as an effect of alcohol except by statistical retrospective studies involving large populations.

These factors have an important bearing on the economics of toxicity testing. The combination of large numbers and long times contributes importantly to the total cost of the screening procedure. The best possible toxicity screening may become, therefore, impossible in economic terms for the company that wishes to develop and market a new drug. It becomes essential to accept a certain element of risk of incompleteness in the advance detection of toxicity. One must therefore do a cost-benefit analysis with respect to the proposed new drug (see Chapters Six and Fourteen). If the drug is merely a variant of an existing one, the advantage of introducing it into clinical practice may not be worth the risk of possible new dangers that have not been detected in advance. In contrast, if the disease is a grave one and the therapeutic goal is urgent, one may be willing to accept a higher element of risk by putting the drug into immediate use even before long-term toxicity screening is possible.

Possibility of Circumvention

A final shortcoming of screening methods is that they are applied only to substances that are deliberately introduced through the pharmaceutical industry as clinically useful therapeutic agents. They do not apply to substances that are not intended for drug use but that may nonetheless be used nonmedically. A striking example was the toxicity of absinthe, which was a popular alcoholic drink at the turn of the century. A more recent example is the toxicity arising from the inhalation of solvent fumes by children and teen-agers who practice glue-sniffing. It is obviously impossible to apply drug screening procedures to all the substances that are used in industry and that under normal circumstances would not be employed for internal use in a potentially dangerous fashion. Another instance is that of sodium glutamate, which is employed as a flavor-enhancing agent in Chinese food. Though this is subject to pure food regulations, it is not ordinarily screened for toxicity as a drug would be, so that there was no way of anticipating the effect it would have on particularly sensitive individuals manifesting what has been designated the Chinese restaurant syndrome. This particularly uncomfortable combination of headache, nausea, flushing and tingling can be produced by extremely large doses of glutamic acid or sodium glutamate, but it occurs in some people even with the relatively small amounts that are used routinely in Chinese restaurants in North America.

Circumvention of drug toxicity testing also occurs in relation to the illicit manufacture of drugs for the counterculture. There is nothing to prevent interested persons from obtaining the necessary information from the scientific literature to permit the underground manufacture of hallucinogens such as MDA or paramethoxy-amphetamine. The program of research aimed at the development of water-soluble derivatives of tetrahydrocannabinol for therapeutic and research purposes could, if successful, generate a similar problem. Substances manufactured and distributed by illicit operators are obviously not subject to drug screening or quality control.

USE AND PREDICTIVE VALUE OF TESTS OF "ADDICTION LIABILITY"

So-called psychoactive drugs—that is, those that affect perception, mood, and behavior—have a high risk of use for nontherapeutic purposes. Such use can generate problems that have been variously designated abuse, dependence, or addiction, according to the varying concepts of the people who classify the drugs and the varying severity of the problem. Accordingly, there has been considerable interest in the development of screening tests for addiction liability. Compared to the overall methods of drug screening, tests of addiction liability are limited and relatively crude. They seek to answer two different fundamental questions: (1) What is the risk that a previously inexperienced subject, exposed to a drug for the first time, will acquire drug-oriented or drug-seeking behavior or psychological dependence? (2) What is the risk that a regular user, employing large enough doses, will develop physical adaptation to the drug, leading to physical dependence as manifested by a withdrawal reaction if drug administration is stopped? To answer these questions, basically two types of test systems have been developed. Ethical and economic considerations impede the wide use of human subjects for screening new drugs with respect to their likelihood of producing drug-oriented behavior; therefore, animal models have been developed for this purpose. There has been less ethical problem in using human subjects for testing new drugs for their ability to maintain physical dependence. The procedures, advantages, and limitations of animal and human models are considered next.

Animal Models

General screening for the behavioral effects of various drugs by techniques such as the Irwin or Bovet-Gatti profiles is used mainly for the identification of the class or type of drug to which a new agent belongs. One attempts to identify it as being amphetamine-like, mescaline-like, chlorpromazine-like, or whatever. The inference is that if it resembles a known drug in its actions, it is likely to have not only similar therapeutic applications but also a similar risk of misuse. The onus would be upon the developer of a new drug to prove any exception to this rule. If a new appetite suppressant, for example, were to demonstrate a spectrum of behavioral effects similar to that of amphetamine, even if less potent, there would be a reasonable suspicion that it would produce amphetamine-like patterns of toxicity and abuse.

The remaining animal models relevant to this question are oriented chiefly toward estimating or predicting the likelihood that a drug will be "abused" by humans. The objective is to study the ability of a drug to generate drug-oriented behavior in experimental animals, free of any preconceptions concerning predisposing or motivational factors such as are commonly invoked to explain "psychological dependence" in man. Full descriptions of the techniques and results obtained to date are contained in a number of excellent reviews, such as that by Schuster and Johanson (1973), and it is unnecessary to describe these in detail here. The basic approach is to insert a cannula into the jugular vein of an animal such as a rat or a monkey and to connect to this cannula the outlet tubing from a pump that injects fixed quantities of drug solution at each stroke. The pump is activated by pressure on a lever to which the animal itself has access. The pump control can be preprogrammed so that the animal will have to make different numbers or groupings of bar-press responses in order to obtain a drug injection. The objective of the study is then to see whether the animal will in fact self-administer the drug when it has the opportunity to do so, and how its drug-administration behavior is influenced by changes in the circumstances and in the pattern of responses that it must make to obtain the drug.

The results of such studies have been, to date, encouraging and in some instances striking. With some drugs—notably cocaine, amphetamine, and opiates —mere availability for self-administration leads rapidly to a high and sustained rate of bar-pressing by the animals. In general, drugs that monkeys will self-administer under these conditions are also drugs that are known to be "abused" by man. One striking exception so far is the group of hallucinogens, such as LSD and mescaline, which the animals do not appear to inject in greater amounts than they would with drug-free saline solution. One difficulty with this technique is that more concentrated solutions of drugs such as morphine may be injected much less avidly by the animals than more dilute solutions. This does not necessarily mean that the more concentrated solutions are less "rewarding," but may simply reflect such a degree of interference with the animal's motor abilities that it is unable to make the necessary bar-pressing responses to get more drug.

It is worth noting, however, that the objectives differ somewhat according to the drug under study, even though the basic techniques remain the same. This probably reflects the impact of cultural or sociopolitical considerations, rather than basic behavioral-pharmacological reasoning. For example, most studies of alcohol self-administration are aimed at determining the conditions under which an animal will self-administer enough alcohol to produce a sustained state of intoxication. The studies with opiates tend to concentrate upon whether the animal will self-administer enough to produce tolerance and physical dependence. The studies with psychomotor stimulants and hallucinogens tend to concentrate entirely on the question of the degree to which the animal's behavior becomes concentrated upon drug-seeking or self-administration. These different questions probably reflect certain underlying assumptions. For example, it is generally assumed that alcohol consumption is not an important phenomenon unless the amount ingested produces intoxication. To a large extent, thinking on opiates is concentrated on tolerance and physical dependence as the major risks. With cannabis, LSD, and other hallucinogens, the concern is with the use of the drugs per se, rather than with addiction as conventionally defined.

These differences illustrate one of the limitations of the animal models—the lack of sound knowledge concerning the extent of overlap between animal and human patterns of drug self-administration. All the studies so far reported have been carried out with known drugs, and all drugs that animals have been found to self-administer were already known to be able to give rise to problems of drug dependence in man. However, some drugs that are self-administered by man are not self-administered by experimental animals, as noted above for the hallucinogens. Is the converse true? Are there some drugs that animals might inject but that humans would not? To date, this possibility has not actually been explored because the method has not really been very widely used in the screening of new drugs. There is some suggestion that this might in fact occur, because monkeys will bar-press much more eagerly to self-inject the very weak narcotic dextropropoxyphene than for morphine. In humans, dextropropoxyphene has extremely low abuse liability, compared with morphine or heroin. It is evident, therefore, that if animals should prove to work to obtain some drugs for which no human abuse problem exists, it would greatly reduce the usefulness of the technique for predicting dependence liability of new drugs in man.

Another limitation is the basic assumption that dependence liability, or liability to provoke drug-oriented behavior, is inherent in the chemical itself. The assumpton is sometimes implicit that "reinforcement" of self-administration by the drug effects is equivalent to "pleasure" or "reward" in man. Such an anthropomorphic interpretation probably accounts for the different orientations noted above in work on such various drugs as alcohol, opiates, and hallucinogens. The apparent assumption is that if humans self-administer these substances, it should be possible to arrange the experimental procedures in such a way as to induce animals to self-administer them also, in corresponding amounts and for comparable reasons. This simplistic approach ignores the fact that some drugs that animals will self-administer, when given at the same doses as those used in self-administration studies, have been shown to produce aversive effects in these animals (Cappell, Le Blanc, and Endrenyi, 1973). An animal can even be trained to self-administer a punishing level of electric shock by an appropriate manipulation of the behavioral training. Therefore, the development of "drug-oriented behavior" depends upon a drug-behavior complex, rather than on the drug alone. In humans, this complex includes cultural and social factors in the user's environment, which helped to shape his drug using behavior. Despite Beecher's observations on the aversive effects of first experience of opiates or the well-known nausea produced by peyote or the unpleasant dizziness that many people experience on first exposure to alcohol, the social context can have a very strong influence in shaping the level of acceptance and the selectivity with which the user comes to ignore unpleasant effects and perceive only the desired ones.

A third important limitation in these methods is the dependence of the drug response on the previous drug-exposure history of the experimental subjects. For example, the aversive effects of drugs such as amphetamine or barbiturates, which were noted above, may disappear after repeated administration of the drug. This probably reflects the development of tolerance to some of the more physiologically disturbing actions of the drug, and possibly the replacement of these by some rewarding or quasi-therapeutic effects. For example, in an animal that has been made physically dependent by repeated administration of opiates, additional doses may serve to delay the development of withdrawal symptoms. In such a situation, a drug that an animal might not self-administer initially may be fairly readily self-administered following a period of obligatory exposure to the action of the drug.

In other instances, a drug that is not self-administered initially may become effective in this sense following a period of self-administration of another drug by the same animal. For example, cocaine is self-injected by rats or monkeys with extreme ease, while alcohol is not; but after a period of self-administration of cocaine, an animal will inject alcohol with relative facility. This situation may give rise to misleading or erroneous conclusions in either direction. An examination of a new drug that initially was not self-administered might lead to the conclusion that humans would not be likely to misuse it. Alternatively, its successful use in self-administration experiments after cocaine might lead to the conclusion that humans would use it nonmedically. Either of these conclusions could be wrong.

There is clearly a requirement for a considerable increase in the sophistication of the experimental methods for this type of investigation. There is need for an increased complexity of models such as the second-order schedules described by Goldberg (1972). Another welcome development is the use of animals in social settings, such as the studies on alcohol consumption by monkeys in group

cages (Cadell and Cressman, in press), for studying the effects of social interactions on the self-administration of drugs. By such developments, it may be
possible to produce animal models that include better approximations of the
sociocultural and environmental influences on drug use by humans. This might
go a long way toward improving the predictive value of animal models in the
testing of new drugs.

Human Models

The best known and most frequently used human model of dependence
liability is the Lexington (Kentucky) test program involving human addicts as
test subjects ("United States Procedures," 1970). Hospitalized addicts who have
been brought to a stable level of physical dependence on an opiate are given test
doses of new drugs in place of the usual one, in order to see whether these will
successfully prevent the opiate withdrawal reaction. If they do, it is assumed that
they are essentially similar in their action to the opiates, and will therefore show
the same liability to misuse. Basically the same approach is used in studies with
primates at Ann Arbor (Villarreal and Seevers, 1972) and elsewhere, and the
rationale is identical. A significant advantage in the use of humans is that they
can describe the subjective effects of the drugs to the observer. No animal model
has yet permitted the recognition of effects comparable to what humans experience as euphoria. The fact that a human subject can describe such an effect is
therefore an advantage for anticipating the likelihood of provoking drug-oriented
behavior in man.

A basic drawback in this human model, however, is that it has been
developed with excessive emphasis on the opiate drugs. By definition, this model
is suitable only for testing new compounds of the same pharmacological type as
those used for producing the dependence in the test subjects. A little work of
this type has been done with sedatives of the barbiturate and other types, but
very little indeed has been done with stimulants, hallucinogens, and other drugs
with a potential liability for nonmedical use. Consequently, the model is used
almost exclusively for screening drugs that may function as substitutes for those
giving rise to presently existing problems. There is no way in which it can be used
to screen for possible new types of problems.

This limitation is also shown in the few studies that have been carried
out with amphetamine, cannabis, and hallucinogens. The procedure has been
used primarily for the study of cross-tolerance among these agents (Isbell, Wolbach, and others, 1961), and the argument is again one of analogy. If a subject
is made tolerant to LSD, and he is then shown to be cross-tolerant to another
drug, it is assumed that the second drug has basically the same type of action
as the LSD and would presumably share the same types of risk. So far, the
technique has really been used only for studying cross-tolerance among known
drugs. Its purpose has therefore been primarily to clarify fundamental similarities
or differences in their mechanisms of action. It could also be used for screening

new drugs; but, again, as in the case of the opiates, it would be suitable only for drugs of the same general type as that used to produce tolerance. The broader use of the cross-tolerance model is improbable because in some cases, such as the barbiturates and related drugs, physical dependence poses too serious a hazard to life, and ethical considerations limit the extent to which the technique can be used. In other cases, such as LSD and related hallucinogens, there is no known development of physical dependence because tolerance arises through tachyphyllaxis or exhaustion of the basic mechanism by which the drug acts. With other drugs that disappear slowly from the body, such as amphetamine, it is possible that physical dependence does occur but that it disappears at almost the same rate that the drug itself is eliminated, so that the manifestations are greatly reduced in intensity (Kalant, LeBlanc, and Gibbins, 1971).

The general concept underlying this human test of drug substitution is very narrow, in that it puts all the emphasis on physical dependence as the cardinal phenomenon of "addiction." This type of screening test, therefore, ignores all the cultural and social factors in the generation of drug-oriented behavior. If one were to screen MDA or LSD by this test, one would come to the false conclusion that they are unlikely to pose a serious social problem. The implication is, therefore, that a positive test (that is, an ability of the new drug to prevent opiate withdrawal symptoms) is useful in predicting addiction liability, but a negative result is considerably less valuable. There are even instances in which members of the opiate or synthetic opiate-like groups have given false negative results. For example, nalorphine and dextropropoxyphene do not substitute for a morphine on this test and yet instances of dependence on these drugs have arisen in clinical practice. It is clear that this type of screening is much too restricted in its applicability to be of general value as a prognostic index of potential drug problems.

Conclusion

Drug screening, both for therapeutic and for toxic or undesirable effects, is a process that can yield only approximate answers. Errors of two types are possible and probable: rejection of potentially useful drugs, and adoption of others that later prove to give rise to an unacceptable level of harm. The probability of errors of either type is related to the diversity and specificity of screening methods employed. These are in turn related to both the state of the art in development of methods, and the economics of product development by the pharmaceutical industry.

In the whole spectrum of screening methods, those pertaining to "addiction" or "abuse" liability are perhaps more limited than those serving any of the other major screening objectives. One important deficiency must be overcome if substantial progress is to be made: the excessive concentration on the physical dependence model of the opiates, which has exerted undue influence on scientific thought in the field of nonmedical use of drugs. Methods capable of screening for other types of drug problems are required, and for this purpose it is necessary to agree on the types of problems which screening techniques must simulate. In this area, there should be greater emphasis on testing drugs not only with intended therapeutic uses in mind, but also in the range of doses by the modes and patterns of nonmedical use.

Another area that deserves greater attention is the screening of different pharmaceutical preparations of the same drug. In addition to screening for "abuse liability" of a given chemical, there may be considerable merit in screening for low-risk versus high-risk *preparations* of the drug. For example, amphetamine inhalers formerly constituted a high-risk preparation because they could be easily obtained (not being intended for ingestion) and easily extracted to yield a large dose for devotees who desired it. Current experimental preparations of a naloxone-methadone combination provide an example of intended low-risk formulations, because the naloxone should prevent an illicit user from getting the desired euphoriant effect by extracting and injecting the drug. Another suggestion is the addition of a tiny amount of an emetic or laxative to oral preparations, so that doses much in excess of the prescribed range would defeat the illicit user's purpose.

Friebel (1973) has stated clearly and dramatically the size of the problem facing those who must conduct screening procedures: "The market life of a newly introduced product averaged about 5 years. Of the drugs at present on the market, 70% were either unknown or unavailable 15 years ago." This fact confronts the screeners with an extremely difficult task, because of the load of new developments with which they must cope. At the same time, the high turnover rate offers an excellent opportunity to eliminate undesirable or unsatisfactory drugs rapidly as replacements become available. The challenge, one hopes, will help to stimulate new developments in drug screening.

Testing and Evaluating Risk of Dependence and Abuse

Hans Halbach

VIII

A number of animal experiments have been designed to uncover and characterize the properties of psychoactive substances (see Bovet, Chapter Six). Some of these experiments—for example, those relating to wakefulness, locomotor activity, emotional and nociceptive reactivity, or social behavior—may have a bearing on the dependence and abuse potential of the substance in question. None of them, however, is immediately and specifically indicative of such a potential. Special techniques have been developed reproducing the human features and conditions of physical and psychic dependence.

TESTING AND EVALUATING

In order to understand the limitations of the conclusions one is able to draw from animal tests it is necessary to distinguish between *testing* and *evaluating*. The purpose of a test is the comparison of a substance of unknown properties with a substance of known properties. It is carried out as an experiment using physical, chemical, or biological methods. Its results are reliable only if they are reproducible. The properties of a substance that make it one liable to produce a state of dependence can be tested in animals and in man. Evaluation, on the other hand, is the appraisal of a human and social situation, that is, the risk of the nonmedical use of a substance liable to produce dependence. Such evaluation takes into account experience, if available, with known situations of a similar nature or other relevant considerations. Evaluation is thus essentially different from the experimental, and hence reproducible, act of testing and consequently less precise, less reliable, and less conclusive. This applies also to behavioral experiments with animals in which effects cannot be measured, but must be assessed by the subjective judgment of the experimenter who must be familiar with the behavioral characteristics of the species studied.

One must be aware of the difference between testing and evaluating in order to understand the contribution that science can make to decision-making in respect to drug-abuse control. For example, the international conventions of 1925 and 1931 as well as the 1948 protocol stipulate the control of substances having similar properties and giving rise to similar abuse as the drugs already covered by those treaty instruments. Thus, testing as well as evaluating is required for any substance considered for control, especially when such controls are stringent and are imposed to prevent abuse, that is, when practical experience with the drug in question is not available ("before the fact" situation). However, in the absence of suitable test and evaluation procedures these treaties like other legislative or social-control instruments are bound to limit the controls to what has been shown in practice to be abused ("after the fact" control).

When the Single Convention assigned to the Commission on Narcotic Drugs the final decision as to controls of certain drugs, this served, in part, to demonstrate that social and other environmental factors were considered relevant for the evaluation of abuse risk, in addition to the results of psychopharmacological testing. Under the Convention on Psychotropic Substances (1971), which is not yet in force, "economic, social, legal, administrative, and other factors" will have to be taken into consideration before a decision on the control of a drug is reached.

The World Health Organization Technical Report #407 (1969) postulated: "If the drug dependence is associated with behavioural or other responses that adversely affect the user's interpersonal relations or cause adverse physical, social, or economic consequences to others as well as to himself, and if the problem is actually widespread in the population or has a significant potential for becoming widespread, then a public health problem does exist. Society must then, among other things, take the responsibility for determining whether or not the drug in question should be controlled."

Pertinent as these conditions and factors are for imposing controls, to the extent that suitable methods to *evaluate* those factors are lacking, social legislation remains limited to inexact estimates of the risks involved and relies heavily on the narrow range of data coming from those research areas that allow only the *testing* of psychopharmacological properties of a drug and, at best, of its behavioral effects.

Before referring to the various tests available for determining the dependence potential of a drug, the criteria of dependence and tolerance must be clear. Note that the terms *addiction* or *habituation* have not been used in this chapter, this for good reasons.

DEPENDENCE

Difficulties in terminology have become increasingly apparent as new drugs have appeared and as the patterns of their nonmedical use have altered. These developments were not adequately characterized by the existing definitions of *addiction* and *habituation,* terms that were generally used, often interchangeably. For scientific and practical reasons, a term was sought that would as an underlying feature embrace all kinds and forms of drug abuse. *Dependence* was elected by WHO to serve that function. The significance and characteristics of drug dependence have been delineated as follows (Eddy, Halbach, and others, 1965):

> Drug dependence is a state of psychic or physical dependence, or both, on a drug, arising in a person following administration of that drug on a periodic or continuous basis. The characteristics of such a state will vary with the agent involved, and these characteristics must always be made clear by designating the particular type of drug dependence in each specific case; for example, drug dependence of morphine type, of barbiturate type, of amphetamine type, etc.
>
> Individuals may become dependent upon a wide variety of chemical substances that produce central nervous system effects ranging from stimulation to depression. All of these drugs have one effect in common: they are capable of creating, in certain individuals, a particular state of mind that is termed "psychic dependence." In this situation, there is a feeling of satisfaction and a psychic drive that require periodic or continuous administration of the drug to produce pleasure or to avoid discomfort. Indeed, this mental state is the most powerful of all of the factors involved in chronic intoxication with psychotropic drugs, and with certain types of drugs it may be the only factor involved, even in the case of most intense cravings and perpetuation of compulsive abuse.
>
> Some drugs also induce physical dependence, which is an adaptive state that manifests itself by intense physical disturbances when the administration of the drug is suspended or when its action is affected by the administration of a specific antagonist. These disturbances, i.e., the withdrawal or abstinence syndromes, are made up of specific arrays of symptoms and signs of psychic and physical nature that are characteristic for each drug type. These conditions are relieved by re-administration of the same drug or of another drug of similar pharmacological action within the same generic type. No overt manifestation of physical dependence is evident if an adequate dosage is maintained. Physical dependence is a powerful factor in reinforcing the influence of psychic dependence upon continuing drug use or relapse to drug use after attempted withdrawal.
>
> Many of the drugs that induce dependence, especially those that

create physical dependence, also induce tolerance, which is an adaptive state characterized by diminished response to the same quantity of drug or by the fact that a larger dose is required to produce the same degree of pharmacodynamic effect. Both drug dependence and drug abuse may occur without the development of demonstrable tolerance.

The nature and significance of drug abuse may be considered from two points of view: one relates to the interaction between the drug and the individual, the other to the interaction between drug abuse and society. The first viewpoint is concerned with drug dependence and the interplay between the pharmacodynamic actions of the drug and the psychological status of the individual. The second—the interaction between drug abuse and society—is concerned with the interplay of a wide range of conditions, environmental, sociological, and economic.

For scientific reasons and also with a view to contemporary national and international programs and legal provisions for prevention and control, the following types of dependence are currently distinguished: morphine (opiate); barbiturate; alcohol; cocaine; cannabis (marijuana); amphetamine; and hallucinogen. Khat (catha edulis) contains an active ingredient of amphetamine character and can thus be assimilated to the amphetamines. There would be no reason not to include other types of substance dependence with ensuing behavioral or toxic reactions considered or judged to present a threat to public health or safety.

The state of dependence, whether physical or psychic in origin and outcome, is the result of the interaction between a chemical agent and an individual (human or animal). It is thus a biological phenomenon that should be amenable to scientific experimental investigation and describable in adequate biological terms. In contrast, the development and pattern of abuse are contingent upon a number of environmental factors: anthropological, sociological, cultural, traditional, economical. Thus the nonmedical use of a dependence-producing drug occurs in response to an interplay of a wide range of endogenous and exogenous factors.

The task of determining, for preventive medical or legislative control purposes, the presence and degree of the dependence potential of a hitherto unknown substance and, hence, the risk of it being abused meets with considerable difficulties. For certain types of drugs, pharmacologists, psychologists, and behavioral scientists have at their disposal a number of tests applicable to man and/or animals. What cannot be tested, must be left to evaluation.

Keeping the distinction between evaluation and testing in mind, we must realize that tests for a possible dependence potential of a substance are fraught with ambiguity. This is because the major component in dependence leading to abuse is psychological and thus less amenable to investigation and measurement than the withdrawal syndrome, which is a manifestation of physical dependence. Indeed, even the measurement of the latter is still being refined.

For drugs of the morphine type it has been possible for some time to assess their physical dependence capacity* in monkeys, using a scale of indicators that allow a semiquantitative comparison between substances in respect of their dependence-producing potential. The transfer to man of the potency ratios observed in the monkey is, however, neither possible nor permissible. For central nervous system depressants of the barbiturate type (which include many diverse substances of different chemical structure), suitable tests are of much more recent date. Their predictive value in respect to the human species is, therefore, not yet as well ascertained as is the case with drugs of the morphine type.

For the assessment of the potential of a substance for producing a psychic dependence, a number of techniques have been developed using infrahuman species, especially monkeys. Because of the relatively recent experience gained with them we do not know to which extent these experiments are valid predictors of the test substance's ability to produce psychic dependence in man.

In order to draw valid conclusions from animal experiments in regard to drug effects on man, one must be sure that the way the drug acts in the animal and human organism is essentially the same. This depends on a number of factors and conditions. The drug may exert its effects on the organism in its original chemical form or it may be transformed (metabolized) by the organism and the product of such transformation is then the active substance. These mechanisms quite often differ between man and animals and among animal species. There are also species differences in respect to the distribution and excretion of the drug as such or of its metabolites, which in turn lead to differences in the concentration (amount) of the active substance in the body. For practical purposes this means that any drug to be tested should be administered to a human subject at the earliest possible stage of the study in order to ascertain how the drug is handled by the human species and to be able to select for further detailed study of its various effects the animal species which resembles man as closely as possible in that respect (World Health Organization Technical Report #341, 1966).

An ethical problem arises from the desirability of early drug administration to human subjects. It may become a dilemma in the case of drugs with a suspected dependence potential. This is one of the reasons why the fundamental requirement of making the choice of the experimental animal species dependent upon its metabolic and pharmacokinetic similarity to man has so far hardly been met. Notwithstanding these considerations, in the monkey, the dog, and the rat, species have been found in which the human phenomena of physical and, in part, psychic dependence can be reproduced.

Nevertheless, monkeys and dogs do differ pharmacodynamically from humans so that animal tests alone without confirmation by clinical observation

---

* Physical dependence capacity is the ability of a drug to act as a substitute for another upon which the organism has been made physically dependent, that is, to suppress abstinence phenomena that would otherwise develop after withdrawal of the original dependence-producing drug.

should not form the basis of arguing for controls unless experience has shown that in the animal species the human phenomena of dependence can be replicated. A case in point is the relative discrepancy between the physical dependence capacity of pethidine and morphinan in the monkey and in man. The monkey is more sensitive to pethidine than man, whereas with morphinan compounds the reverse is observed. Whether this is due to metabolic or pharmacokinetic differences is not known. There could well be other discrepancies of this same sort, which, if not properly elucidated, could lead to incorrect generalizations about the physical dependence liability of drugs for man.

The demonstration of tolerance has occasionally been used to characterize a dependence-producing drug. In the present context, *tolerance* is defined as the adaptation of the organism to the effects of a drug in the sense of decreasing sensitivity so that increasing dosages are required to obtain the initial drug effect. The mechanisms by which tolerance is brought about are manifold, for example, by changes in the pharmacokinetics of the drug or by diminished responsiveness of neural mechanisms. In view of the fact that the human and animal organisms develop a tolerance, sometimes very rapidly and to a considerable degree, toward a great variety of substances, the demonstration of tolerance is by no means proof of a potential for dependence development though it may hint to such a possibility. Besides, dependence on a drug can develop with or without tolerance.

When studying the dependence potential of a drug, one must distinguish between those types that produce a physical dependence and those that do not. For the former, that is, drugs of morphine and barbiturate type,* a number of test procedures in animals and man have been worked out that permit the demonstration of the development of physical dependence.

Physical dependence results from the distortion of physiological processes after more or less prolonged administration of a drug, so that the presence in the body of an adequate amount of the drug is necessary for the maintenance of physiological equilibrium. The mechanism of physical dependence is not fully understood. It is demonstrated by the appearance of characteristic signs and symptoms after withdrawal of the drug. The withdrawal syndrome differs between drugs of the morphine and barbiturate type. An essential characteristic of any withdrawal syndrome, irrespective of the type of drug, is its alleviation or disappearance when the level in the organism of the drug that originated the dependence is restored. A withdrawal syndrome is also produced when the dependence-producing action of the drug is counteracted (neutralized) by means of a specific antagonist. Such antagonists (nalorphine, naloxone, levallorphan) are known in the morphine group, but not in the group of barbiturate-type drugs.

There are two categories of tests for physical dependence. (1) In so-called substitution tests, the organism is made dependent on a prototype drug—usually morphine or barbital—by its regular administration in sufficient quantities (in-

---

* The distinction between these drug types is made on account of their pharmacological properties—not the chemical structure—morphine and barbiturate serving as prototypes.

creasing when tolerance develops) over a sufficiently long period of time. Then, the prototype is substituted by the test substance. If no abstinence symptoms occur, the latter has a physical dependence capacity the degree of which can be compared with that of the prototype on the basis of the respective dosages required for comparable effects. (2) In the "direct test," the test drug is administered regularly in doses adjusted to the development of tolerance. The outbreak of typical abstinence phenomena after sudden withdrawal of the test substance proves its dependence-producing capacity. Where specific antagonists exist—and this is the case in the morphine class only—this test may be supplemented by administration of such an antagonist, which would precipitate a typical abstinence syndrome. These considerations are valid in principle for central nervous system depressant substances of both the morphine and the barbiturate type, but in practice there are important differences between them.

Techniques have been developed for the study of physical dependence of morphine type in monkeys, dogs, guinea pigs, rats, and mice (Halbach and Eddy, 1963; World Health Organization Technical Report #287, 1964; Friebel and Kuhn, 1965). Whereas the tests in lower animals are mainly exploratory and useful for screening purposes in drug development to detect the presence or absence of dependence-producing properties, the results obtained with morphine-like substances in monkeys are qualitatively quite similar to those in man and may also show a quantitative relationship to the respective effects in man—which, however, cannot be relied upon in attempts to transfer data from animal tests to man. When unequivocally positive, that is, indicative of dependence liability, results may, in the view of the World Health Organization Technical Report #407 (1969), be used as a sound basis for evaluating the liability of an agent to produce physical dependence in man. This view is supported by subsequent confirmation in man of positive evidence of physical dependence in monkey tests.

For the detection of physical dependence on drugs of barbiturate type, tests with monkeys and dogs are available. (World Health Organization Technical Report #287, 1964; Yanagita Takahashi, 1970). These methods are more recent and the experience gained with them so far would appear not to be sufficient to credit them with the same predictive value as in the case of morphine-type drugs. In addition, the structural variety of substances of the barbiturate type is enormous; it ranges from the chemically simple chloral hydrate or paraldehyde to the complex structures of modern psychoactive substances. The wide chemical, metabolic, and pharmacodynamic differences in this group should be expected to entail great differences in respect to the capability to produce dependence with ensuing difficulties as regards comparison and prediction relative to man.

Whereas concordance is generally observed between the demonstration in the monkey of physical dependence on a morphine-type drug and the dependence potential in man there are some exceptions with barbiturate-type drugs. For example, carisoprodol and tybamat, both so-called tranquilizers and congeners of meprobamate, substitute for barbital in the dog, but with neither of them are withdrawal symptoms obtained in the direct test nor are they evaluated as having abuse potential in man. Meprobamate, however, has given positive results in both tests and is known to produce physical dependence in man. One sees that a drug substituting for barbital in the animal test cannot automatically be considered as one producing dependence in man.

An expert conference convened in 1969 by the U.S. Bureau of Narcotics and Dangerous Drugs and the Food and Drug Administration emphasized the need for additional experimental work with barbiturates in animals and man to establish reliable techniques for predicting abuse. The conferees concluded that the methods for testing the major tranquilizers were much less advanced than for barbiturates; that the major tranquilizers diminished responsiveness to stimuli in animals and that animals will not self-administer these drugs; no methodology for predicting abuse liability of these drugs had been developed yet and with the minor tranquilizers there seemed to be specific difficulties. The conferees being unable to make specific recommendations for testing methods in the area of tranquilizers made a plea for establishing data on the reliability and validity of new methods that might be developed.

Whenever experiments with higher animals give doubtful or negative results (especially in the presence of relevant pharmacological evidence or resemblance to known dependence-producing agents), studies with human subjects are imperative. The World Health Organization Technical Report #142 (1958), while recognizing the progress made in initial screening procedures for detecting dependence liability, nevertheless considered that observations in man are still required for the final judgment as to the safety of any new compound intended for introduction into general medical use.

Contrary to the recognized practice of clinical pharmacology, where human studies only follow animal experimentation, dependence tests can be applied initially to human subjects under appropriate safeguards. Indeed, they antedated the broad application of animal tests. The often-voiced objection that the subjects in question, that is, hospitalized, incurable former addicts, are not representative of an average population would appear to be offset, in part at least, by the advantage of their being especially alert to the specific psychological effects to be investigated.

Tests for physical dependence capacity of presumed morphine-type drugs conducted in human subjects (be these addicts or patients needing certain drugs because of their medical condition) are decisive. In humans, the degree of physical dependence as manifested in the abstinence phenomena can be measured, for example, by the size of the pupils, blood pressure, body temperature, and so forth. Thus a semiquantitative comparison is possible between drugs in respect to their strength to produce dependence. The extent of clinical dependence studies of morphine-type drugs exceeds by far those of the barbiturate type. Only two representatives of the latter (secobarbital and pentobarbital) have been experimentally investigated in man and those on a limited scale. Further, since the abstinence phenomena following withdrawal of a barbiturate-type drug in a state of high dependence are potentially deadly, no experimentation can be conducted in human subjects that involve abrupt withdrawal of a drug of barbiturate type.

Of the drugs considered to be commonly abused and included in international control instruments, only those of morphine and barbiturate type are, in principle, capable of producing a state of physical dependence characterized by a specific withdrawal syndrome. Cocaine, cannabis, amphetamines, and hallucinogens lack this capacity. The abstinence phenomena after withdrawal of amphetamines have been claimed to be characteristic of a specific state of dependence, but they may as well be interpreted as rebound phenomena, that is, physiological responses to the drug-altered state such as fatigue following upon the drug-induced insomnia.

A much stronger component in abuse than physical dependence is a state of psychic dependence. It is characterized by behavioral responses, which include a compulsion to take the drug on a continuous or periodic basis in order to experience its psychic effects and to avoid discomfort caused by its absence. Indeed, such psychological features appear to be the most powerful factors associated with abuse. Therefore it is of paramount importance for all types of drugs to be able to estimate liability for such psychic dependence.

Methods are being developed to study the behavioral aspects of drug dependence in animals. Most often primates are used. In self-administration experiments, monkeys can administer the test drug to themselves in fixed quantities by various routes and under variable environmental conditions. The latter can be designed to imitate certain real-life situations, for example, stress. These methods provide information on the animal's response to the drug in respect to liking, choice of alternatives offered, and the degree to which self-administration is repeated (Schuster and Thompson, 1969). By such means, the drug-seeking behavior of the animal is open to study as is the reinforcing effect of a drug on such behavior under various conditions that are, hopefully, analogous to human situations and behavior. So far it has been possible to imitate in the monkey drug-seeking behavior analogous to that in man for cocaine, amphetamines, and alcohol as well as morphine and barbiturates (Deneau, Yanagita and Seevers, 1969). Understandably, self-administration of a drug comes to a halt when its narcotizing sedative effects predominate, that is, when the animal takes so much it goes to sleep.

For practical purposes, it is usually assumed that drugs that are more repetitively self-administered by animals under a greater variety of conditions have a high potential for abuse in humans. Nevertheless the World Health Organization Technical Report #407 (1969) stated: "These methods are yielding interesting and suggestive data, but none has yet reached a level of refinement and reproducibility that would make it acceptable as yielding conclusive evidence of the possibility of man developing psychic dependence on a new agent."

Psychic dependence on hallucinogenic substances such as mescaline, LSD, and psilocybin is usually not intense even though a wide variety of motives and outcomes are associated with their use. Animals do not usually self-administer these drugs. In animals, LSD and other hallucinogens can produce an increase in body temperature and provoke certain behavioral patterns. For example, in the "open field" test, such drugs lead to exploratory activities and increased emotionality as measured by defecation and preening. Whether or not one would claim parallels between these animal effects and the hallucinogenic properties in man, it is reasonable to conclude that animal tests with hallucinogens do not tell much about how humans will behave when using them.

In conclusion, it would appear that the more remote a drug is from the morphine type, the less present animal methods are able to predict the risk of abuse associated with dependence. Perhaps this is so because dependence on and abuse of morphine-type drugs have aroused the attention of the scientific world and the public much earlier than the problems caused by other types of dependence-producing drugs.

Not only the abuse potential of a drug but also the direct consequences of its use for the user himself and for society (or the "risk to public health") must be considered when making a decision on the need for and extent of drug control. The car driver in a state of oversedation by morphine- or barbiturate-type drugs can be as dangerous to himself and others as the person who becomes aggressive in an amphetamine-produced paranoid episode. For the study of such direct psychotoxic effects, animal experiments can yield much information, but the full picture will have to be obtained through clinical studies with humans. The latest international control instrument, the Convention on Psychotropic Substances, takes cognizance of the variety of direct drug effects referring to drugs considered for control as those with "central nervous system stimulation or depression, resulting in hallucinations or disturbances in motor function or thinking or behaviour or perception or mood."

The account of the contribution animal experimentation can—or cannot —make to the process of decision-making would be incomplete without reference to the obligation of WHO, under the Convention on Psychotropic Substances, to assess also the degree of usefulness in medical therapy of a substance considered for international control. *Usefulness* is not necessarily tantamount to *efficacy*, and its evaluation is fraught with still more ambiguity than the assessment of efficacy.

The assessment of the therapeutic value or, more precisely, efficacy of a drug involves the skills of many disciplines including toxicology, pharmacology, clinical pharmacology, biometry, biostatistics, and epidemiology. Yet, the scientific approach toward evaluating therapeutic efficacy is of very recent date. In certain cases and under certain circumstances, the less scientific trial-and-error procedure cannot be excluded entirely from the process of evaluation. An efficacious drug considered useful in one geographical area may be considered less so in others where lack of experience or certain local circumstances could interfere with its appropriate administration or effects respectively. The assessment of usefulness might become still more difficult if a comparison with existing drugs should be required as might be the case under the terms of the Convention on Psychotropic Substances. To compound the issue, situations are known in which new therapeutic properties were detected in a drug after it had been used in medical practice for some time. For example, methaqualone was developed as an antimalarial drug, whereupon its value in treating arthritic conditions was discovered; today methaqualone is used as a hypnotic only, but at the same time it is widely abused and controlled accordingly because of its barbiturate-like liability to produce dependence. It is thinkable that with other substances events might occur in the reverse order beginning with their use as a hypnotic or sedative followed by the discovery of other perhaps more valuable therapeutic properties.

SUMMARY

Animal tests are available to detect and characterize the dependence potential of psychoactive substances. The actual risk of abuse must, however, be evaluated taking into account experience with similar drugs as well as the prevailing social and environmental factors.

When studying the dependence potential of a drug one must distinguish between those that produce a physical dependence (morphine and barbiturate types) and those that do not (cocaine, cannabis, amphetamines, and hallucinogens). Although its mechanism is not fully understood, physical dependence can be demonstrated by characteristic signs and symptoms after withdrawal of the drug. The withdrawal syndrome differs between drugs of the morphine type and those of the barbiturate type. It is alleviated when the level in the organism of the drug that originated the dependence is restored. In the morphine class, specific antagonists exist the administration of which precipitates a typical abstinence syndrome in an organism physically dependent on drugs of the morphine type.

For the study of physical dependence of morphine type, tests have been developed using monkeys, dogs, guinea pigs, rats, and mice. Tests with lower animals are mainly exploratory and useful for screening purposes. Results obtained with monkeys are comparable with those observed in humans and, when unequivocally positive, may be used as a sound basis for evaluating the liability of an agent to produce physical dependence in man. For the detection of physical dependence of barbiturate type, tests with monkeys and dogs are available. Experience gained with them so far would appear insufficient to credit them with the same predictive value as in the case of morphine-type drugs. Further, the wide chemical, metabolic, and pharmacodynamic differences in this group of substances is likely to entail great differences in respect to their capability to produce dependence. The WHO Expert Committee, while recognizing the progress made in screening procedures for the detection of dependence liability, considered that observations in man are still required for the final judgment as to the safety of new compounds.

The demonstration of tolerance has occasionally been used to characterize a dependence-producing drug. Since, however, the human or animal organism can develop tolerance toward a great variety of substances and since dependence can develop with or without tolerance, the demonstration of the latter is no evidence of a potential for dependence development.

Psychic dependence (characterized by behavioral responses including a compulsion to take the drug on a continuous or periodic basis in order to experience its psychic effects and to avoid discomfort caused by its absence) is the most powerful factor associated with abuse, and it is of paramount importance to estimate liability for such psychic dependence. To this end, most often primates are used. In self-administration experiments, monkeys can administer the test drug to themselves under variable conditions designed to imitate certain real-life situations, for example, stress. It has been possible to initiate in the monkey drug-seeking behavior in respect to cocaine, amphetamines, and alcohol as well as morphine and barbiturates. Drugs that are more repetitively self-administered by animals under a greater variety of conditions are assumed to have a high potential for abuse in humans. Nevertheless, according to the WHO Expert Committee, these methods cannot provide conclusive evidence as to the possibility of man developing a psychic dependence on the agent in question. Psychic dependence on hallucinogenic substances is usually not intense. Since animals do not usually self-administer these drugs, animal experiments with hallucinogens are of very limited predictive value as to how humans will behave when using them.

Besides the abuse potential of a drug, the immediate, possibly toxic, consequences of its use must be considered when making a decision relative to control. Such direct psychotoxic effects can be studied in animals, but clinical observations are indispensable.

In keeping with the Convention on Psychotropic Substances, a drug considered for control must be examined also in respect to its therapeutic usefulness, which is not necessarily tantamount to efficacy, depending on geographical and other conditions. If a comparison with existing drugs should be required, as might be the case under the terms of the Convention on Psychotropic Substances, the assessment of usefulness might become rather difficult.

Experiments and Surveys on Drug Dependence

C. R. B. Joyce

IX

It might be supposed that the necessity to use sound methods in the study of drug use is so self-evident and their employment so easy that advocacy of their use is unnecessary. However, lack of clear definitions has (as always) led to a failure to carry out good experiments; poor experiments have not yielded hard information, and the resulting vacuum has been filled by vigorous emotional involvement. The consequent emotionalism has often interfered with the task of definition.

DEFINITION, PERCEPTION, AND HYPOTHESES

Various systems of definition in the field of drug dependence and abuse have been widely published (Eddy, Halbach, and others, 1965; Kalant, LeBlanc, and Gibbins, 1971) or are discussed elsewhere in this volume. Definition as such will therefore not be discussed here. However, it is certainly useful to emphasize the fact that definition depends upon perception. The discussion by Petrie (1972, pp. 70–71) of the relationship between measurement and interpretation of such psychological phenomena as aggression or masculinity can easily be applied to drug dependence.

One of the major problems is whether we are to see certain kinds of human behavior as essentially aggressive, or we are to see aggression as

aberrant and caused by some lack of genetic determination or up-bringing.
. . . If aggressive behaviour is 'natural,' then aggression can be counted
as one of the basic physiological drives and used in explanations of other
aggression-related behaviour. If aggression is not natural, then it must be
explained in some way by other drives or stimuli which are themselves
assumed to be natural.

Turning from aggressivity to masculinity-femininity, Petrie points out that

categories of femininity presented by dominant male culture are not based
on basic biological or physiological characteristics, but are rather the
result of the cultural picture the adult male has of what a truly feminine
human being should be like. . . . Even after one attempts to determine
empirically what attributes can be attributed [sic] to upbringing, . . . the
very categories in which the experiments are carried on are themselves
male-culture-bound. For example, it is at least plausible to entertain the
hypothesis that some of the physiological differences one finds between
male and female and which show less strength on the part of the female
are traceable to differences in the amount and kind of physical exercise
our culture deems important for the two sexes. . . . Do we start by seeing
human beings and determining what differences there are, or do we start
by seeing [different categories] and determining what similarities there
are?

It is essential to consider closely the nature of the question that is being
asked, for this will affect the experiment designed to answer it. Where we speak,
for example, of the liability of a drug to cause dependence, we should state clearly
whether we are attempting to define the risk for a particular individual, or for
a particular kind of individual, or whether we wish to assess the average risk
for an unselected group; or whether we are trying to predict the risk that a new
substance will be liable to induce dependence. The estimates, and the experiments, will differ, depending upon whether we extrapolate from risk rates for
chemicals that are in widespread use or whether we are proposing to obtain
appropriate evidence from experiments with the new chemical itself. Distinctions
of all these kinds are often omitted. Only on the basis of confirmed estimates is it
possible to make predictions about related problems, and only when such predictions have been tested can we know whether the methods designed to estimate
the risks were valid.

Problems can be and have been caused, sometimes by failure to define or
by assuming that the definitions used were so generally understood as not to
need explicit statement, and sometimes by combining two quite different purposes (individual prediction and population prevalence) into a single survey.
The admirable compendium on the dependence liability of "non-narcotic" drugs
prepared by Isbell and Chrusciel (1970) on behalf of WHO for the Vienna

Conference is an example of the latter. The column headings of their summary tables of central nervous system depressants, stimulants, hallucinogenics, crude plant drugs, and precursors are respectively chemical formulas, synonyms, symptoms of intoxication, tolerance, psychic and physical dependence, "pharmacological notes," major dangers of abuse, and bibliographic references. In explaining how the ratings of "abuse-potential" (column 9 in their tables) were made, they say: "A rating of 'high' in column 9 indicates that the substance can create strong psychic dependence and that extensive abuse has occurred or is judged likely to occur if the drug was readily available. A rating of 'moderate' indicates that the drug creates a less intense degree of psychic dependence and that some degree of abuse has occurred or is judged likely to occur if the drug was readily available. A rating of 'low' indicates that the drug creates only mild psychic dependence and that only little or no abuse has occurred or is deemed likely to occur. If 'None' appears in column 9, the compound is judged not to be a drug of dependence" (p. 7).

The point to notice is that each scale point is arrived at conjunctively: *"psychic dependence . . . and . . . abuse"* (my italics) is involved each time. Psychic dependence is an individual phenomenon, extension of abuse is a group phenomenon. Although the authors are rightly careful to eschew pseudo-quantification in their work, they have here committed the error of basing a vital series of evaluations upon the addition of noncommensurables. Though you may *wager* all Lombard Street to a china orange, or a kingdom for a horse, it is not possible to *add* one to the other.

The difficulty is compounded by the fact that many of the estimates of individual risk are eventually found to be based upon experimental work in animals. It is true that animals can be made experimentally dependent upon drugs in "social" ways that may be analogous to human involvement (Thompson, 1968); it is also true, but little known, that spontaneous dependence has been described in animals other than man (Nilsson and Lindroth, 1959). However, the well-known differences of pharmacological responses between guinea pigs, monkeys, mice, and men are so great (Glick, Jarvik, and Nakamura, 1970; Fennessy, Heimans, and Rand, 1969) that inference would be hazardous even if mankind were genetically as homogeneous as the strains of subprimates normally used in laboratory work. The more complex series of human motivations and other psychological apparatus increase individual variability to an even greater extent, and to make prediction from a hundred rats or ten monkeys to a nation of men even more hazardous. For example, mice are apparently extremely susceptible to benzomorphans (such as pentazocine), judged by a specific jumping test (Saelens, Granat, and Sawyer, 1971), whereas rhesus monkeys are hardly so at all (Eddy and May, 1966). Since human beings differ widely in their susceptibility, too, some being liable to become dependent upon one or many drugs and others apparently not at all, which is the "right" test? Which man is the rat and which the monkey?

In fact, the official "United States procedures for screening drugs: testing for dependence liability in animals and man" (National Academy of Sciences, 1970), though willing to interpret results from experiments on monkeys or humans to determine physical dependence liability of morphine type, is more cautious in interpreting experiments in dogs to determine physical dependence liability of barbiturate type. It has at present no models at all for investigating psychic dependence liability in animals, nor (in consequence) any programs for investigating dependence liability of kinds of drug other than those of morphine or barbiturate type. Recent attempts to extend the techniques available for these purposes are, however, described by Yanagita (1973) and Yanagita and Takahashi (1973).

Another, but also admirable, survey of the dependence liability of narcotic analgesics (Martin, 1966) underlines the extent to which untested assumptions and moral judgments compromise the apparently clear statement of scientific objectives: "Two basic problems concerned with the assessment of the abuse potentiality of drugs that affect the functioning of the brain will be given major consideration. The first and general problem is concerned with identifying and establishing the characteristics of drugs that make their abuse probable *and their control desirable.* The second and immediate practical problem is concerned with the development and validation of methods for measuring characteristics of centrally acting drugs *which have been adjudged to be undesirable* and for classifying drugs that have these properties" (p. 155, my italics). An even more basic problem than those identified by Martin is to define what is meant by *abuse, desirable,* and *undesirable.* Of all the criteria for classifying drugs, that proposed by Martin is probably one of the most subjective. Moral judgments cannot be separated from scientific work, nor is it desirable that they should be. But all assumptions should be tested and moral judgments should always be explicitly stated. As Delisle Burns insists, everyone working on the central nervous system should state his prejudices and expectations in advance, since these to a large extent determine his hypotheses, his experiments, and his findings (Delisle Burns, 1958). My own experience has mainly been in the fields of human laboratory pharmacology and clinical trials, so it is from these that my examples will most frequently be drawn. However, I believe that the argument that follows can be applied with little modification to other disciplines, such as those of the animal laboratory or the social survey.

EXPERIMENTAL DESIGN AND STATISTICAL INFERENCE

Scientific investigation seldom proceeds by hypothesis to experiment to observation to conclusion and restatement of hypothesis, as is commonly believed. Nonscientists perhaps make more use of the classical procedure than do scientists; for example, in deciding whether or not to carry an umbrella or to take lobster Thermidor rather than a plain omelet. Though the application of scientific method to the study of social phenomena is difficult, and some phenomena (economics, for example) studied by social scientists may not in fact be amenable to scientific study in the traditional sense at all, it is surprising how seldom scientific method is used for social studies where it is legitimate, feasible, and indeed essential to do so.

Each of us as his own scientist makes predictions about phenomena he observes in his immediate environment that he knows are either under his own control or at least, although capricious, not completely unpredictable, especially if the results of failure to use appropriate methods will fall upon his own head— perhaps literally. Drug dependence, on the other hand, is, even in those countries where it is most frequent, still a phenomenon of low incidence. Most cases are therefore physically more distant from the average individual than are people infected by an influenza epidemic. But whereas influenza epidemics have been studied scientifically and something is already known about etiology, methods of control, and future development, drug dependence is widely believed to be mysterious in origin, immediately dangerous, and unpredictable in its developments. Attitudes to cholera infection perhaps represent an encouraging half-way point. The causative organism and manner of spread of cholera have been known for a relatively long time. Prevention has long been possible, in theory, but until recently treatment for the infected has been uncertain and often ineffective. With increased understanding of the physiopathology of the disease, however, the panic that formerly accompanied its appearance should also soon subside. As with influenza, cholera, or environmental pollution, one should consider how drug dependence may be prevented, controlled, or treated. Although, as with infectious diseases, the only sure way of prevention (eradication of the causative agent) is probably not feasible, it is essential to study the patterns of disease to determine the causative agents (drugs, like bugs, are necessary but not sufficient causes of the disease they bring about); their interaction with other factors in patient, environment, and society; their manner of spread; and their response to control and treatment. Unlike influenza, drug dependence spreads by contacts that are only partly linked in time and place. Such contacts involve motivations, expectations, attitudes, and perceptions. To make predictions about the risk of infection (that is, of becoming drug-dependent) that are valid either for the group or the individual therefore involves experimental design and statistical analysis of some sophistication. The importance of using scientific methods in relation to drug dependence has, most exceptionally, been emphasized in the interim report of the Canadian (Le Dain) Commission of Enquiry into the Non-medical Use of Drugs (1970), but no systematic accounts of its application appear to have been given. Let us, therefore, begin somewhere near the beginning.

Necessary features of any experiment, whether it is in the animal or human laboratory, or in the field, include the following: (1) a clear statement of the phenomena to be studied, and as far as possible the conclusions that are permissible even if the phenomena change during the experiment; (2) correct selection of the sample to be studied; (3) appropriate measures to control the experimental conditions; (4) proper choice of the measuring instrument to be used and choice of correct methods for analysis; (5) adherence to protocol and the use of legitimate inferences; and (6) decision-making.

Description of Phenomena

First, the question to be answered must be so stated that it can be asked in the same way by every investigator (physician, social psychologist, or market researcher) and (if the behavior studied is a verbal response) can be understood in the same way by every individual who is to answer it. Second, it must be developed in such a way that any answer can be directly compared with answers by other respondents to the same or other questions to which it is logically related and with which it may be combined in some composite score or function, such as an intelligence quotient or a measure of intraversion. This can be achieved in part by providing alternative precoded answers or a visual analog scale or an exact specification of the laboratory method to be used. Even without crossing national or other cultural barriers, these requirements can pose problems. Also, the passage of time during an investigation may change the meanings of questions or answers or the behavior of respondents. For example, during an investigation of drug use on an American campus some years ago (Blum and Associates, 1969b), it proved necessary to change the way of referring to LSD users to "heads" rather than, as previously, "acid heads" because the language of the drug-using respondent group was changing; it was considered necessary to change the language of the question in order to maintain the consistent language of the answer. *Gay* as an adjective applied to personal behavior has strikingly changed its meaning in the past few years.

Even in crossing from one English-speaking culture to another, such problems multiply. For example, *sick* (American) means *ill* in English, but can be interpreted as *fed up* or, in other words, *annoyed*. *Mad* in American means *angry* or *cross* in English but *mad* in English means *crazy* in American, and so on. The examples given are so obvious that they are usually dealt with satisfactorily. However, even if the definition is agreed upon, evaluative problems may not be so easily resolved; *aggressiveness* tends to be a valued quality in America, a pejorative trait in England. Thus the scores on questions measuring such traits not only may be different, but also will in part at least be measuring different things. A useful review by Gaber (1972) discusses the dangers in survey question-framing and some ways of reducing them, and there are of course many more detailed texts on survey research, construction of questionnaires, and so on (Wittenborn, 1972; Armitage, 1971). Some unexpected difficulties arise with the latter: for example, "position effects" are so marked that respondents have a tendency to structure their series of responses in a definite order of "yes" and "no" replies, even if no specific questions at all are asked (Whitfield, 1950)! This kind of difficulty will be exacerbated when, as is certainly the case with drug dependence, the vocabularies of many different disciplines are involved

(Bross, Shapiro, and Anderson, 1972). The problem is not necessarily easier with what are customarily regarded as the harder data presented by measurements of pulse rate, blood pressure, and the like. In one careful experimental comparison of nurses' measurement of pulse rate, for example (M. L. Jones, 1970), the error rates reported, with simultaneous standard electrocardiograph recording for comparison, ranged from about −10 percent to +50 percent, with an average error of about +10 percent. Errors decreased to about half these rates with training to graduate level; but, surprisingly, the errors were larger the longer the period over which the measurements were made: estimates were more accurate if made for only 15 seconds than for 30 seconds or 60 seconds.

These examples have illustrated the concepts of reliability and validity of the measuring instrument to be used. "Reliability," in Wittenborn's (1972, p. 83) words, "refers to the verifiability of a [measure]. Validity refers to the pertinence of the [measure] for the avowed purpose." In other words, a reliable measure must give virtually the same answer under identical conditions and a valid measure varies appropriately, within acceptable limits, with the intensity of an intrinsic, measurable, part of the behavior of interest.

For example, in a recent study by Blum and his associates (1972a), items from interviews with parents and children on social, medical, and other questions were first correlated with other measures of the children's use of drugs and then combined in a complex score. These measures were then used both to "predict back" to the original sample and to predict forward—a far harder test—to the drug use of a new sample. The success of this established both the reliability and the validity of the methods developed.

However, such results (like any others) are demonstrably valid, in the absence of further experimentation, only for the group on which their validity has been demonstrated. This kind of tautology is responsible for much lay (and often scientific) impatience with scientific method; but neglect of the logic involved is responsible for much misplaced confidence in the transferability of results from one epoch or nation to another, or even from one classroom to another of the same school. As N. C. Smith (1970) is among many to point out, exact replication in a second experiment as identical as possible with the first is an essential but almost invariably neglected part of scientific discipline: If "the goal of scientific research is to render established truths, . . . the neglect of replication must be viewed as scientific irresponsibility."

Replication, or repeating the experiment in exactly the same way, will be seen as all the more essential if it is realized that apparently significant experimental results will be obtained that are *really* due to chance once in twenty times although they were *statistically unlikely* to have been due to chance. Yet, as most people—authors, editors, and readers alike—are more excited by positive than negative results, it is highly likely that many spurious results have been embedded in the literature because they were not replicated before publication. It is highly probable that reports are prematurely reported with disturbing (but unknown) frequency, that this accounts in part for the proliferation of journals (which might perhaps even be reduced to a proportion approaching 5 percent of their present number if adequate replication were practiced), and that the frequency with which one worker greets the achievement of a positive result by a colleague with the cry "whatever you do, don't repeat it" is so high as to be neither an accident, nor funny.

Such considerations lead us to a discussion of sampling, because each experiment that is actually done is only one sample from all those that might have been done.

Sample Selection

In a statistical sense, a population consists of all those individual cases that exhibit the phenomenon of interest. Thus a population may be numerically quite small—babies born of heroin-dependent mothers in Britain in 1972, for example. Even so, it is seldom possible to study an entire population: either this is not accessible, or it would be too time-consuming or too expensive to do so. One is almost always obliged to take samples. Any sample must be representative —that is, it should contain all the features, in appropriate concentration, that are related in the same way as in the population itself to the phenomena it is desired to study. Since in any situation beyond the most elementary these are seldom either fully or even partially known, this theoretical requirement often causes difficulty. The difficulties are lessened by random sampling in which the opposite solution is adopted—to avoid as far as possible any systematic relation with any possibly important feature. In survey experiments, these methods correspond to the distinction between quota (or stratified) and probability sampling. The two techniques can be combined in series. In the former, each subgroup believed to be relevant is represented in a sample deliberately constructed to have the same proportions as those of the tested population. In the latter, a random sample is taken (1 percent, 10 percent, or whatever) from the whole population within as comprehensive a frame as possible: for example, a register of electors, taxpayers, or other more or less comprehensive list. Even if such a frame is available, quota samplings are more expensive; but they have the advantage that dropouts or nonrespondents (who often cause a serious problem in probability samples) do not occur, or can be appropriately replaced. On the other hand, although quotas may adequately represent the separate incidences of factors of primary importance, they may not correctly represent the incidence of *interactions* between two or more of the factors. For example, a sample might be constructed to resemble exactly the population from which it is drawn in containing 75 percent whites, 25 percent blacks, and 50 percent women with 50 percent men. However, such a sample might be composed of 50 percent white and 0 percent black women, even though the population contained 20 percent white and 30 percent black women. Crude quota samples may thus fail to represent the more complex interactions likely to be more important than the primary factors in the population (see, for example, Blum and Associates, 1969a and 1972b).

Probability sampling, on the other hand, is cheaper, and large samples can be collected conveniently and quickly if sampling frames are available. But such frames are often difficult to construct without introducing bias (telephone directories underrepresent, even in these days, lower socioeconomic groups, and electoral registers underrepresent immigrants, who may, depending upon circumstances, be better—or worse—educated than the average in the neighborhood). Both these errors are likely to distort results severely in the field of drug dependence (and in spite of popular folklore, not everyone eventually passes Piccadilly Circus or Times Square); and dropouts or nonrespondents, who are unlikely to be typical, cannot be replaced. The causes of dropout are most probably related to important systematic factors that are unidentified, at least at the beginning of the study.

Representativeness and Inference. If the final sample is not representative, however it was originally constructed or drawn, in terms of age, sex, nationality, economic class, or whatever the relevant point may be, it will not be possible to draw valid conclusions from it to the population as a whole. Even if it is representative, generalization must follow either statistical or logical principles. The latter require that close attention be paid when sampling to recording at least a description of such "unbalanced independent variables" (Neufeld, 1970) as weather, place, or time of day, so that if there are differences in the results of replications these can be plausibly, if not definitively, interpreted in terms of differences between factors that differed between the situations. For example, a failure to replicate in Britain American observations on the consequences of long-term use of heroin would be inexplicable if, among other aspects, the differences in composition of the injected materials had not been recorded: pure heroin in Britain; heroin of uncertain concentration and diluted with a variety of other substances, some themselves pharmacologically active, in America.

Time. Adequate sampling is particularly difficult when studying phenomena that take a considerable time to develop, as drug dependence does. The composition of the sample itself changes with time, as may the controlling variables, in particular the interactions between them. For example, mice incorporate progressively less radioactive amino acid in their liver protein, then later in an experiment they are taken from their cages to be treated (McArthur, Dawkins, and Smith, 1971). Speculations about the reason for this are beyond the present text, though they may depend on interactional factors studied by ethologists (Chance, 1968). Similar factors may affect metabolism, though they have been little studied, in interactional situations involving human beings. These difficulties are met in part by balanced serial sampling through time and the analytical procedures known as cohort study (Armitage, 1971; Feinstein, 1972a, b). Here again it is as vital to study those who drop out as those who remain in, because determination of the reason for dropout is often the most revealing part of the study. In other words, full dropouts can seldom be permitted if a study of drug use is to be valid and meaningful.

Sample Size. A sample must not only be adequately composed but also be of adequate size. The optimal size sample is the population as a whole, but this is clearly impractical. Some help can be given by the statistician in suggesting realistic sample sizes short of this, using criteria related to the frequency of the phenomenon, say, death from overdose of alcohol, that is under study. Even if there are no deaths at all in a given sample, the statistician can estimate the *limits* within which the frequency of death will probably lie in the population (Diem, 1962) or the probable difference in frequencies observed when samples of different size are being compared. The sample size, the expected frequency of the phenomenon in a single group, and the size of the difference in frequency that it is desired to detect between two groups are related in such a way that if any two of these are known, the third can be calculated. For example, if the frequency with which the drivers involved in a sample of fatal car accidents in, say, the United States had consumed a stimulant or sedative drug within the previous six hours is known to be 40 percent, the statistician can estimate the number of fatal accidents in another country that must be sampled to show that the involvement of drugs is say 5 percent or 20 percent smaller.

We have now introduced the vitally important principle of comparative experimentation.

Comparative Experimentation. All experiment—even personal—is in fact comparative, although the principle is often rejected by those who should know better. The idea of comparison does not necessarily include that of simultaneity, but historical comparison should be allowed only in the case of phenomena that are subject to rather little uncontrolled disturbance, such as those studied by astronomers. Thus, though the figures for dependence upon opiates in the United Kingdom between the two World Wars were so stable as almost to have justified their use as a reference standard, the change that began in the middle 1950s—whatever the reason for it—effectively abolished any possibility of using British data in this way. As far as scientific biology is concerned, the dependent variable (the measure of effect) is usually subject to a great deal of variation due to causes that are poorly understood or difficult to control. This uncontrolled or random variation (sometimes also called experimental error) must be estimated to see whether the deliberately modified experimental factor (the so-called independent variable) has caused more or less variation than might have been expected to occur by chance.

It is therefore always necessary to compare two or more groups treated in or selected to differ in different ways. One "treatment" is often an attempt to do nothing but leave the course of nature undisturbed. For ethical reasons, this is sometimes impossible (that is, any illness must be actively treated if a treatment of proven value already exists), but an appropriate comparison can almost always be set up. The statistical work done usually takes the form of trying to *disprove* the so-called null hypothesis (that there is no difference between the treatments). Probably the most intelligible reason for doing this is that the null hypothesis is usually the simplest that can be stated, and simple hypotheses can be disproved more easily than complex ones. Many experiments are inconclusive or lead to argument because the hypothesis tested was not sufficiently simple to enable the experiment to be appropriately designed. It can be seen that as soon as two or more comparative groups are involved, it becomes of crucial importance to ensure that their composition is identical in every relevant respect except that of the experimental treatments being compared, otherwise any differences observed may really be due to irrelevant ways in which the groups differed. The principles of sampling from a population already discussed need to be applied with equal care to the construction of groups for comparative experiments. In this, the principle of randomization, by which is meant that any equivalent participant is just as likely as any other to be allocated to one or other of the treatments being compared, is vital. Systematic allocation, whether conscious (or, as is frequently the case in inadequately controlled experiments, unconscious) plays havoc with the interpretation of results and frequently renders interpretation completely impossible.

Measures of Control.   All the foregoing instances, and those to be discussed below, are in fact examples of controls. The purpose of control is to enable the factors under experimental study to be measured as accurately as possible. The main principle is that if the effect of a given factor is suspected to be large as well as interesting, its value should be varied deliberately and exactly so that the effect of this controlled variation can be estimated over a wide range: if this is not possible the value should at least be held constant; if however, the effect, though large, is considered uninteresting, it should be reduced as far as possible, since it is very unlikely that it can ever be eliminated altogether. Whichever of these procedures is adopted, it is of the greatest importance to measure accurately not only the level at which the independent variable itself is operating (the stimulus or dose), but also the behavior that results (measured as the dependent variable or response). Since more than one such independent variable will often be important, even after a careful selection has been made, a so-called "factorial" design is often used, in which the effect of the presence or absence of factors such as emotional deprivation, parental alcoholism, and the like, can be compared, as can that of more readily quantifiable variables such as number of siblings, age, schooling, or even anxiety level. Since the number of subsets rises as the number of factors and levels are multiplied together, and since some confirmation is needed, a duplicate comparison of two ways of treating a group in which two factors are important, each at two levels, involves a minimal sample size of $2^4 = 16$. Even this will certainly be inadequate, but the apparent necessity to achieve samples of a size larger than can be obtained in practice is in fact overcome by technical devices that are described in statistical texts (Armitage, 1971; Cochran and Cox, 1957). Further, if other relevant data can be collected in a complete and systematic way, they can be used to improve the sensitivity of the measurements of behavior by the technique of covariance analysis. Thus, for example, by estimating the number of tablets actually consumed by patients taking part in a controlled comparison of two active drugs and a placebo, it was possible to obtain a much more sensitive measure of their relative efficacy and toxicity (Joyce, 1960).

Statistical Significance and Practical Importance. Whatever statistical techniques are employed, the experiment must be so designed as to compare the effect of the deliberate manipulation of factors intended to cause variation with the accidental variation expected to occur if the experiment had had no effect at all. If the estimates of deliberate and accidental variation do not differ to any great extent, there are no grounds for thinking that the experimental procedure had any effect that matters. It is obviously necessary to define what is meant by large and small differences; but first the important distinction between concepts of *statistical* and *practical* significance must be made clear. The former are defined by strict mathematical procedures so that the likelihood that an event is due to chance can be estimated by the statistician for the clinician, sociologist, or other applied worker who has provided him with the data in the first place. The latter has to say whether the statistically significant differences observed make sense or nonsense, or whether they are of any practical importance even if they can be sensibly interpreted.

The statistician often puts his conclusions in a form that allows an estimate to be made of the limits within which the true value of the variable of interest (again, with a defined degree of probability) lies, above and below the value actually observed. Thus, while it is rather unlikely that the frequency of cannabis use among American West Coast college students is exactly 32 percent, a statement that the probability that the true frequency lies within 23 to 41 percent is much more plausible and more informative. If two such groups are compared, it may be more interesting to know that they are unlikely to represent samples from the same population than that their absolute rates of use are, say 16 percent and 32 percent.

Whether statistical probabilities are to be trusted, in fact, as the basis of real-life decisions, is for the practical worker to decide. Whether the decision will be implemented, of course, is another matter altogether. At least a knowledge of the methods described here should enable the responsible agent to learn something of the way in which the evidence has been obtained and interpreted. There is a symbiotic relationship between the statistician and the applied worker; and, like all such relationships, it frequently gives rise to stress and misunderstanding. For though it may have been impossible to demonstrate statistical significance in a set of observed data, the worker may feel that the result is "there," if only it could be disinterred. This is a legitimate feeling, and a useful one, if it leads to better designed or more appropriate experiments. So long as this is not the case, however, it leaves the worker or his commentator where he was had the experiment not been performed in the first place. The usual dogmatic statements and immutable opinions, though impressive to others who share them, are not a substitute for evidence. Sometimes even the mighty lapse. Caught by his editor in a failure to document a quotation, a fellow contributor intones hopefully: "Despite the urging, indeed importuning, of several delegations of . . . editors, the author has been unable to discover when or where [the authority quoted previously] said this. In any event, the reader *may rest assured* that he did so."

"Blind" Experiments.   One general, and vitally important, measure of control should not be forgotten. This is the use of "blindness" wherever possible to reduce the possibility of bias either by the experimental subject or by the investigator. It is particularly necessary to make the greatest efforts to reduce bias, especially where this appears to be impossible. The requirement applies with equal force to judgments about laboratory and clinical data. The concept of blindness derives from clinical research, especially in the comparison of two or more treatments. Since even the most fair-minded of us usually has some hypothesis, or at least prediction of outcome, in mind (if only that both treatments will be equally useless) and since it has been repeatedly shown that expectations influence outcomes, it is most important that no one involved in the recording of the results or, preferably, in the presentation of the treatment to the subject, should know the identity of the treatment he receives. Of course, this cannot always be achieved. Particularly in social experiments, not only will the subject know the nature of the treatment that he is receiving but also he will often be aware that there are alternatives and he may well know their nature too. In such situations, the important aspect of control is that the *judge* of the effect is ignorant of the treatment received by those he is judging and preferably of the hypothesis under test as well. This is particularly difficult to achieve with sophisticated subjects, such as the eight former-addict federal prisoners at Lexington, Kentucky, who may even become so adept as to be able to predict the last five of eight treatments to which they are to be exposed after they have compared notes about their experiences of the first three (H. F. Fraser, personal communication, 1960). Similarly, anomalies observed in the air encephalograms of habitual cannabis smokers (Campbell, Evans, and others, 1971, 1972), for example, are more likely to be judged due to cannabis if it is known that they smoke cannabis habitually, if their consumption of other drugs is ignored, and if no comparison is made with a nonsmoking control group or the comparison is with an inappropriate control group (the resulting radiographic pictures being judged for abnormality by experts who do not know which came from smokers and nonsmokers).

Choice of Measuring Instruments

Attitudes and Behavior.   In addition to the errors introduced by biasing or even omitting relevant questions altogether, it is possible that a measuring instrument, although designed with care and accuracy, may not serve. It may be quite inappropriate—as, for example, the attempt to measure state, or situational, anxiety by using such measures of trait, or intrinsic anxiety, as the Taylor Scale; or trying to estimate intellectual or social extraversion separately by using the Maudsley Personality Inventory, which does not make such a differentiation.

Or the difficulty may be fundamental: although it is the measurement of the *behavior* which is of interest, one is often compelled to fall back upon measurements of *attitudes*. A comparison of the efficacy of facts and information versus "horror-show" movies in persuading schoolchildren not to start experimenting with drugs is best made by studying their subsequent drug-taking behavior for an adequate time, rather than asking them about their intentions immediately after exposure. Even if the attitudes are stable in their expression, they are quite likely to be singularly poor predictors of actual behavior when the respondent finds himself in the real situation about which he has previously been only hypothesizing. It is for this reason that a great deal of research on preventive measures, such as education or suspended sentencing, fails to give information of real value: what matters, when the treated junkie leaves the hospital or the susceptible teen-ager has finished with his programmed textbook on drug dependence, is not what each *says* he will do, but what he actually does. However, careful design of attitude questionnaires to avoid such conflicts of values that lead to apparent inconsistency of response can substantially increase the correlation with subsequent behavior (Schuman, 1972).

  Test Batteries and Analysis.   Clearly, the measurement must correlate highly with the behavior; or, more accurately, the limits within which the behavior predicted on the basis of the measurement can vary must be as narrow as possible. This is often exceedingly difficult to achieve with a simple measure, even in more objective sciences, so a battery of tests is commonly employed instead. This, however, leads to another dilemma. If the items of a test battery are chosen in such a way as to correlate highly with each other, it is arguable that there is no need to use a battery at all. If they are all measuring the same thing, each is as good as another. To this it can be replied that repeated measurements do give a more reliable estimate—the most likely next performance of a baseball or cricket player is estimated more accurately from his average up to that point in the season rather than from the first five games he plays. On the other hand, a test battery designed to uncover as many *different* facets of the behavior as possible will not relate strongly, as a whole, to any single factor; nor, as a rule, is the picture presented by a set of correlations particularly easy to interpret.

  For these reasons, and to retrieve as much information as possible, various more complex methods of statistical analysis have been introduced. Their purpose is to reduce the mass of data to a small number of intelligible factors. The factors extracted in this way have to be interpreted by examining the extent to which they relate to the original tests. Thus, though the way in which clear patterns of association seem to emerge is often surprising, the label used to describe the factor is a matter of personal decision by the experimenter. Even if this appears appropriate and reveals new insights, it remains subjective and represents a risk that value judgments and verbal bias will surreptitiously reenter by the back door after being forcefully expelled from the front.

  The multiplicity of methods that have been evolved is due to the desire to reduce the possibility of subjective interpretation, to utilize as much information as possible and to generate factors that are most easily interpretable. A recent paper (Guertin, 1971), however, using the hypothetical hard data provided by physical measurements of body build to compare eight different techniques of multiple regression analysis, concludes that "the different methods lead to the same results."

Prediction, Association, and Causation. Hence it matters little which is used to *describe* the phenomenon. The most valuable techniques for *predicting* outcome—of treatment, a way of life, or the dependence-inducing liability of a new drug—however, are those related to discriminant functions. Here, the various measures found to correlate with outcome are again combined into a single score. The optimal cut-off point (or points) is found that separates the distribution of scores into two or more segments in such a way that the number of misclassifications is reduced to a minimum: either when the equation is used to "back-predict" into the sample upon the characteristics of which it was based, as in the case of the Blum study already quoted (Blum and associates, 1972b), or, as is always necessary but seldom done, into a new sample. It must be said that this subsequent use of such a function almost invariably disappoints—the variation is so great and the population characteristics differ. Apart from the extent of un-controlled variation, this failure may be due to the fact that the apparently correlated phenomena are themselves not causally linked but are both effects of a common cause. It appears unnecessary even to think of this possibility when two or more curves (such as those for per capita alcohol consumption and per capita motor-car accident rate) move across the page in close parallel; possibly helpful to remember it when the curves in question describe numbers of television receiver licenses issued and prosecutions for drug offenses, and absolutely essential to do so when the curves for first admissions to psychiatric hospitals and per capita consumption of bananas are seen to follow each other's every inflection. Had the alleged demonstration that bananas contained a powerful psychotogen been correct, the category of this last association would have changed from the third (that is, obviously fortuitous) to the first (that is, almost certainly causal). The examples chosen are real and illustrate the need to be flexible in the interpretation of statistical association. The relationship over smoking and pulmonary and other forms of cancer, though still not decisively settled, has at times been interpreted as due to association with a common, intervening personality variable or set of variables. But Seltzer's (1972, p. 243) attack on the Royal College of Physicians' Report (1971) is not concerned with an intervening variable of this or any other kind; instead, he attacks the interpretations of epidemiological data on methodological and statistical grounds, some of which have been referred to previously above: "Data as presented are found to exhibit geographical and populational restrictions, age restrictions, and unexpected changes in classification of diseases; they also omit a crucial time period and assume certain unverified trends in smoking habits."

Replication. Whatever method is used for description or prediction, any investigation showing a statistically significant result should be replicated at least once. There is no immediately apparent logical reason for this; it may even appear to be completely unnecessary. If it has been demonstrated that an experimental observation in a well-conducted experiment had only a small likelihood of being due to chance (say the odds were 1 in 100), its successful replication with the same level of probability raises the combined likelihood that chance (that is, uncontrolled factors) was responsible to $(1:100)^2$, or 1 in 10,000. Although the combined odds arising from the successful replication on *two* subsequent occasions of an experiment that originally gave a likelihood of only 1 in 20 that chance was responsible are $(1:20)$ or 1 in 8,000, that is, smaller than those in the first case, most people would probably feel that the latter result is far more impressive. And rightly so, for it is in fact never possible to do *exactly* the same experiment on a subsequent occasion. If nothing else, time has changed or at least run away, and the population studied will have changed, so that samples drawn from it will have changed too. Thus the demonstration of the same phenomenon on three occasions is in part a demonstration of its probable occurrence in three populations, and this is usually more exciting than its occurrence in two, even if the overall odds are less impressive.

However, social or behavioral experiments are too seldom repeated even once. This is in part because it is even more exciting to go on and do something different, but also because uncontrolled variation is great and the likelihood of being able to obtain a second outcome at the same level of probability as on the first occasion is certainly less than fifty-fifty. Many of the behavioral science journals publish a substantial number of reports (almost always by other authors than those of first instance—itself a clear indication that a different population is being studied) that are, either in title or in essence, failures to replicate the original work. There could be and should be many more, especially in the supposedly harder sciences.

Protocol

The experimental protocol is the name given either to the plan of what it is intended shall be done or to the description of what actually was done. Ideally, the two should coincide. Adherence to the intended plan is one of the strictest rules in every experiment or inquiry. If the need to change protocol is foreseen as a possibility, the circumstances under which such changes are permitted should be defined as far as possible a priori—this is often easier than might be supposed, since it may well involve no more than clear rules for the exclusion of data that are invalidly collected, contaminated, or ambiguous in previously defined ways. The definition of so-called stopping-rules is automatically involved in the special kind of technique named sequential analysis (Armitage, 1971). In this method, the results from individual observations or pairs of observations are looked at, not at the end of the experiment but as they come in, in order to terminate the experiment at the earliest possible time: that is, when agreed levels of likelihood have been reached. These are suitably adjusted for the fact that repeated testing of samples that grow in size by accretion of new items inflates the probability of occurrence of differences of any specified size that are really due to chance. The method is more economical, on the average, than an equivalent fixed sample design. Sequential analysis is generally suitable only for problems, such as quality control, with an outcome that can be stated in terms of a single variable. The potential danger that the information continually fed back to the experimenter in the course of the study will change or confirm his beliefs and hence modify the outcome is certainly greater with such designs, although this fact does not appear to have been recognized. Though the initial interest of medical circles (Armitage, 1971) in sequential analysis has faded, its emphasis on the necessity to state protocol explicitly and then follow it should be more widely copied. All departures from protocol should be reported: any publication with no such reports should be regarded with grave suspicion.

Inference.   Once the evidence has been collected and analyzed according to decisions previously made, inference comes into play. It is assumed that the experimenter's logical apparatus is of adequate standard and is matched by his integrity. It would be invidious and exhausting to give instances of the betrayal of such expectations: indeed, the temptation to do so must be firmly resisted. One may perhaps propose the following "law": the frequency with which scientific logic is violated increases with the square of the distance that a scientist ventures from his basic discipline.

Inference in Social and Epidemiological Studies.   Statistical inference from social or epidemiological investigations presents additional problems. In general, control in the sense described above is often difficult to achieve, and so such determinations as are made require particularly careful estimation. This applies to the incidence of the phenomena involved, the characteristics to be used as predictors (for example, of the frequency of marijuana smoking, if the "escalation" from marijuana to heroin is under study) and the behavior or disease being predicted (for example, mainlining heroin). It is often suggested that to calculate the possible enhancement of the risk of acquiring a heroin habit due to previous use of marijuana requires some kind of prospective study, in which either one large sample representative of the entire generation being observed, or two smaller matched samples, one smoking and the other not, is followed through time to a predetermined point. It is expected that at this point, a sufficiently large number of individuals will be using heroin to enable the relative risk associated with (not *necessarily* due to) previous smoking to be calculated. However, it has already been mentioned in connection with quota sampling that prospective studies can be prohibitively uneconomic, especially if the behavior examined occurs but rarely. Further, matched samples are prone to become unmatched as time goes on, because many nonsmokers tend to transfer themselves into the smoking category and some individuals (probably fewer) transfer in the opposite direction as well. The similarities with the behavior of women using oral contraceptives suggest that models based on such studies may be useful (Vessey, 1971).

Cornfield and Haenszel (1960) point out that retrospective studies can, in fact, give the same information much more economically than prospective ones where the total proportion of the population developing the behavior during the period under study is small; if this is so, this proportion can be dropped from the equations used to calculate the risk without leading to error. It is ironic that whereas it might therefore have been possible to use retrospective studies to obtain an accurate estimate of the relative risk attributable to pot-smoking when this behaviour was itself stable at a low level (say, before 1955 in Britain) it would have been unwise to do so subsequently (say, from 1965 to 1970) at a time when the number of heads was exponentially increasing. One may predict that, if present trends continue, it should be possible (as with work on the association between smoking and lung cancer) to use retrospective studies once again some time in the 1980s. An apparently independent and simpler development of the method of Cornfield and Haenszel (1960) by Cole and MacMahon (1971), applied to matched ("case-control") samples enables the risk attributable to a given factor to be calculated either for exposed individuals or for the population as a whole. The method can also be used to estimate the extent to which multiple etiological factors interact, additively or by potentiation. Such approaches appear to be of particular value if, for example, the denominator is total drug consumption (however measured) and the numerator is total adverse drug reactions. These quantities are difficult to obtain even for drugs legitimately produced, prescribed, and consumed.

The large-scale neglect by workers in the field of drug dependence of quantitative epidemiological methods can hardly be justified by the softness of their data. For example, the "truth" of the reports of marijuana and heroin use made by subjects in a series of retrospective studies could at least be assumed, in order to obtain several different estimates of the incidence, prevalence, and risk factors mentioned above. This approach hardly seems to have been used as yet (Hughes and Crawford, 1972). With the advent of many comprehensive public health schemes, for example, the Kaiser-Permanente system in San Francisco (Friedman, Collen, and others, 1971), that use rapid data accumulation and tabulation, the acquisition of complete observations on prescribing and drug-related medical events becomes a reality, and some of the causally associated factors in the development of drug dependence may emerge from obscurity. The British and international systems of reporting suspected adverse drug reactions (Finney, 1971), though they uncover only the tip of the iceberg, have proved fertile in generating experimental inquiries to substantiate postulated associations (for example, of contraceptive estrogens with cerebral and other thromboses), or, more frequently, to disprove them (for example, the nonteratogenicity of the antidepressive imipramine).

"Ice-floe" methods such as those that could be based upon the Kaiser-Permanente system would prove similarly stimulating if the passion for collecting data on a massive scale (and for reporting all statistical associations, even if these are no more in total than would be expected to occur by chance) could be complemented by intelligent interpretation as a prelude to specific enquiry. Both iceberg and ice-floe systems could be made relevant to the improvement of pharmacotherapy as well as the study of drug dependence by incorporating checks on the possibility that nonprescribed drugs were responsible for an effect apparently due to prescribed drugs, especially when so much information is available with regard to age, geographical distribution, and the like. The use of epidemiological models should also help to evaluate and predict the comparative success of alternative control methods.

An attractive feature of some recent epidemiological work is that it incorporates social and other behavioral measures. Waaler and Piot (1970), for example, use a "social-time-preference parameter" (r) in their comparison of the effectiveness of case-finding and treatment versus BCG vaccination in the control of tuberculosis. "A high value of r can be visualized as corresponding to a close planning horizon, a lower value of r to a more distant one. . . . A planner with a high . . . r would favour case-finding and treatment, and a planner with a low . . . r would tend to emphasize BCG vaccination" (p. 1). Thus the methods used for investigation, the models constructed to help the study, and the implicit or explicit ideas held by those involved are once again inextricably interwoven.

A Priori and A Posteriori Reasoning.   One point at least deserves special consideration. This is the importance, and validity, of a posteriori reasoning. Although, logically, there would appear to be no difference between a hypothesis stated before conducting an experiment and the same hypothesis stated for the first time after examination of the data, the two situations differ from the point of view of statistical logic. As mentioned in connection with sequential analysis, repeated testing inflates the probability of obtaining an apparently significant result that is really due to chance. Inspection and rearrangement of data enable one, almost inevitably, to find some association that is statistically significant; the other associations that could have but in fact did not produce significant results are ignored. The correct procedure, as always, is to replicate the experiment. This can be done with a certain economy relative to the initial experiment, since the hypothesis to be tested now has a direction ("A is significantly *greater than* B" instead of "A is significantly *different from* B") and the power of the experiment to reject the null hypothesis, if the sample size remains the same, is doubled. Alternatively, the size of the sample can be reduced if the power is held constant.

Decision-Making

Even when the evidence has been collected, however, and the inferences have been made, the decisions taken may be illogical. Illogical decisions may be taken because the real determinants have not been studied or cannot (perhaps because it was felt that they could not) be entered into the model. Thus, as Lee

(1972) says: "Other products found to be dangerous to man would be—and have been—taken off the market on the basis of only a fraction of the evidence linking cigarettes to lung cancer." It is therefore profoundly disappointing, when a major requirement of the measures proposed for the international control of psychotropic substances is that the potential danger to public health must be compared with the potential therapeutic (or other) benefit, that virtually no official attempt has been made (for example, in Isbell and Chrusciel, 1970) to establish even the most elementary rules for the way in which this information is to be combined. Rules of this kind have been stated for hazards associated with the therapeutic use of drugs without too much difficulty in a preliminary way; as, for example, by Friedman (1972, p. 17): "Priorities for investing resources in further studies or analyses must take into account the magnitude of the potential public health problem involved. Estimates of the magnitude must consider at least four factors: (1) the extent of usage of the drug, (2) the degree of risk that might be attributable to the drug, (3) the seriousness of the untoward event and (4) the conditions treated by the drug." A more sophisticated development of these principles is clearly needed.

Much has been made of so-called cost-benefit—or, more optimistically, benefit-cost—analysis, and Kaplan (1971) has used this approach to survey alternative ways to incorporate marijuana into social mechanisms. Lind describes the technique in Chapter Fourteen of the present book. Another interesting technique (Howard, 1966, pp. 3–11) of decision-analysis is based on assessments of the probability of alternative outcomes in real uncertainty situations by different individuals or groups who have different experiences, expectations, or expertise. The method uses consensus-seeking procedures that themselves result in fuller exchange and subsequent use of information. Simple propositions are used to elaborate the decisive procedures: "Decision-making requires the study of uncertainty. . . . Uncertainty can only be studied formally through probability theory. . . . Probability is a state of mind, not of things. . . . Probabilities measure our state of knowledge about phenomena rather than the phenomena themselves." Further: "All prior experience must be used in assessing probabilities. . . . [Nobody has] 'no' information about an event that [is] important to him. . . . Decisions can only be made when a criterion is established for choosing among alternatives." Decisions must be distinguished from outcomes: A *decision* is good if it is "based on a logical evaluation of the information available . . . and . . . consistent with the goals of the [institution]," whereas an *outcome* is good "if it represents a situation highly valued by the organization." The object of good decision-making is to maximize the chances of reaching a good outcome. This will be achieved because "a decision is not a mental commitment to follow a course of action, but rather [its] actual pursuit." The procedures, which involve the calculation of individual risk preferences as a preliminary to setting up the "profit lottery" or statement of the possible benefits and possible risks attached to the alternatives available, often reveal that one alternative demonstrates a significant degree of superiority to, or "dominance" over, the others, so that the number of alternatives that need to be considered can be enormously reduced if, indeed, they cannot be eliminated altogether. An indisputable benefit, which Howard believes may indeed be the most important contribution of decision-analysis, is that the concepts involved often come to provide a common communication language between individuals or groups with very different backgrounds. This seems an important consideration in such a field as drug control, where medical, psychological, economic, disciplinary, judicial, and political considerations and personalities interact, or fail to interact effectively.

Combining Information. Information from different sources must be combined if the base on which descriptive or predictive statements can be erected is to be enlarged. Combinatory methods are therefore needed both for the traditional kinds of problems with which the first part of this review was concerned and for the decision procedures just described. Methods of combining information involve either the *planning* of a series of experiments that enables the relevant hypothesis to be stated more and more precisely, and the corresponding probability that chance is responsible to become less and less; or equivalent, but much more difficult, procedures after the conclusion of all experimentation, often by different workers using different hypotheses and methods.

As a simple example of serial planning, we may mention the application of sequential analysis (Armitage, 1971) to attitude and other surveys, enabling sampling to be stopped as soon as sufficient evidence has been collected to decide either between alternative hypotheses or that a difference between hypotheses is unlikely (Peel and Skipworth, 1970). A more complex technique is the application of successive testing screens, limited by time or other economic factors, to the selection of new products (for example, drugs) with potential usefulness (Finney, 1971). Finney points out that although increases in the number of screens "always make possible some improvement in the performance of the screening . . . gains from an increase above . . . 3 or . . . 4 are small." This is encouraging for those who regard the effective screens for drug-dependence liability testing as only three in number: animal, clinical, and social.

Light and Smith (1971) review techniques of post hoc combination of results in relation to educational research, but their proposals are certainly applicable to other fields. They note four general appoaches: listing all the data, averaging across data, excluding data that do not fit, and "taking a vote," or accepting only results in the predominating direction. However, as they point out, the legitimate inferences from a set of, say, 100 apparently "similar" experiments of which 2 gave significant results in the positive direction, 2 significant results in the negative direction, and the remainder no difference, are very different from another set of 100 in which, say, 30 went in one direction, 30 in the other, and the remainder gave no difference. Yet the conclusions drawn from both sets are often identical: "that the results were randomly distributed and no real difference was demonstrated due to treatment or other factors." Insofar as their own proposal seems to be a rather sophisticated example of the method described by

Howard (1966) as weighing, multiplying, and adding of divergent prior information, it may perhaps be legitimately applied to descriptive statistics, but may be a less efficient way of using the information for decision-making.

The techniques are primarily concerned with decision-making about, or on the basis of, group phenomena. From the medical or judicial point of view, it is also necessary to make decisions about individuals (differential diagnoses, prediction of the outcome of alternative treatments, and the like). Though some of these problems can be handled by such deductive techniques as those mentioned above, the development of inductive methods, based upon so-called Bayesian statistics, is becoming increasingly powerful (Lusted, 1968). As adequate and comparable information about different whole samples (countries, age groups, personality types, drug users with different preferences) accumulates, it should eventually be possible for the social decision-maker, too, to predict the consequences of alternative courses of action by similar methods.

Conclusion

It is probable that all experiments are imperfect, but that some are less imperfect than others. It appears to be a minimal obligation of the policy-maker to familiarize himself sufficiently with ways of evaluating imperfection, and with techniques of combining the information from what remains. Whether his concern be with detection, prevention, treatment, or cure, he may then be in a position to make recommendations or initiate policies that are as valid as possible and—no less important—as easy as possible to replace with better ones immediately these become available.

SUMMARY

Social action should be based upon policies that have been framed to take account of the best evidence available at the time, as well as of the best estimates of their own consequences. These considerations involve the concepts of evaluation and prediction. Depending upon its nature, evidence can be evaluated in different ways—scientific, legal, or even theological. Broadly speaking, any method of evaluating evidence depends, in one form or another, upon that evidence being judged to be plausible, relevant, reliable, and important. Methods of scientific evaluation use rather strict definitions of plausibility, relevance, and reliability. The decision of importance is a more subjective matter, or is at least based upon common sense or common consensus of experience. Nevertheless, a close parallel can be drawn between the employment of scientific methods of inquiry and the formulation of a constructive, fair, and workable social policy. If the parallel appears not to be close but to diverge, this is most probably due to unfamiliarity with the principles of scientific investigation, attention to which is likely to be rewarding.

The definition of a policy resembles the statement of the object of an experiment. What is it intended that the policy, or the experiment, shall achieve? The scientist states his objective in precise terms and the policy-maker should do the same. Just as the scientist's purpose is not to "see if this drug works," but, for example, "to examine the effectiveness of a (specific) drug in relieving the pain of surgical trauma without giving rise to phenomena, such as hallucinations or euphoria, associated with the presence of liability to induce dependence"; similarly, policies should not be aimed at "suppressing" or even "controlling" drug dependence, or illicit traffic in drugs, but should rather state a more precise objective—as, for example, "the reduction of the percentage of those (in a specified population) dependent (in a defined sense) upon heroin" to an exact figure: or "the optimal employment (of a specified fraction) of the community's resources upon detection or prevention of drug offenses or rehabilitation of those physically dependent upon (specified) drugs."

After stating an objective, the scientist states his hypothesis: that if he carries out such-and-such an action (for example, modification of the formula of a chemical in a certain way), the consequence will be so-and-so (for example, loss of hallucinogenic activity), within certain limits that he also defines; otherwise, he will not consider that the relationship between cause and effect has been demonstrated. The formulation of hypotheses in this way sometimes occurs when social policies are framed—but all too rarely; and it is exceptional, when a social hypothesis of this kind is not substantiated, for the policy to be abandoned, modified, or replaced. Once a policy has been initiated, it tends to resist change or evolution. It may be suggested that any policy should incorporate its own self-evaluating machinery (and its own self-destruct mechanism if the result of the evaluation is negative). Not until the objective has been defined and the hypothesis or hypotheses set up, is it possible to see clearly what kinds of subjects (animals, patients, experimental volunteers, or the like) will be most suitably chosen in order to find the answer, or to decide upon the appropriate kinds of measuring instrument (biochemical, pharmacological, psychological, or clinical, for example) to be employed. Of course, the feasibility and economic consequences of choices will interact with the hypotheses and a process of mutual modification will often be necessary. Then it will be possible to decide upon the number of experimental objects required in the samples in order to detect differences of a specified size between the consequences of proceeding in various ways, and to choose the appropriate experimental design and method of analysing the results.

All such investigations should be comparative, and steps should be taken to eliminate or control known or suspected causes of difficulty in the conduct or interpretation of the experiment. It is particularly important that bias due to prejudices and the like of the subjects, or even of the experimenter, be he physician, sociologist, or chemist, be prevented from influencing the work, especially where, as in matters affecting drug control, emotion is often allowed to replace the need to gather evidence, or to cause disregard when it has been collected.

It is particularly important that every effort be made to avoid systematic bias, distributing it instead over the different treatments or groups to be compared by the twin principles of randomization (of the subjects) and blindness (of the judge of the effects). If this is done, confidence that a given result is meaningful rather than haphazard (or the contrary) can be greatly increased. It can never, however, amount to certainty, whatever the strictness with which the control measures are adopted.

As noted above, the importance of even a meaningful result requires judgment by those who are affected by it, or who need to make use of it, and at this stage prejudice can again vitiate the best-controlled enquiry. It is usually necessary, in any case, to reach an agreement about such matters between several individuals, often coming from different disciplines; and a related problem is the addition or comparison of evidence from several different sources, using different techniques, or even reaching different results although they have ostensibly been designed to study the same problem in exactly the same way.

Methods of reaching valid conclusions in such circumstances are beginning to be available, but it can also be recommended that the policy-maker or decision-taker obtain sufficient familiarity with the logical (not necessarily technological) methods of scientific inquiry to enable him in consequence to reject some purported evidence with confidence, and to feel a proper degree of skepticism about accepting that which remains.

Use, Abuse, and Dependence on the Basis of Clinical Observations

P. H. Connell

X

The clinical evaluation of the presence of drug use or, in the case of new drugs, possible drug use, is a complex process that makes use of certain disciplines and techniques. To understand the difficulties and complexities, it is necessary to set out in detail the evaluation of a "patient" in a clinical setting and then to expand the theme into nonclinical settings, in the sense that evaluation may be needed outside the strictly clinical services—that is, in the community at large or in other institutions such as schools, factories, and the like.

CLINICAL EXAMINATION

The traditional examination of patients who complain of symptoms that may be produced by organic disease includes careful history-taking that covers such points as the symptoms (for example, pain and when it started), the quality of the symptoms (for example, sharp or dull pain), the radiation of the symptoms (for example, whether it moves from the front to the back or from the shoulder down the arm), what makes the symptom better or worse, whether the symptom prevents normal life, and so on. A full inquiry into previous illnesses and family history of illness is necessary.

Once the history, which often indicates special areas for e[...] has been taken, a physical examination is carried out, which, in [...] physical disease, involves observation (for example, seeing if the che[...] ing symmetrically), palpation (feeling for lumps, vibration, and th[...] cussion (seeing if the chest is normally resonant), and auscultatior [...] the breath sounds are normal and are equal on both sides). In the examination [...] special systems, such as the central nervous system, appropriate tests are used by the clinician to demonstrate defects in muscle tone, skin sensitivity, balance, hearing, sight, taste, smell, and so on.

In the majority of instances some abnormality will be found but not always, so normality on physical examination does not necessarily mean actual normality. Hence x-rays of the chest, blood counts, and many other methods are used to demonstrate disease processes that do not necessarily show up even when the physical status of the patient is carefully examined clinically by the physician.

EXAMINATION OF MENTAL STATE

Almost all physical disorders produce some change in the mental state of the patient. These may be of a general nature, such as general anxiety about loss of the feeling of being well, or they may be more specific, particularly in those who have personalities that include emotional reaction to stresses or mild anxieties of a specific nature.

In the practice of psychiatry, the physician must always bear in mind the possibility of an organic basis for the condition, whether it be aches or pains or tension and restlessness. For instance, the disease thyrotoxicosis may present as nervousness, tension, restlessness, and irritability, due to the overactivity of the thyroid gland and to overproduction of its hormones. However, this is an infrequent cause of the symptoms of the large numbers of persons who suffer from excessive nervousness, tension, and the like.

Dealing now with patients whose illness is not due to physical causes, one can consider the problem of examining the mental state of a patient who has complaints, or about whom relatives or even society has complained, about his behavior or change in his normal state.

It must be recognized, at the outset, that the examination of the mental state is less precise than the examination of the physical state. If all patients were able to talk freely about everything the doctor wished to raise in his diagnostic assessment the task would be easier, as indeed it would if all patients were as knowledgeable as the physician about the kind of symptoms that may denote psychiatric illness. In some ways, the situation is rather like that of a detective who has no evidence that a crime has been committed examining an individual who has not committed a crime but feels that it is a crime to be "weak" and to give in to fears, and therefore denies the fears. For example, the patient may feel that it is a crime to have sexual problems (which may be causing anxiety and tension) or, alternatively, he may admit to things too readily (like untrue confessions).

Many lay persons attribute to psychiatrists a precise ability in examination that is far from justified. It is often the view, particularly among those involved with legal aspects of behavior, that one has only to ask a direct question and one will get a valuable and helpful direct answer. There is also the contrary view, among lay persons, that a psychiatrist is easily hoodwinked and naïvely accepts the veracity of anything the patient says. This also is untrue.

The examination of the mental state involves many areas and can be briefly and incompletely summarized as follows:

Talk—flow of talk, use of strange or incomprehensible words, repetition of words or phrases, and so forth.

Thought—general content of thought, concreteness, thought disorder, thought blocking, bizarreness of ideation, presence of abnormal thoughts such as delusions or hallucinations, obsessive-compulsive ideas, and the like.

Orientation—awareness of who he is, the day, the year, where he is.

Behavior—quiet, inhibited, restless, aggressive, and so forth.

Mood—tense, anxious, depressed, fearful, agitated, euphoric, elated, or whatever.

Insight—the patient's own opinion of the cause of his complaints.

This is not just a question of bombarding the individual with stereotyped questions. There is a considerable art in achieving the appropriate empathy with a patient that will allow him to describe many aspects of his mental state. Much vital diagnostic material is lost to those who attempt to carry out examinations of the mental state under pressure of time or before an atmosphere of reasonable confidence has been built up in the person being examined.

To carry out this examination effectively, therefore, the psychiatrist must use the art, that he has learned throughout his training, of achieving appropriate empathy with the patient so that there is a maximum chance of obtaining information about areas of mental activity that are vital for diagnosis and that cannot emerge if the patient has not enough confidence in the psychiatrist. Often more than one interview is required for a comprehensive evaluation.

Furthermore, it is even more important, in the field of psychiatry, that data are obtained from another informant who knows or who has known the patient well enough and during a sufficiently long period to be able to contribute observations about previous personality, changes in behavior, and factors that seem to have led to or influenced such changes.

The principle diagnostic categories can be summarized:

Neurotic states—In these conditions the patient complains of tension, anxiousness, often relating to fears of physical illness, and sometimes of phobias relating to specific situations, but also of physical symptoms such as palpitations, dry mouth, sweating, and the like, and sometimes sleep disturbance. A particular neurotic state known as an obsessive-compulsive state manifests symptoms of compulsive thought or behavior (for example, rituals) or both, the carrying out of which eases the degree of tension and anxiety.

Depression—In this condition there is a sad mood, often accompanied by sleep disturbance, feelings of worthlessness and that there is no future, and so forth.

Schizophrenia—In this condition, of which there are several types, there may be delusions, hallucinations, paranoid feelings, and ideas of influence.

Personality disorders (including antisocial aspects of behavior).

Mental handicap (mental deficiency, mental subnormality).

Organic states (including psychiatric abnormalities produced by brain tumors, brain damage, epilepsy, drugs, endocrine disorders, and the like).

CLINICAL EXAMINATION AND EVALUATION OF DRUG USERS

Special problems confront the clinician in terms of the diagnosis of drug-taking—particularly in those instances where there is no direct reason to suspect the taking of drugs. These difficulties can be summarized as follows:

1. Drugs, and particularly drugs of dependence, can be and often are, used to ameliorate symptoms of nervous and mental disorder or disturbance.
2. Some drugs of dependence may themselves produce symptoms of nervous and mental disorder as simple side effects or as complications due to excessive dosage.
3. Most persons who are drug dependent do not wish the examining doctor to discover this and are unlikely to be truthful in their statements if areas are explored that may reveal their dependence on drugs.
4. Even if there is some inkling that the patient may be taking a drug, and the patient admits his use, it is very unusual to obtain an accurate history of the dose, amounts, and frequency of drug-taking.
5. Many individuals who become dependent on drugs are suffering from a personality disorder that may contain such features as unreliability, untruthfulness, manipulativeness, and paranoid ideation.
6. Since much drug dependence is maintained by illegal recourse to supplies of the drug, fears concerning the law, punishment, and so on, complicate the examination as compared with that of a patient who is suffering from a physical illness and asking for help. This factor is particularly important in attempts to delineate sources of "infection" and mapping out the "epidemiology" of the situation.

7. For similar reasons, particularly those relating to the law, it is often difficult to gain accurate data from other informants concerning the patient.

8. Some drugs (such as amphetamines or LSD) produce a psychosis that, particularly in the case of amphetamines, may be identical to a form of schizophrenia called paranoid schizophrenia. In the 1950s many cases of "amphetamine psychosis" were labeled paranoid schizophrenia and sent to mental hospitals for treatment of this condition since it was not known at that time that excessive amphetamine use produced the same symptoms. Again, it was thought, in the case of those known to be using amphetamines, that the drug had lit up a "latent" schizophrenia though now it is known that this general statement is untrue.

9. Some drugs (particularly central nervous system stimulants, such as amphetamines) produce signs and symptoms of anxiety states, which have often led to initial treatment for anxiety state. Only much later has it been discovered that the patient was taking amphetamines.

10. The recent development of the practice of multiple drug use among drug-taking groups makes it even more difficult to pinpoint definitive effects referable to one drug in the absence of knowledge about the drug taken.

It is particularly important to take a history from another informant, especially when the patient is still living at home and parents or siblings can supply details of changes in behavior and the present behavior of the patient.

PHYSICAL EXAMINATION

In lay circles, and some medical circles, there is often a belief that drug-taking can be diagnosed by physical examination. This belief is a myth and requires exploding. It is true that one diagnoses drug-taking of some drug or other if there are signs of injection marks over veins, in particular, and commonly on the antecubital fossa (in front of the elbow), the back of the wrists, legs, or wherever veins are accessible to the self-injector. However, this does not tell which drug is being taken and, unless the physical examination is very thorough indeed, injection marks can be missed and the individual thought not to be taking drugs. One example of this which came to notice was that of a female patient who was examined in the usual sites of injection and later found to be injecting into the breast veins. The examiner had failed to require that she strip completely for the examination!

In opiate dependence, there will be constricted pupils which continue to be constricted during the drug use. Tolerance does not develop to this effect. It needs a trained person to diagnose the contricted pupil: a classroom of students on a bright sunny day will have constricted pupils even though none are taking heroin or other opiates. However, the pupil does not markedly dilate when the individual dependent upon opiates is placed in relative darkness. Certain other tests can be used to confirm the diagnosis.

Amphetamines can cause various symptoms and signs due to their effect on the sympathetic nervous system (Connell, 1968). Thus dilated pupils, raised pulse rate, dry mouth, palpitations, tremor of the limbs, restlessness, and so forth, can be produced. None of these symptoms are diagnostic of amphetamine-taking. In clinical psychiatric practice, they are usually due, in fact, to the presence either of an anxiety state requiring psychiatric treatment or to the simple anxiety resulting from coming to see a doctor. Again, the often quoted finding of dilated pupils in amphetamine users can lead, in the school situation, to much distress, since dilated pupils can be caused by anxiety or, much more commonly, to a rather ill lit room or to a dull day without sun.

The use of other drugs, such as sedatives and tranquilizers, cannot be diagnosed by physical examination unless toxic doses have been taken and there are signs of overdose such as slurred speech, ataxia, and the like. Those symptoms, in someone not smelling of drink, should always suggest the presence of drug-taking as part of the differential diagnosis, which will also include various organic neurological disorders.

In summary, the detection of drug use by clinical, including physical, examination, is an imprecise exercise. In many cases, the well-trained and astute psychiatrist, by the technique of his examination of the mental state, can obtain data that may suggest the possibility of drug-taking and often, by special techniques, can obtain an admission of drug-taking from the patient. However, even this does not necessarily provide the full picture of drug use.

LABORATORY AIDS TO DIAGNOSIS

In recent years, the development of chromatography, especially thin-layer chromatography and gas-liquid chromatography, has introduced a new factor in the detection of drug taking. It is important to recognize the full meaning of such tests and the snags involved. Urine is the usual biological fluid tested because it is convenient and because some drugs of dependence cannot yet be easily detected in the blood or plasma but can be detected in the urine.

Individuals who are manipulative and who do not want to be discovered as drug users use various methods to avoid detection. These include bringing a bottle of someone else's urine; males may secrete a bottle of urine under their clothing with a tube leading to the underside of the penis. Even though they may be supervised when passing urine, they may thus still escape detection. Close supervision of the passing of urine is essential; in its absence a negative result does not necessarily denote that the individual is not taking a drug. Various attempts have been made to obviate the indignity involved in these circumstances, such as taking the temperature of the specimen produced, but these are compromise solutions to the only effective solution—close supervision.

Urine Testing

It has been demonstrated that the reliability of urine testing depends upon a number of factors. The most reliable results are likely to arise from laboratories working in close cooperation with the clinical services, the staff of which know what is being done clinically and feel interested and involved in the clinical situation. In such instances, very high reliability can be obtained with the use of thin-layer chromatography, gas-liquid chromatography, and other methods.

Conversely, the least reliable results are likely to arise from central and distant laboratories that do large numbers of tests on a routine basis and that are not involved with the clinical service or the personnel of the clinical service. In such situations the reliability may be as low as 45 percent.

It is wise for laboratories to bank the specimens so that repeat testing can be carried out if the clinician desires. Hydrolysis of urine and repeat testing for morphine are often valuable if the results are initially negative for morphine (heroin is detected as morphine). Fuller consideration of these matters can be found in De Angelis (1972, 1973), May (1972), Montalvo, Scrignar, and others (1972) and Lewis, Petersen, and others (1972).

As has just been noted laboratory testing may be unreliable. However, all that may be inferred from even a highly reliable positive test is that, at the moment represented by the time at which the urine was voided, the individual had, in his body, the drug or drugs detected. The test gives no information as to (1) the dose of the drug taken or (2) whether the individual is dependent on the drug and taking it continuously or whether he is merely a sporadic user or whether this was the first and only time he had taken the drug.

In Britain, for instance, where those dependent on opiates are medically maintained on such a drug, it has been shown that it is unwise to prescribe heroin to any individual unless there have been three consecutive positive urine tests over a period of time. Failure to keep to this principle may result in converting a sporadic user to a continuous user or, to be blunt, a drug-dependent person (Gardner and Connell, 1971).

Whatever the institutional setting, whether penal or medical, it is very difficult and probably impossible to ensure a completely drug-free environment at all times. Drug dependent persons are adept at making arrangements to circumvent even the most stringent control regimes.

Daily testing of urines of drug-dependent persons is an expensive and time-consuming process, not only for the laboratories but also for the supervisory staff. There is no definitive work on the value of daily urine testing in the management of drug-dependent persons in an institutional setting. A research project at the Bethlem Royal Hospital, London, designed to evaluate this problem, is nearly completed and will soon be submitted for publication (Connell and Bowman, 1973). It suggests that daily screening in this unit is not worth while in terms of the number of positive results obtained when compared with the number of tests carried out; that other methods of evaluating the possibility of drug use (such as employing the Lexington Questionnaire on patients or making use of observations by nurses) are of no value in this setting; and that the value of urine testing in terms of cost benefit is limited to testing at particularly relevant times in the individual's life, such as after a weekend pass or a day pass; after he has had visitors or when the "grapevine" suggests that it would be wise to examine the group of patients.

Certain drugs, notably LSD and cannabis, are not detectable by urine testing. The inhalation of drugs such as morphine or heroin, also, do not necessarily lead to positive urine tests.

Ideally, the clinician requires the development of laboratory side room tests that can be carried out by relatively unskilled personnel and that will provide a result within half an hour so that action can be taken. Such a tool is still not available but appropriate investment of money, resources, and personnel may well produce it.

Nalline Test

A test was developed to demonstrate the presence of narcotic use; it involved the injection of Nalline (a narcotic antagonist) and the measurement of the consequent change in pupil size in those taking heroin (Way, Elliott, and Nomof, 1963). The acceptance by some courts of a positive Nalline test as legal proof of re-addiction, and a series of papers, including those by Grupp (1968; 1970a, b, c, d; 1971), fully discussing this test are referred to by Lewis, Petersen, and others (1972). These authors note that "later evidence indicates beyond dispute the inadequacy and inaccuracy of results of the Nalline test, and thus the prematurity of the Courts' uncritical hospitality to its results."

LIMITATIONS OF CLINICAL EVALUATION AND DETECTION

It will be understood, from the foregoing, that even with well-trained and skilled psychiatrists and with laboratories that are reliable, the clinical evaluation of the presence of drug-taking is much less precise than one would wish.

The unreliability of laboratory findings has already been mentioned but it must also be recognized that there are far too few psychiatrists and general physicians who are trained in the field of drug use and drug effects. The undergraduate training of doctors contains little, if any, special training in the evaluation of drug use or drug dependence and postgraduate training in psychiatry rarely contains more than a superficial content in this field. In the field of general medicine such training hardly exists.

One can therefore conclude that, due to the difficulties of accurate diagnosis and detection of drug dependence by fully trained personnel and with the backing of reliable laboratories and the paucity of such personnel and facilities, in the general field of medicine, the diagnosis of drug use, abuse, and dependence in individuals remains at a generally low level of accuracy and precision. In fields outside clinical services, such as schools, universities, factories, and elsewhere, the precision is likely to be even less.

Nevertheless, well-trained staff, the use of a standard method for recording observations (including questionnaires), and the support of first-class laboratory facilities can contribute greatly to the detection and definition of drug-dependent and drug-using individuals (Gardner and Connell, 1971, 1972), particularly if standard methods are used by all clinics (Bransby, 1971).

EVALUATION OF DRUG TAKING AND DEPENDENCE

Quite apart from the evaluation of the individual in terms of his involvement in drug-taking, whether sporadic or continuous, and of which drugs he is using, there is the wider field of the evaluation of drugs themselves in terms of dependence-producing liability, their methods of spread, and the general epidemiology of the problem.

In October 1968, a main task of the World Health Organization Expert Committee on Drug Dependence was the consideration of "Drug Dependence and Abuse: Evaluation and Criteria for Control" (World Health Organization Technical Report #407, 1969). The Committee recognized "that authoritative data and criteria were required in order to determine the degree of hazard and the need for control of drug abuse, whether or not new international control regimes were established" (p. 5). It also noted that "the criteria would have to be kept under continuing review in the light of rapidly developing scientific knowledge and accelerating social change" (p. 6).

In considering the problem, this committee noted that "If such a drug abuse or dependence is likely to be, or is known to be, only sporadic or infrequent in the population, if there is little danger of its spread to others, and if its adverse effects are likely to be, or are known to be, limited to the individual user, there is no public health problem. Such forms of abuse may be prevented or managed by adequate information and appropriate medical care. On the other hand, if the drug dependence is associated with behavioural or other responses that adversely affect the user's inter-personal relations or cause adverse physical, social, or economic consequences to others as well as to himself, and if the problem is actually widespread in the population or has a significant potential for becoming widespread, then a public health problem does exist."

Noting that evidence concerning the presence and degree of psychic dependence was drawn mainly from case histories, subjective statements, and general observation, the Committee stated that "more reliable evidence may be obtained from a controlled, double-blind, quantitative procedure for the measurement of subjective effects and behavioural responses." Ethical considerations relating to such studies are considered later in this chapter.

In considering criteria for determining the need for drug control and evaluating the risk, the WHO Committee noted that "sound decisions on control measures can be taken only if reliable and comprehensive data are available. Very often the quality and quantity of information are inadequate. Reliable, comprehensive data can be provided by a single discipline, but often a multidisciplinary approach is required. Sociological, psychological and epidemiological approaches, with their specialised techniques and experience, will be particularly important" (p. 7). Going on to stress that research into the attitudes toward drugs, their patterns of use and abuse are important in terms of possible legislative, educational, and therapeutic strategies, the Committee also noted that "at a practical level highly mobile emergency teams trained in such disciplines will have an important part to play in assessing the relevant facts, such as the real extent of the problem, the epidemic risk, and possible methods of spread, and will provide information useful in developing corrective strategies along public health lines. The value of data obtained from cross-sectional and longitudinal studies of drug-dependent persons needs stressing, as does the fact that there are very few adequately conducted studies of this kind" (p. 12).

It must be recognized, however, that the implementation of these sound recommendations and observations by the WHO Committee would be costly: Trained personnel to carry out the studies are in short supply, and attitudes to drug-taking and sociocultural patterns change quite rapidly so that continuous assessment is required. Trained personnel would include epidemiologists, psychologists, and laboratory workers, as well as psychiatrists and other physicians. There are unlikely, at the present time, in most countries, to be a sufficient number of these; nor, even if this were not the case, would it be likely that large enough numbers would wish to devote themselves entirely to this field.

The value of the epidemiological approach can be documented. In a paper on prevalence and early detection of heroin abuse (De Alarcon and Rathod, 1968), the aims were "(1) to discover if there was an undetected pool of heroin users in the community, and (2) to test various methods for the early detection of cases." The survey was carried out in a New Town some thirty miles from London which had a population of 62,130, of which 41 percent were under twenty years of age. The study covered both sexes in the age groups fifteen through twenty. Data were collected from the probation service, the police, and patients (actual heroin users). A jaundice survey was carried out in all general practices in the town. There were also surveys of cases seen by a casualty department and of direct referrals. This valuable study showed what could be done by psychiatrists in this field and concluded that "routine channels by which heroin users are referred for treatment are inefficient early detectors of the disease," and "more patients could be brought into treatment earlier by using the screening methods described."

A further incidence study of the same population (De Alarcon, 1969), using, for operational purposes, the model of a contagious illness, showed how the disease was transmitted. Many valuable public health data were gathered.

A further pay-off of these studies, which collected standard data over time, was the demonstration of the effectiveness of a voluntary withdrawal of methedrine ampuls (for injection), which led to the sudden disappearance of a serious problem with this drug (De Alarcon, 1972).

Others have also made important findings using an epidemiological and contagious disease model (Hughes, Barker, and others, 1972; Hughes, Senay, and Parker, 1972; Kosviner, Mitcheson, and others, 1968). That such an approach can lead to intervention and the termination of a localized heroin epidemic, resulting in a heroin-free community has been described (Hughes, Senay, and Parker, 1972; Zacune, Mitcheson, and Malone, 1969).

In all these studies, the need for a multiprofessional approach is apparent and for cooperation among the investigators and a wide variety of social agencies. The psychiatrist is in a particularly advantageous position as a member of such a team in view of his background, training, and his image as one who is interested in treating illness.

ETHICS OF RESEARCH

It will be clear from the foregoing that many areas in the field of drug abuse merit research.

Ethical problems are raised in a general sense when information is given to a doctor under the normal confidentiality that exists in a doctor-patient relationship, when material is presented to a doctor that involves the commission of a crime—such as possession of an illegal drug or possession of a drug obtained illegally. This clinical problem is usually solved by adhering to the code of confidentiality between doctor and patient so that no data relating to criminal matters are given to others who do not operate under such a code, except when serious matters such as capital offenses are in question, when the social responsibility may be caused to outweigh the doctor-patient ethic by, for instance, direct instruction to a doctor in court by a judge.

This medical ethic is not easily understood by nonmedical persons and can be the cause of considerable friction between the medical and law enforcement agencies unless close collaboration and understanding of the different frames of reference can be brought about. Thus, for instance, I personally would not, on receiving a request for the names of all my patients who lived in a certain area where there had recently been a murder, give these names. If, however, I were asked by the police if I had a specific person in my ward and the name and address of the person was given to me, and the reason for wanting it was clearly stated, I would answer the question.

The problem in this area that confronts the doctor is the difficulty in effecting and maintaining adequate trust and confidence in the patient on which to base therapy. Drug abusers, and particularly drug-dependent persons, only too easily convert to a hostile, noncooperative attitude if they consider that the doctor or paramedical personnel have "informed" on them.

As far as research on drugs and their actions is concerned, it is vitally important that drugs that may be of benefit to mankind, including analgesics, tranquilizers, and central nervous system stimulants, are fully investigated before being freed for general use. Much important and valuable work is first done in the laboratory; but when one comes to the field of clinical drug trials, international and national discussion has caused certain ethical principles to be laid down. The extension of these principles to the trial of drugs of potential dependence has been reviewed (Connell, 1973). A number of publications have appraised this area ("Declaration of Helsinki," 1964, "Medical Ethics," 1972; Medical Research Council, 1963; Royal College of Physicians of London, 1967; World Health Organization Technical Report #403, 1968).

As far as the United Kingdom is concerned, the Medical Research Council report (1963) drew a distinction between "procedures undertaken as part of patient care which are intended to contribute to the benefit of the individual patient, by treatment, prevention or assessment, and those procedures which are undertaken either on patients or on healthy subjects solely for the purpose of contributing to medical knowledge and are not themselves designed to benefit the particular individual on whom they are performed." In the case of patient care, the report notes that "the question of novelty is only relevant to the extent that in reaching a decision to use a novel procedure the doctor, being unable to fortify his judgment by previous experience, must exercise special care." It is advised that if any doubt exists the opinion of an experienced colleague should be obtained.

If the procedures are not of direct benefit to the individual, the person should "volunteer in the full sense of the word." By "true consent" is meant consent freely given with proper understanding of the nature and consequences of what is proposed. Assumed consent, or consent obtained by undue influence, is valueless; and, in this latter respect, particular care is necessary when the volunteer stands in special relationship to the investigator, as in the case of a patient to his doctor, or a student to his teacher. Acceptable evidence of consent is, in general, obtaining "the consent in the presence of another person. Written consent unaccompanied by other evidence that an explanation has been given, understood and accepted is of little value."

The report of the Royal College of Physicians (1967) accepted the findings of the Medical Research Council report (1963) but considered that "because of the wide varieties of research formal codes can only provide general guidance, and their applications to specific problems must often remain a matter of opinion"; and that "it is of great importance that clinical investigation should be free to proceed without unnecessary interference and delay. Imposition of rigid or central bureaucratic controls would be likely to deter doctors from undertaking investigations and, if this were to happen, the rate of growth of medical knowledge would inevitably diminish with resultant delay in advances in medical care."

The special case of minors and those psychiatrically ill was also referred to, and more recently it has been recommended that all institutions that carry out research on patients or volunteer human subjects should have a special local ethical advisory committee that can scrutinize research projects.

The general points made above clearly apply to the area of the clinical evaluation of drugs (World Health Organization Technical Report #403, 1968) and with special force in the case of the clinical evaluation of drugs with dependence-producing propensities. It is one matter for individual members of society to take huge amounts of drugs not controlled as yet under legislation, as a matter of choice, and, by inadvertent consequence, demonstrate that psychosis can result (Connell, 1958), but it is another matter for such large doses to be given to patients or volunteers deliberately, to investigate the effects of the drug.

Certain issues can be defined in this difficult area. Pharmacological, biochemical, and animal experimentation do not necessarily answer the question "Is this drug certain to produce a dependence problem if given to humans?" Therefore, it is necessary to try to estimate, if there is a risk of dependence, how large the problem of dependence in humans is likely to be. In the absence of a definitive answer, it must next be asked if clinical research is essential to assess the possible harm and dangers of such drugs. If the answer to this question is in the affirmative, the problems relating to clinical research with such drugs must next be considered.

There are a number of problems relating to the clinical use of drugs of dependence potential, especially where little or no physical reaction follows withdrawal. Some of these can be summarized:

1. Although the large majority of persons who become dependent on such drugs have psychiatric problems or defects of personality, there is no guarantee that the "normal" person will never, whatever the stress, become dependent on such drugs (Connell, 1970).

2. There is no accurate way of evaluating which persons who have psychiatric problems or defects of personality (the vulnerable groups) will, if exposed to the risk, become dependent on such drugs. Many such persons who have had access to such drugs and tried them avoid becoming dependent.

3. The methods available to assess individuals in terms of their psychiatric and personality status and drug-dependence liability, imprecise as they may be, are time-consuming and require comprehensive assessment of the individual and also information from other informants.

4. Global studies of large numbers of supposedly "normal" individuals are unlikely to reveal significant numbers of persons who show indisputable evidence of dependence liability.

The group of individuals who are "experts" in this field, in that they have already demonstrated dependence liability, are addicts themselves. Research, therefore, that utilizes this "expertise" may be important and even essential in the evaluation of certain types of drugs. Nevertheless certain problems are to be ventilated in this case, too.

1. There may be a risk that such research will tend to 'light up' previously existing tendencies to drug dependence and tend to cause a relapse to drug taking and a poorer prognosis. Work in Uppsala (Götestam and Gunne, 1972) suggests that, in the case of amphetamines, this fear is groundless and even that the persons who participated in the research, all

previous amphetamine addicts, did better on follow-up than controls or those receiving only one dose of amphetamine. This finding cannot be considered as conclusive, and the follow-up lasted for only six months. Nevertheless, it does suggest that the fears may not be as substantial as all that.

2. Research on drug dependent persons is often difficult because personality traits of unreliability, untruthfulness, manipulativeness, and paranoid ideation are frequently found.

3. The problem of utilizing "volunteers" in a prison setting requires considerable thought in terms of the basic issues of undue influence, rewards, and other factors covered in the general statement of ethics relating to clinical trials.

My personal views in this difficult area have been stated (Connell, 1973) and can be summarized as follows:

1. I regard clinical research on drugs of potential dependence hazard as being a major and essential part of the total field of investigations of drugs, whether new or old, in terms of dependence liability and other dangers to mankind.

2. In no instance, particularly in the case of new drugs, should it be possible for the individual taking part in the trial to find out the name of the drug being tested. Thus, if a drug is found to have a pleasant or other sought-after effect the individual should not be able to seek it afterward.

3. I have no objection to rewards for those taking part in such clinical research as long as these do not constitute "undue influence" and do not cut across the need for impeccable methodology in the design of the research. In group settings whether hospital or penal, the reward must not, in my view, create a "status" that conflicts with general management considered to be of benefit to the individual or group, whether in terms of a therapeutic community approach or in respect of general management within a penal system. Whether group requirements are not present or not infringed, there is a case for regarding the previously drug-dependent person as an expert who is entitled to a fee.

4. There is also a case for regarding such research as "procedure of direct benefit" (see Medical Research Council report, 1963) in that it may demonstrate, on an individual basis, possible dangers to that individual in terms of future dependency risk should the drug in question be issued widely for clinical use.

5. There would seem to be a case for regarding such research as being related to "benefit by protecting from a future hazard" (see Medical Research Council report, 1963, on Vaccines), in that general observations may be made indicating the need for banning or strictly controlling a drug if issued for general clinical use.

6. I fully endorse the need for the highest ethical standards in the field

of clinical trials and the measures, referred to earlier in this chapter, to secure such standards.

SOCIAL IMPLICATIONS OF DRUG USE

There are many social implications of drug abuse and it is not intended here to do more than mention some of them.

The question of safety and productivity is clearly relevant. This would include such areas as screening applicants for employment—particularly in potentially hazardous occupations—not only in blue-collar jobs but also in white-collar groups. (See Chambers and Heckman, 1971.) Such activities as car-driving, plane-piloting, and many more are of considerable public concern. The extent of these problems in terms of drug use is unknown; and until some framework is set up that enforces evaluation—even if limited to laboratory evaluation of the presence of drugs in those involved in accidents or found dead—there is unlikely to be national or international progress so that any advances must depend upon individual research teams.

Many serious social consequences attend drug abuse. In the young, for instance, there is often the problem of deteriorating academic and social performance, interference with the normal processes of emotional maturation, disruption of family relationships, and the problem of "dropping out" of traditional society. In the older drug-dependent persons, as in the case of the alcoholic, there are family tensions and disruption of family life, financial stress, deterioration in work record, and so on. Again, because of the illegality factor of drug abuse and dependence there is involvement with antisocial and criminal elements of society and possible pressure toward antisocial activity and antisocial personality development in the younger age groups. Those who become involved in drug abuse, particularly those who become dependent upon drugs, often have a powerful drive and need to convince others of the desirability to take drugs. Thus the risk of contagion and seduction to drug use is ever present, and the vulnerable are always at risk.

The direct effects of drugs, particularly of central nervous system stimulants, may lead to uninhibited, aggressive, and "mad" behavior, the latter sometimes being consequent upon the development of delusions, hallucinations, and persecutory ideas.

Finally, the statement is often made, though it has still to be proved, that the use of drugs by young persons to solve normal problems of growing-up will prevent normal maturation and lead instead to the creation of immature, inadequate personalities. If this is true, it would in my opinion represent a real danger.

CONTROL OF DRUGS IN A RESIDENTIAL SETTING

It will be clear from the foregoing that it is still not possible to be absolutely sure that a residential establishment is free from drugs, even with skill, knowledge, and special expertise, including the use of particular investigatory procedures such as examination of the urine for the presence of drugs.

Much discussion has taken place as to whether to treat drug-dependent individuals in special units or whether to treat them on a 'dilution' principle, in general psychiatric wards. Inasmuch as such individuals are attention-seeking, do not admit illness or personal problems readily, and often manifest features of behavior that are, to say the least, aggravating to other patients and to staff, it seems clear that to treat such a person in a general psychiatric ward presents difficulties that, in many instances, would lead to hostile attitudes from other patients (who may be neurotic, schizophrenic, or whatever), and from staff— hardly a beneficial therapeutic milieu. Taking into account, also, the fact that general psychiatric nurses and general psychiatrists have no special training in or knowledge of the problems of drug dependence, it is most likely that in such general wards there will be little chance of controlling for the presence of drugs. Furthermore, if such wards contain other young people, not at this time involved with drugs, there is the danger that the drug-dependent young person will subvert others to drug use that, in such a setting, may remain undiscovered for some long time. A survey of 332 young voluntary patients in residence in a psychiatric hospital showed that 60 percent employed abusable drugs while hospitalized (Blumberg, Cohen, and others, 1971). For these and other reasons it seems inescapable that the treatment of young drug-dependent persons is best carried out in special facilities staffed by persons with a special training and special interest in helping them.

The highest level of control of drugs can take place in such a treatment facility by the use of special methods of investigation, by skilled observation, and by being aware of the danger periods such as visits from a friend or relative; return from passes out, and so on. In such a setting, apart from cannabis and LSD, there is little chance of drugs being available for more than a short period of time—that is, the time needed to demonstrate their presence. It is well known that in penal settings it is just as difficult to control for the presence of drugs and, in nonspecialized penal settings in particular, the expertise of staff and availability of screening methods may be low thus making it more likely that drugs will be available.

COMPULSORY NOTIFICATION AND REGISTERS

There has been much discussion about the advantages and disadvantages of compulsory notification of drug-dependence to a central agency. The general opinion seems to be in favor of this administrative arrangement because of the possibilities for keeping in touch with sufferers and more accurate assessment of "cure," prognosis, incidence, and prevalence. The World Health Organization Expert Committee (World Health Organization Technical Report #460, 1970), has recommended such a procedure but has emphasized, as do all who discuss this difficult issue, that such data should be confidential and should not be available to law enforcement agencies.

In the United Kingdom, compulsory reporting of addicts is provided for in the Dangerous Drugs Act (1967). This requires that any doctor coming into a professional relationship with an addict, or a person suspected to be an addict, to the drugs controlled by the Single Convention (1961), shall report him to the Chief Medical Officer at the Home Office.

Whatever the arrangements for storage, many would consider it impossible to be absolutely sure that the data are kept entirely confidential. Such provisions, as a legal requirement, are therefore not likely to be adopted widely, particularly in the United States. In countries that have a small problem and a reasonably reliable system of recording data with highly trustworthy staff, compulsory notification can clearly be a very helpful tool in general efforts to deal with drug-dependent persons, both in providing treatment and also in reaching a more realistic appraisal of the total problems on a long-term basis. To give a full picture of the extent of abuse, sporadic users would also have to be notified. This clearly presents difficulties.

The use of a narcotics register in New York has been described, however (Amsel, Fishman, and others, 1971; Conwell, Fishman, and Amsel, 1971), and its value in following up a cohort of adolescent addicts has been discussed. This is one of several attempts throughout the world to set up central data banks under appropriate safeguards.

In 1971, the Misuse of Drugs Act was passed, and it was implemented in 1973 with the passing of necessary regulations. This act brings together previous Acts, schedules drugs in a different way, and allows for placement of drugs on a schedule or a change from one schedule to another, thus avoiding the need for a new act. It also contains provisions for dealing with overprescribing doctors, for permitting research on banned drugs such as cannabis, and for a change in penalties for possession of drugs.

EVALUATION OF NEW DRUGS

The evaluation of new drugs in terms of toxic effects is carried out in initial studies in animals where such matters as the minimum lethal dose and the relation of this to the therapeutic dose (that required to produce the desirable effect) are quantified. Thus, for instance, a drug the therapeutic dose of which is only a little less than the average lethal dose in laboratory trials on animals is likely to be too dangerous for clinical use in humans but a drug whose therapeutic dose is, say, one-fiftieth the average lethal dose is much less likely to be dangerous and warrants further study if it is to be used in humans.

Countries have different administrative arrangements for securing the safety of drugs; and, in order to minimize risk, the criteria of safety tend to become more and more stringent. Clearly, a drug that has clear-cut harmful and toxic effects in laboratory and animal experiments will not be sanctioned for use in humans. The thalidomide tragedy represents an occasion on which, even with complex and apparently comprehensive screening techniques and safety regulations, a drug slipped through and was freed for human use. However, such clearcut and harmful effects shown clinically to be *directly* caused by a *specific* drug or agent are rare, and the clinical situation is usually much less precise when attempts are made to attribute a specific effect to a specific cause. A few single-case reports of untoward effects (such as anemia in an individual taking a drug) are inconclusive since one has to take into account the incidence of anemia in the population (a high incidence) and other etiological factors before implicating the drug. There is a tendency to rush into blaming a drug for a given harmful effect on quite inadequate evidence.

Drug dependence has been studied intensively and extensively in terms of concepts of physical dependence and psychological dependence. In the former instance, abrupt withdrawal of a drug of dependence from a dependent animal or human will lead to an abstinence syndrome in which the symptoms are characteristic of the drug used. Thus, animal and human studies have been carried out to compare a new drug with a drug well studied in terms of abstinence phenomena to classify the drug in terms of its dependence liability. Opioids have been extensively studied using morphine and diamorphine (heroin) as the comparison. A new drug that, either in terms of chemical structure or pharmacological effects (sedation, analgesia, and the like), is similar to morphine is tested on animals. If it suppresses the abstinence syndrome when given to an animal or human abruptly withdrawn from morphine, the new drug will probably represent a risk of producing dependence in proportion to the efficiency with which, dose for dose, it suppresses the withdrawal syndrome. The World Health Organization (Technical Report #407, 1969) has termed this phenomenon physical dependence capacity (PDC), which is defined as follows: "The ability of a drug to act as a substitute for another upon which an organism has been made physically dependent, i.e. to suppress abstinence phenomena that would otherwise develop after abrupt withdrawal of the original dependence-producing drug."

There are therefore a number of levels at which drugs can be classified including the following:

The chemical level—similarity of chemical structure

The pharmacological level—similarity of effects on animals or on humans such as central nervous system stimulation, central nervous system depression, analgesic effect, and the like

Physical dependence capacity (PDC)—see above

Clinical observations—noting untoward effects, the occurrence of dependence, the social setting, and so forth, and classifying in relation to the drug; for example, dependence of the barbiturate type or of the amphetamine type or of the opiate type

The World Health Organization (Technical Report #407, 1969) notes that "techniques for detecting the development of physical dependence are much more advanced than those for detecting psychic dependence." The former, which have been used in monkeys, mice, rats, and dogs, have been well reviewed (Halbach and Eddy, 1963). Even with the development of such techniques and methods, there are considerable problems in the definitive classification of new drugs. For instance, drugs such as pentazocine show agonistic effects (similar effects to morphine) and also antagonistic effects (preventing the effects of morphine), so that clear-cut classification of this widely used drug is difficult. Assessment of dependence liability will require careful study and documentation of individuals reported as showing untoward effects.

Documentation of untoward effects of drugs is carried out by submitting case reports of such effects to professional journals (with a variable delay before publication), by letters to journals (usually less delay), by informing the manufacturer of the drug (drug companies appreciate receiving well-documented reports of untoward effects), or by some more organized method of data collection. Many countries have set up procedures that encourage the report to a central agency of untoward effects observed in patients receiving drugs. The World Health Organization (Technical Report #498, 1972) describes the Swedish and the United Kingdom drug monitoring systems and urges the setting up of similar national centers. It stresses the need to improve the effectiveness of existing national centers and to identify the contribution that national centers should make to the international system. The report states that the "prime objective of drug monitoring systems is to diminish the time necessary to recognise that a drug produces an adverse reaction and to determine the importance of the reaction."

The success of such voluntary systems depends upon the interest, efficiency, and care of doctors who send in reports. Ideally, every doctor who suspects that a particular reaction might be attributable to an identifiable drug should report to the central agency. It will require continued education of doctors to achieve widespread cooperation in such reporting. The reclassification of drugs as dependence-including is largely supported by such evidence, but the reclassification of drugs previously thought to cause dependence, though no less important, is obviously a more difficult matter. The success of such systems depends upon the quality of the data sent in (the quality of the adverse reaction form to be filled in is also relevant) and the ability of the center to carry out further inquiry since an individual will often be receiving more than one drug.

An evaluation of spontaneous reports of all adverse reactions to drugs (not only drug dependence, which was very rare) (Inman and Evans, 1972), which took a random sample of such reports received during the eight years of operation of the British central register, noted that there were seventeen deaths, twenty-six serious reactions, and thirty-nine reactions of moderate or only minor severity in the sample. Of the reactions, 78 percent were considered to be "probably" drug-related and 13 percent "possibly" drug-related. The conclusion was that "the reports are of value in the detection and evaluation of drug safety."

In the case of drug dependence, the situation is more complex, as has been stressed earlier in the section on clinical examination. The clinical detection of already existing dependence, particularly in young people, in relation to a specific drug, is a complex exercise in which laboratory tests are part of the evaluation. A new drug, allowed to be sold by a retailer without the requirement of medical prescription, is likely to come to the notice of doctors only if individuals, increasing the dose because of developing tolerance, show untoward reactions that bring them to the doctor. The doctor, however, in the absence of any "body of knowledge" about such effects, is unlikely to attribute these to a drug unless they are similar to well-documented effects reported in relation to other drugs. Warning as to a dependence liability would therefore first come from retail chemists and the manufacturer's sales charts. For example, when in the mid-1950s amphetamines were placed on a restricting schedule in the United Kingdom, the subsequent steep rise in the sales of amphetamine inhalers (which had not been included in the schedule) alerted the producing company, which subsequently withdrew these inhalers from the market.

In the case of a new drug released for sale only on medical prescription, evidence relating to dependence will be provided by the demands of the patient for increasing doses because he claims that the drug is losing its effect, by reports of forged prescriptions, and so on. Such data are notoriously slow in reaching the light of day—thus the need for improving reporting systems.

Carefully conducted controlled clinical trials, which not only examine the efficacy of a drug in relation to its hoped-for therapeutic effect but also examine the possibility of the development of liking for the drug and euphoriant action or of the development of abnormal mental symptoms, are clearly of some value; but, as pointed out elsewhere in this chapter, the size of the population at risk of developing drug dependence in a general study of the efficacy and unwanted effects of a drug given for a specific symptom or for its psychotropic effects is likely to be small. In consequence, research on known vulnerable persons is important.

Public and professional insistence on control and caution in allowing new drugs to be released for therapeutic use is understandable, but there is little realization that decisions relating to drugs have to be based upon evaluation of complex data that may be inadequate to give categorical answers to questions relating to risk. Even if approval is delayed for special trials or further research, this may still not provide precise data on which highly accurate decisions relating to risk can be made.

Few deny, however, that such administrative controls on new drugs are helpful, in terms of not only banning drugs that clearly represent a risk but also freeing drugs that just as clearly do not. The difficulty, particularly in the case of psychotropic drugs, is that clear evidence is often lacking and thus, by excessive caution, man may be denied a drug which could be extremely valuable. Further discussion of the risk-benefit question is to be found in Wade (1973), as well as in Chapter Eight of the present book. If the introduction of drugs that have been successful in curing tuberculosis had been postponed for two years, for example, there would have been 45,000 additional deaths during the period and 90,000 extra cases of the disease. Clearly, risk-benefit questions must be answered in terms of the size of the benefit as well as the size of the possible or actual risk.

Finally, in relation to benefit, it should not be forgotten, as Bovet reminds us in Chapter Six, that if fears are to take precedence over more positive attitudes toward drugs and regulations relating to them, the research that leads to the discovery of new drugs of benefit to mankind may be discouraged or so wrapped round with restrictions that new discoveries become fewer and fewer; and those rare individuals whose intelligence, application, and devotion to research in this field produce new drugs will find it not worth while to continue.

Epidemiological Methods

N. H. Rathod

XI

Increasing social interest and concern about use of drugs by man is a relatively new development. Issues concerning the extent of such uses and their effects have become sufficiently clouded with emotions as to make distinction between fact and fiction difficult. And yet, clarification is essential if acceptable and effective social policies are to emerge. Many kinds of reliable evidence are needed to achieve this, for example, pharmacological, clinical, social, and epidemiological.

We examine here the contributions (actual and possible) of epidemiological techniques in our understanding of some aspects of drug use. The main function of epidemiology is to study an illness or a behavior as it affects groups of people. Its unit of observation, therefore, is the group, or population as it is called. This may be the actual population of a country or a specified group of people in it. Unlike the clinician, the epidemiologist does not concern himself with the individual and his illness. The scope of epidemiology is broad; and, according to Rogers (1965) it extends to "the study of all factors (and their interdependence) that affect the occurrence and course of health and disease in a population."

At this point it seems appropriate to make brief references to some of the basic requirements of research as they apply to epidemiology.

RESEARCH REQUIREMENTS

It is necessary to state clearly the objective in view, for example, to determine proportion of people using a particular substance, the frequency with which it is used, or the amount consumed over a unit of time, or to determine the proportion of the population that is dependent on a substance, excluding other users. Each different objective leads to a different answer. In consequence the need for clarity is great.

Purposes are different from objectives. Both dictate the choice of methods and instruments. It may be that the purpose is to draw attention to what proportion of people are breaking the law by using illicit drugs. If so, it is necessary to find out the number of people who are participating in this illegal activity. We may further look into their other criminal activity to determine whether drug users are basically criminals. If, on the other hand, we want to alert the community to the health hazards associated with drug use, then we will have to look for quite a different type of evidence (for example, jaundice, other infections, and mortality). If we want to use the data for other social purposes, then the choice of information required may be different still (for example, employment, public records, alienation from family and peers).

Terminology in epidemiological research is responsible for considerable confusion. It suffers from lack of precision (for example, terms such as *abuse, dangerous,* and *problems*). Meanings vary with the context and often tell us more about the views of the authors than the terms themselves. Terms are freely transferred from one discipline to another without regard for distortion of meaning. For example, pharmacologically, cocaine is a central stimulant, but for legal purposes it is referred to as a narcotic as under the Single Convention. Terms (for example, *addiction* and *dependence*) are used interchangeably, and criteria of addiction or dependence are ignored. Thus as early as 1964, the World Health Organization (Technical Reports #407, 1964; #287, 1964) observed that these two terms "are used interchangeably and often inappropriately. Very commonly both lay and legal language tend to apply the term *addiction* to any and every type of misuse of drugs outside medical practice with the connotation of serious harm to the individual and the society." The situation is not much different today. In 1964, the WHO abandoned the term *addiction* and adopted the term *dependence* instead. However, interestingly enough, its sister institution—the UN Commission on Narcotic Drugs—still continues to adhere to it, and so do many scientists. In view of this situation, it is very difficult to know how many of the "addicts" reported by governmental agencies are really "dependent" on the named substance, and how many are just occasional users. In this chapter, the terms *addict* and *addiction* are used in quotes to alert the reader not to be misled.

Epidemiological data should provide accurate measures of the chosen parameters in the given population—for example, degrees of use of a substance in the complete population or subgroups identified by distinct criteria such as age, sex, and social class; being imprisoned or being under treatment; and so forth. The study of each person in a population ensures that the data collected are representative of the population in question, but when the numbers are large this technique is not practical. Appropriate sampling methods, however, provide a reliable and practical alternative. First, the population to be studied must be clearly identified. Second, we must ensure that, as far as possible, the sample is representative of the population in question. This is done by making the sample big enough and, more important, by using techniques that will give every member of the population an equal chance of being included in the sample. When the population is homogeneous (for example, all males or all females between the ages of fifteen and twenty-five), we can use the technique of random selection (not haphazard selection) or that of systematic selection by picking out every Nth member of the population. When, however, the population is not homogeneous (for example, a large town with mixed ethnic groups), the method of stratified sampling is more suitable. Various groups of strata are first identified and then the technique of random sampling is applied to each group. As each sample can speak only for the population it represents, any temptation to generalize or to extrapolate the findings from one population on to another should be strongly resisted. Sample selection may be a tedious and an unexciting exercise but as credibility of the results so much depends on sampling it is a pity that authors often do not pay enough attention to it. This is not an uncommon failing of many epidemiological studies, as is observed by Dorothy Berg (1970) and Smart and Fejer (1971) in their detailed surveys of many epidemiological studies on drug use in the United States and Canada respectively.

We must briefly discuss methods and instruments of measurement in collecting data. Methods used should procure maximum response rate. The lower the response rate, the less the value of the exercise; for example, Binnie (1964) sent a questionnaire on drug use by post to 5,000 university and college students in the Midlands in the United Kingdom and received a response rate of only 48.5 percent, thus grossly undermining the value of the study. Perhaps a pilot trial on the appropriateness of the method might have been worth while. As for instruments—questionnaires, interviews, and screening techniques are the commonest devices used; and it is essential to test their reliability and validity. Not infrequently this is not done; reliability and validity are taken for granted. It is refreshing to come across accounts wherein these aspects are given serious consideration (for example, Costell, Lewis, and Phillips, 1971; Whitehead and Smart, 1972).

Reliability refers to consistency of response—validity refers to the consonance between what one thinks one is measuring and what is being measured. Here problems arise. Respondents may tell lies or labor under fantasies of using a substance or may genuinely believe they have used a chemical, when the substance they have used did not contain the alleged chemical. For example, Whitehead and Smart (1972) quote a study by Whitehead and Brooker wherein 106 patients under treatment were given a drug-history questionnaire containing names of two fictitious "drugs." Of the subjects, 7½ percent admitted to have used these fictitious chemicals. Marshman and Gibbins (1969) found that one-third of illicit samples of chemicals did not contain the alleged chemicals, but the users who bought them believed otherwise.

Kok and colleagues (1971) also analyzed 119 samples of substances that were obtained by drug users on the black market in Amsterdam. Only 56 contained the claimed and pure substance and 48 did not contain the claimed ingredient.

Measures used to assess validity depend on the nature of the exercise. Chemical analysis of body fluids or clinical signs including evidence of injecting may be suitable in individual cases but not in conducting mass surveys. In these circumstances, the independent opinion of a knowledgeable and responsible person is used to check the credibility of the users' response. This, however, presupposes that the independent witness is alert enough and knows what behavioral or other signs to look for. These cannot be guaranteed. In our own research (Rathod, de Alarcon, and Thomson, 1967) we found that parents were not aware of the relevance of certain behavioral changes associated with drug use.

Bias in interpretation of the findings (and even in designing an experiment) is not unique to scientists. The scientist is a creature of the society he lives in, and this makes it very difficult for him to be neutral about prevailing social attitudes and fashions. As Ingleby (1970) puts it, "In a traditional paradigm, science is treated in its own terms as something which can be abstracted from the people doing it, but in the human sciences above all we need to study not only propositions but the minds in which they are formed—not only scientific procedures but their meanings as social acts. We need to know what ideologies are before we can hope to discern their influence in science."

USES OF EPIDEMIOLOGY

Assuming that bias can be controlled (Rosnow, Rosenthal, and others, 1969)—through rigorous attention to sampling, methodology, and testing of instruments of measurement and use of appropriate statistical methods—one can consider the uses of epidemiology.

Morris (1964) has set out seven uses: historical, community diagnosis, vulnerable group, working of health services, individual risks completing the clinical picture, identification of syndromes, and search for causes. Much of his classification will be used in what follows.

In our reference to drugs in this chapter, they are grouped into three broad categories: (1) Drugs that are available on medical prescription: barbiturates and nonbarbiturate hypnotics, tranquilizers and antidepressants, stimulants and appetite suppressants. (2) Drugs that are available without prescription: alcohol and analgesics such as aspirin. (3) Drugs whose use is legally restricted and/or whose possession without special authority is an offense: opiates and opiatelike narcotics (heroin, morphine, physeptone), hallucinogens like LSD; cannabis and stimulants like amphetamines. These are often confusingly referred to in some countries as "dangerous drugs," or "narcotics."

Self-administration of certain substances is as old as civilization itself. Tobacco, alcohol, opium, and, in some countries, cannabis, have been used liberally for many centuries. Recent pharmacological discoveries have put at our disposal an increasing number and variety of chemicals that alter moods, perception, and consciousness, for example, barbiturates and other hypnotics, stimulants, tranquilizers, antidepressants, hallucinogens, and analgesics.

In this section we examine the changing patterns of consumption of the above-mentioned categories of substances to indicate their relationship to indiscriminate or harmful administration. As far as possible, information derived from official sources is used in an attempt to achieve uniformity and in the hope that comparison between countries may be possible.

Tobacco is perhaps the most widely used drug of dependence all over the world (Beese, 1968; World Health Organization Technical Report #407, 1969); and cocaine also is widely used (in the form of coca leaves) in regions such as South America (Mariategue, 1970). These and similar drugs have not been included in this review because as far as the author is aware, their use patterns have not shown any significant changes in the past few years.

Prescribed Drugs

Since their introduction in 1903, barbiturates have been used extensively as hypnotics and sedatives. The total quantity of barbiturates prescribed by general practitioners in the United Kingdom per year increased from approximately 41,000 kilograms (90,000 pounds) in 1951 to approximately 73,000 kilograms (162,000 pounds) in 1959. Estimated numbers of prescriptions of barbiturates and other hypnotics in England and Wales rose by more than 20 percent from 18.1 million in 1961 to 22.2 million in 1970 (Department of Health and Social Security, 1972). Commenting on the use of hypnotics, Dunlop (1970) observes, "Very roughly these represent sufficient tablets to make every tenth night's sleep in the United Kingdom hypnotic induced." Similarly, according to Sharpless (1970), "Since 1954 over 360,000 kgm (approximately 800,000 lbs.) of barbiturates have been produced in the United States every year (enough quantity to fill 33 x 60 mg. barbiturate capsules for every person in the United States)." In Canada the import or production of barbiturates for home consumption rose from about 532 million unit doses in 1964 to more than 556 million in 1968. The standard dose varied from between 30 and 100 milligrams, depending on the type of barbiturates used (Department of National Health and Welfare, 1970). None of these increases can be explained in terms of rise in population. Chile reported the sale of 11,137,474 units (units not defined) of barbiturates in the first six months of 1969 (Secretary General, 1964–71).

However, in the United Kingdom most of the increase in the prescription of hypnotics and sedatives in recent years is due to prescribing of nonbarbiturate hypnotics, for example, nitrazepam, methaqualone, and glutethimide. Prescriptions for these increased by more than 144 percent, from 2.9 million in 1965 to 7.1 million in 1970 while those for barbiturates declined by 24 percent (Department of Health and Social Security, 1972). A similar trend has been observed in the United States, where gluthethimide became the next most frequently prescribed hypnotic after barbiturates (Sharpless, 1970).

Since the introduction of chlorpromazine in 1952, tranquilizers and anti-depressants have found increasing popularity in the treatment of a variety of psychological disorders, in which tension, overactivity and/or depression were predominant features. The more commonly used tranquilizers belong to the phenothiazine and benzodiazepine group of drugs, and monoamine oxidase inhibitors and the tricyclic group of drugs are among the more popular anti-depressants. These drugs are sometimes referred to as psychotropic drugs.[*]

The number of prescriptions for tranquilizers in England and Wales rose by more than 250 percent, from 6.2 million in 1961 to 17.2 million in 1970, and that for antidepressants by more than 300 percent, from 1.4 million to 6.4 million during the same period. According to Camps (1971), prescriptions for sedatives and tranquilizers increased from 112,990,000 in 1963 to 130,931,000 in 1967 in the United States. Again, this large rise in the use of tranquilizers and anti-depressants is not paralleled by increase in populations. Copperstock (1971) in Canada found 99 prescriptions for psychotropic drugs per 100 adults in 1965. The comparable figure for the United States in 1969 was 133 per 100 adults. With a population of less than 10 million, sales of meprobamate in Chile were in the range of 117,376,674 units (not defined) for the first six months of 1969 (Secretary General, 1964–71).

Not only are these drugs widely prescribed but also many patients remain on them for long periods. It is difficult to say whether or not this is a recent trend. Surveys of prescriptions for psychotropic drugs used in general practice over the last six years in three different urban areas in England show that between 1.3 and 2.3 percent of the practice population was on barbiturates for more than a year (Adams, 1966; Johnson and Cliff, 1968; Parish, 1971). A similar trend for tranquilizers was found in one study (Parish, 1971).

Indiscriminate use of these drugs is not uncommon, as judged by the increasing frequency of their use in self-poisoning (Lerner, 1970). Many studies over the past ten years, also in the United Kingdom, bear this out (Jones, 1969; Kessel and Grossman, 1961; Lawson and Mitchell, 1972; Mathew, Proudfoot, and others, 1969; A. J. Smith, 1972). During the period from 1965 to 1970, prescriptions for barbiturates dropped by 24 percent and concurrently the use of these drugs in self-poisoning declined from more than 50 percent of patients to between 26 and 30 percent. The reverse is equally true. We have already referred to the multiple rise in the use of tranquilizers and antidepressants over the past decade. Lawson and Mitchell (1972) in a series of more than 900 patients, observed that during the same period the proportion of people using these drugs for self-poisoning increased from 4 percent to more than 20 percent. Similar trends have been observed in Canada (Whitehead, 1971), where the known cases of self-poisoning with barbiturates rose from 197 to 478 and those with

---

[*] The Vienna Psychotropic Convention refers to a much broader group of drugs than the ones noted here. One suspects the convention would have done better using the term *psychoactive*. The criticism of the very name of the convention serves to illustrate how profound the problems of drug classification are.

tranquilizers increased from 63 to 973 between 1961 and 1967. These examples show that indiscriminate use *(abuse) of drugs is directly related to national trends in prescribing, that is, to availability and social acceptance.*

An observation by the Dunfermline workers (Lawson and Mitchell, 1972) was the manifold increase in the use of combinations of drugs (poly-drug use). This is a common pattern in North America as well. Intravenous use of barbiturates by "addicts" is a relatively new but not uncommon phenomenon as is described by Mitcheson, Davidson, and others (1970). Bransby (1971), in an analysis of records of 2,187 heroin, methadone, and cocaine "addicts," found that between 21 and 28 percent were currently using barbiturates. Camps (1971) found traces of barbiturates in 31 percent of autopsies on heroin addicts. Frequent use of barbiturates in self-poisoning by alcoholics is by now well recognized.

It is not easy to find reliable data on the numbers of those dependent on tranquilizers and antidepressants. The Secretary General (1964–71) of the United Nations Commission on Narcotics became concerned about the abuse of psychotropic drugs in various regions of the world and requested 140 countries to provide statistics; 74 countries replied. The Commission felt that no meaningful conclusions could be drawn for lack of data. Most countries did not keep statistics related to these drugs. In the United States, 200,000 to 400,000 people, that is, approximately 1 to 2 persons per 1,000 of the *whole* population, are estimated to be "addicted" to hypnotics and tranquilizers (Secretary General, 1964–71). This figure gives an underestimate as most persons who use these drugs over long periods are adults. In South Africa, the problem is growing (figures not given). In Czechoslovakia, 12,000 are said to be "addicted" to hypnotics and tranquilizers, the rate being similar to that in the United States, that is, one per thousand of the whole population. In the United Kingdom, about 1 percent of the population are possibly long-term users of hypnotics and tranquilizers (Johnson and Cliff, 1968).

Amphetamines, phenmetrazine, methylphenidate, and fenfluramine are some of the drugs belonging to this group. Amphetamines, introduced in 1935, have been prescribed to lift depression, combat fatigue, and suppress appetite. Their use to ward off fatigue and sleep among soldiers during World War II was not unknown. The patients receiving these drugs on prescription are predominantly women between the ages of twenty-five and fifty (Abraham, Armstrong, and Whitlock, 1970; Kiloh, and Brandon, 1962; Parish, 1971).

In a study based on scrutiny of prescriptions in 1966, Kiloh and Brandon (1962) found that between 2.5 to 3.4 percent of those for whom drugs of any kind were prescribed by the National Health Service were receiving amphetamines. Many patients used the drugs to excess and adopted various illegal means for procuring excess supplies.

Until 1961 their use in the United Kingdom was widespread, but since then the number of prescriptions for this group of drugs has declined by 44 percent, from 6 million to 3.4 million in 1970.

As to their illicit use, among heroin "addicts," between 40 and 50 percent state that their illicit use of drugs started with amphetamines. In April 1968, following uncertainty among users about the continuing availability of heroin in the United Kingdom pending new drug legislation, there was an upsurge of self-injections of methylamphetamine, and 364 persons were reported to the Home Office as dependent on this drug. From then on, supplies of methylamphetamine were restricted to hospital pharmacies and general availability was greatly reduced. A sharp decline in the number of known injectors followed, so that today it is rare to find them.

In Canada, the Commission of Enquiry into the Non-medical Use of Drugs (1970) noted that the availability of legal supplies of amphetamines increased from 60 million standard doses in 1964 to 100 million in 1966, declining to 56 million in 1968. These figures do not apply to the volume produced and distributed illegally in Canada. Prescriptions for stimulants in the United States increased from 22,909,000 in 1963 to 26,340,000 in 1967. Although stimulants are believed to be widespread, there are no available estimates on the incidence of stimulant "abuse" in the United States.

In Japan, illicit use of amphetamines was widespread in the middle 1950s, and nearly 50 percent of the 55,000 regular users were assessed as "addicted" (Camps, 1970). The officially reported number of known "addicts" recorded by the Secretary General (1964–71) of the United Nations Commission on Narcotics is 4,000.

In a recent study in Australia (Abraham, 1970) no amphetamine users were detected in a survey of general practice in Queensland, although 1 percent of the patients under psychiatric care were either regular users of amphetamines or were dependent on them. The Secretary General (1964–71) of the United Nations Commission on Narcotics records a total of 108 people said to be abusing stimulants.

In 1968, Goldberg (1968) published a comprehensive review of drug "abuse" in Sweden. He found that the sale of amphetamines increased fifteen-fold from 1938 to 1942, from 400,000 to 6 million tablets a year. In 1942 and 1943, 3 percent of the adult population, that is, 200,000 persons, in Sweden were using amphetamines. Instances of abuse soon became evident. Warnings about the spread and legal restrictions were followed by decrease in consumption. Methylphenidate and phenmetrazine soon supplemented and partly replaced the amphetamines, and in 1959 an estimated 33.2 million doses of these drugs were consumed. Another warning followed, and the number of prescriptions for all stimulants fell by 29 percent in 1961. Commenting on the situation in 1968, Goldberg (1968) estimated that although the legal supply of stimulants was probably no more than 1 million doses per year, the illicit supply was 20 to 40 million doses per year. A study of persons arrested in Stockholm (Bejerot, 1971) showed a ten-fold increase in the number of intravenous users of these drugs in Stockholm in the youngest and oldest age groups between 1965 and 1970. Official estimates, as submitted to the United Nations in 1971, stand at 9,000 (Secretary General, 1964–71). According to the Secretary General (1964–71) of the United Nations Commission on Narcotics, "The abuse of stimulants injected intravenously is fairly widespread in the Scandinavian countries; Czechoslovakia, France and the United Kingdom have also reported some cases, but in Czechoslovakia abuse of amphetamines by drug addicts is usually oral." In Czechoslovakia, 18,000 persons were estimated to be "addicted" to stimulants in a population of less than 15 million people.

Drugs Available Without Prescription

Aspirin and similar analgesics based on acetylsalicylic acid are household "remedies" freely available over the counter. In the United Kingdom, sales of acetylsalicylic acid compounds increased from 1,923,000 tablets in 1954 to 5,775,000 tablets in 1958. In the United States, more than 20 million pounds (more than 9 million kilograms) of the drug are purchased every year, that is, equivalent to 44 million tablets every twenty-four hours ("Clinical Toxicology," 1970). Widespread consumption—mostly self-administered—continues despite its known hazards to health resulting from excessive or continued use (Woodbury, 1968). Aspirin is also used as a drug of self-poisoning in 14 to 18 percent of cases in the United Kingdom.

Alcohol is freely available in the Western regions of the world and forms perhaps the commonest drug of "addiction" in many countries. Indications are that the per capita consumption of alcohol and concurrent misuse and "addiction" are on the increase. For example, Jongsama (1971) cites evidence showing that in the Netherlands the annual per capita consumption of beer has risen by more than 120 percent, from 23 liters in 1959 to 51.1 liters in 1969; of spirits from 1.05 liters to 1.88 liters, and of wines from 1.61 liters to 4.31 liters during the same period. Zacune and Hensman (1971) also report similar trends in Britain. Between the years 1960 and 1969, the consumption of beer increased from 85.5 liters to 98.7 liters; of spirits from 1.8 liters to 2 liters and of wines from 2.3 liters to 3.7 liters. This trend has persisted despite increase in price of alcoholic beverages (*Report of Departmental Committee on Liquor Licensing,* 1972). Mariategue (1970) reports a similar situation in many Latin American countries. According to the Alcoholism and Drug Addiction Research Foundation (1969), per capita consumption of alcohol in the Canadian population over the age of fifteen years has increased by 25 percent between 1951 and 1967. In 1967, the consumption was 1.83 imperial gallons. If we accept de Lint and Schmidt's (1968) evidence showing a meaningful relationship between alcoholism and per capita consumption, then it is reasonable to assume that alcoholism is likely to increase as the per capita consumption increases, and indications point this way. In many European countries and in North America, about 2 percent or more of the population age fifteen and over is assessed to be consuming excessive alcohol (that is, more than 150 milliliters of absolute alcohol) every day (World Health Organization Technical Report #516, 1972).

Legally Restricted Drugs

These are usually classified as narcotic drugs or dangerous drugs and include opiates (morphine, diacetylmorphine, methadone), cannabis, and hallinogens such as lysergic acid diethylamide, peyote and mescaline.

Use of opiates, although traditional in the oriental world, is recent for the Western countries. In the early part of this century, opiates were commonly used in patent medicines (for example, paregoric), and they were widely prescribed as analgesics and for other maladies such as diarrhea. (Codeine, a derivative of opium, is still widely consumed as an analgesic and is freely available over the counter.) Most dependency on opiates was iatrogenic (that is, originated as an "addiction" as a complication of medical prescribing), and such "addicts" were usually middle-aged and often middle class. Intravenous use and dependence through self-administration (the so-called "nontherapeutic addicts") were limited to a small and identifiable group. A similar minority also smoked opium. This picture has changed since the 1950s, and new trends are observed. These trends take the form of increasing nonprescribed use, use by intravenous route, individuals starting use in middle or late teens, and the use of a variety of opiatelike substances such as diacetylmorphine, methadone, and morphine instead of raw opium. In the United States, illicit use and subsequent dependency has been concentrated in lower-class males living in urban areas. Supplies are largely procured through illicit sources, making criminal acquisition of money as well as drugs an integral part of use of opiates. In this context, it is well to bear in mind that these drugs are legally proscribed in most countries and their availability through legal channels is severely restricted.

Widespread use of cannabis in Western society began in the early 1960s. Although the drug has been liberally used for centuries as an euphoriant and relaxant in the Middle East and Far East where it grows wild, it is only in the last decade that an ever-increasing number of people, mainly the younger generation, in the West have started ingesting this drug (World Health Organization Technical Report #516, 1972; #478, 1971). The supplies in the West are of necessity illegally procured and no legitimate supply is permitted.

LSD is the most commonly used hallucinogen. It was introduced to medicine in the 1940s mainly as an aid to psychotherapy, to further and deepen insight. It can also cause considerable distortion of perception and mood. This effect is unpredictable. It is now widely believed that, as in the case of stimulants, its hazards to health are grave and its therapeutic role dubious. The revelation has unfortunately come rather late in the day because the use by self-administration is already prevalent among the young.

Various international narcotic conventions expect governments to keep records of the number of people addicted to opium, and yearly reports are submitted to the United Nations. The obligation to do the same for cannabis is difficult to comply with because "addiction" to this substance is hard to detect. The following examples are mainly based on the summary of the annual reports of the governments submitted to the United Nations Narcotic Commission, published by the United Nations Economic and Social Council under the heading of "Drug Abuse, Note by the Secretary General" (Secretary General, 1964–71), and are supplemented with relevant data from other sources.

The nonprescribed use of raw opium has been and is most widespread in certain countries east of the Mediterranean (for example, Iran) and Southeast Asia (for example, Burma, Laos, Thailand, Malaysia, and Hong Kong) (World Health Organization Technical Report #516, 1972). The usual mode of use is by smoking. In Iran, with a population of 30 million, there are 8,500 registered opium users, and the estimated number of unregistered users at minimum is 150,000. In the Southeast Asian region, the rates of users may be up to 22 per 1,000. In India, there were an estimated 309,000 "addicts" in 1966 (World Health Organization Technical Report #516, 1972). In Iran, with the ban on poppy culture and nonprescribed use of opiates in 1955, some opium users switched to heroin and a new small group of relatively young heroin users appeared. Poppy culture was resumed in 1969, and opium was made available to those dependent on it.

In the United States, the most commonly used drug is "diacetylmorphine" (heroin); and, according to Winick (1965), the Federal Bureau of Narcotics claimed that there were 46,266 narcotic "addicts" in 1958 and that, between 1958 and 1962, 6,840 new ones were identified each year. In 1969, the total number had risen to 68,088 (approximately 40 percent increase) and 65,915 of these were "addicted" to diacetylmorphine. In 1969, there were an estimated 35 people addicted to opiates per 100,000 of overall population. Most of these "addicts" were from large cities. The proportion of younger addicts increased from 20 percent under twenty-five years of age in 1968 to 26 percent in 1969. The male/female ratio was between 4 and 5 to 1. By 1972, the Bureau was estimating between 400,000 and 600,000 heroin addicts.

In Canada, according to the Division of Narcotic Control, the number of "addicts" rose from 3,395 in 1961 to 4,060 in 1969 (Department of National Health and Welfare, 1970). Of these, 2,175 were using diacetylmorphine. Again, as in the United States, only a negligible number became dependent as a complication of medical treatment. It is claimed that for many years the known narcotic users have made up about 0.02 percent of the overall Canadian population. Most of the illicit "addicts" were under thirty-four years of age. Of the 4,943 addicts in 1970, 4,655 were "criminal addicts" and the male/female ratio was approximately 2:1 in 1964 (Secretary General, 1964–71).

In 1969, 6,089 persons were indicated as "addicts" to morphine in Brazil in a poulation of more than 90 million. In other countries in the American continent "addiction" to opiates is relatively rare. The same is said to be the case in most European countries, except in the United Kingdom.

In the United Kingdom, the total number of "addicts," according to the Home Office (1972), increased from 442 in 1958 to 2,881 in 1969 (that is, to just over 0.05 percent of total population). Latest statistics show no increase for 1971. Again, as in the other countries, almost all of them became "addicted" through self-administration, and the commonest drugs were diacetylmorphine or methadone. Until 1968, methadone accounted for 20 percent of the cases, but by 1971 the proportion rose to 70 percent. This was mostly due to severe restriction on availability of heroin, and increased prescribing of methadone as a substitute for heroin. Although the number of new known users declined recently, it is early to forecast future trends. The increase in methadone is partly an artifact of prescribing or even overprescribing through treatment centers. In 1968, "treatment" centers were established; by 1969, the number of methadone "addicts" increased from 486 in 1968 to 1,687 in 1969. The majority of "addicts" are under thirty-four and the male/female ratio is 4 or 5 to 1. Latest figures do not show a decline in the number of opiate "addicts." In other parts of Europe where opiate "addicts" were not known to exist some years ago, for example, France in 1967 (Secretary General, 1964–71), indications are that the situation is changing. In France, 185 persons addicted to opiates were reported in 1969.

In Denmark, there were 4,357 addicts in 1963. No figures are given in the summary of reports to the United Nations for 1971. The preferred drugs were pethidine, methadone, and morphine. User characteristics were not similar to those in Canada, the United States, and the United Kingdom. Housewives were the most predominant single group and, except for 100 cases, all were above the age of thirty-one.

In Brazil, cannabis was claimed to be the most frequently used drug—the number "addicted" being 7,025 in 1969 (Secretary General, 1964–71). In the United States in 1967, the highest proportion of cannabis smokers was 34.9 percent in the university population; 5.6 percent for the high school population (Secretary General, 1964–71). In Canada, the number of cannabis users is on the increase—2,830 in 1968, 5,000 in 1969, and 10,017 in 1970 (Secretary General, 1964–71). On the other hand the Canadian Le Dain (1970) Commission states that the total number of cannabis users in high schools and universities may be as much as 215,000. According to the report of the U.S. Secretary of Health, Education, and Welfare ("Marijuana and Health," 1972), "Based on converging evidence from several recent surveys we estimate the total number in the United States who have ever used marijuana to be 15 to 20 million. (No estimate can be made of current users.)" They go on to say that the percentage of college students who have used marijuana rose from 31 percent in 1970 to 44 percent in 1971. A similar trend of increased use of marijuana is suggested for Canada (Commission of Enquiry into Non-Medical Use of Drugs, 1970). The potential market for cannabis on the American continent can be guessed by seizures of the drug, which increased from 77,938 kilograms in 1967 to 199,907 kilograms in 1969, more than 150 percent increase (Secretary General, 1964–71). Fifteen to twenty million users are estimated by the National Commission on

Marijuana and Drug Abuse (1973). In Europe, "Cannabis seems to be the drug most widely used." Ten countries mention such abuse in their reports. The main features of cannabis abuse are the increasing number of consumers and that the users are mainly young people (predominantly students). The number of users runs into thousands in many European countries, for example, France, Republic of Germany, Greece, Finland, Sweden, and Norway. As for the United Kingdom, the Advisory Committee on Drug Dependence (1968) says: "We would find no basis for constructing estimates of our own. It is clear from the convictions recorded that such use of cannabis as there is, is widely spread throughout the country." Epidemiological surveys in the United Kingdom have been scarce and do not provide sufficient data to warrant general estimates. The seizures in Europe reported by the United Nations Narcotic Commission went up from 1,348 kilograms in 1967 to 6,048 kilograms in 1969—an increase of more than 350 percent.

Data on the use of LSD are very meager, but various surveys in different countries suggest that a sizable minority of students at all levels have used or are using LSD (Jongsama, 1971; Whitehead, 1971; Secretary General, 1964–71; Hindmarch, 1972).

Although it is hazardous to draw any firm conclusions about consumer trends on the basis of amounts of drugs seized, it is reasonable to use this information as one of the indicators of consumer preference for illicit drugs. In this context, it is of interest to note that the total amount of certain drugs seized throughout the world shows a more or less continuing and consistent pattern for the four years between 1966 and 1969. Amounts of raw opium, morphine, and cocaine seized have declined, and those of heroin, cannabis, and stimulants have increased. Regional differences can indicate local preferences. For instance, although the seizure of opiates and cannabis has increased both for the American continent and Europe, those for cocaine have increased substantially for the former, but have remained static for Europe (Secretary General, 1964–71).

OTHER TRENDS

It is reasonable to assume that over the past two decades there has been a trend toward substantial increase in the consumption and the number of consumers of a variety of drugs affecting the central nervous system. Numerically, the use and indiscriminate use of freely available as well as prescribed drugs is of greater magnitude than those of legally restricted drugs, for example, opiates. This is partly because the users of the former group of drugs constitute the majority of those of age thirty or over, while the younger generation (age fifteen to thirty) seem more inclined to use illicit substances—or to be unlawful in other ways. The number of young people who use illicit drugs is increasing at a faster rate. Broadly speaking, women outnumber men in the use of the medically prescribed drugs. The reverse is true for most of the illicit drugs. The majority of the users of illicit drugs start the experience as adolescents or youths, the reverse being true for those who use prescribed drugs. Other trends include the cultural diffusion of drugs, whereby people supplement drugs traditionally accepted in their society with those used in other cultures—for example, increased use of cannabis in the West, of alcohol in Indo-Pakistan sub-continents, of heroin in Thailand and Iran (World Health Organization Technical Report #516, 1972). It is also observed, especially in the United States, Canada, and the United Kingdom, that the use of opiates and hallucinogens has transcended barriers of social class and economic status. This is diffusion across socioeconomic class lines. As one watches the gradual introduction of illicit and licit use to lower age groups (elementary schools in the United States and Mexico, for instance) and of the extension of cannabis experimentation in older groups, one can identify the diffusion of use across age categories as well.

There are national differences in terms of the most preferred manufactured drugs (for example, stimulants in Sweden, heroin in the United States). The reasons are not clear, and trends are rarely static even within the same country. The use of multiple drugs at the same time or in sequence is common both among illicit users and those who limit themselves to freely available and/or prescription substances. If attention is to be focused on behavior rather than particular drugs, this poly-drug use is a profound feature of the modern world.

The assumption of increased consumption for tranquilizers, hypnotics, and antidepressants is based on increased prescriptions or amounts produced for home consumption. For other drugs, the data are based on official statistics relating to seizures by Customs and Excise (Commission on Narcotic Drugs, 1971) or records of arrest and convictions and reports to government agencies. Survey data, especially in North America, are also available. All these methods deal with different populations and provide different results. No small wonder that uniform interpretation is rendered difficult. Seizures indicate only the level of demand and not the amounts consumed. Arrests and convictions are equally misleading; they do not discriminate between various degrees of use. They often relate to offenses—not the offenders—so that recidivists may swell the figures spuriously. On the other hand, if evidence of surveys is to be believed, the arrests identify only a minority of illicit users. Arrest and seizure data offer only a limited set of estimates of use. Official statistics are based on cases reported to central agencies. As notification is not compulsory in many countries (for example, the United States, South Africa, Hong Kong, and others), there is no way of knowing the response rate from the informing agencies. Second, "diagnosis" and "case finding" are very much at the discretion or ability of the enforcement agencies. In their official reports, there is no discrimination among degrees or styles of use of a particular substance; reports are of an either-or variety. To lump once only users, occasional users, and those who are drug-dependent together can be ridiculous if the objective is to assess varieties and correlates of use. In consequence, official statistics are of limited usefulness, and comparisons between countries are difficult. Nevertheless, the combination of official statistics with health records and survey data does allow estimates of trends in illicit use. Whether the observed worldwide increases are due to more people using the drugs in smaller quantity or due to per capita increase and prolonged use is not clear. This applies particularly to the prescribed drugs and to those available over the counter. We need to know this, for if it is the latter there is much more cause for concern. Most of these drugs have proven dose-related toxicity and are likely to lead to adverse outcomes when use is prolonged and in an increasing quantity.

Although it is only fair to point out that usage of certain drugs such as barbiturates and amphetamines has in some countries decreased in recent years, this decrease is often more than compensated by the substitution of more recently discovered drugs, some of which are less harmful, for example, barbiturates by other hypnotics such as nitrazepam or methaqualone, major tranquilizers by the so-called minor tranquilizers such as diazepam and chlordiazepoxide, heroin by methadone, and amphetamines by other stimulants such as phenmetrazine or methylphenidate. Whether this occurs because of the medical attitude or simply is proof of the wisdom of the medical dictum that drugs can only be replaced by other drugs is uncertain. The reality seems to be what Sir Aubrey Lewis (1968) calls "here we go round the mulberry bush."

It is risky to view the abuse of any particular drug in isolation and without reference to the abuse of other drugs in the community. Danger lies in the overemphasis of hazards of one drug or group of drugs (for example, cannabis and heroin), with relative neglect of the dangers of others (like alcohol and hypnotics); this can lead to unbalanced policies. To illustrate: not until 1968 did the International Commission on Narcotics at its twenty-third session consider that the abuse of psychotropic substances "had attained disquieting proportions in several regions of the world," and found "that Governments have very few statistics available." This illustrates the fact that use of "illicit" or dangerous drugs has received disproportionately greater attention and action, and the hazards of prescribed and freely available drugs have been relatively ignored.

COMMUNITY DIAGNOSIS

Epidemiology provides intelligence for the health services, community diagnosis being an essential part of this service. It provides information on two basic aspects of community health—prevalence rates and incidence rates. Prevalence refers to actual numbers of all the existing cases identified as suffering from a particular phenomenon (for example, "addiction") at a certain point in time (point prevalence), or over a specified period (period prevalence). Incidence refers to all the new cases identified during a particular period (usually a year). Rates for both are calculated by dividing the total number of cases by the relevant total population at risk and multiplying the fraction by either 1,000 or 10,000 and are expressed as rates per 1,000 or 10,000. Without prevalence and incidence rates it is very difficult to assess the size of, and "trends" in (for example, increase or decrease in new cases), a particular illness, or to assess the effectiveness of social and health policies. The term *case* in this context does not necessarily refer to an individual but may be used to denote a chosen aspect of drug use, for example, occasions of use, occasions of overdose, occasions of arrests or of infections, and the like, in the selected but complete population, for example, those who use drugs by injection.

Both prevalence and incidence rates can be calculated by direct or indirect methods. Direct methods use data based on the actual number of all known cases. Statistics based on the number of people convicted of violating drug laws and those "addicts" coming to the notice of the health service are widely used in drug "addiction," and are examples of the direct method. Another direct method is that of surveying a specified population and then seeking out all cases within it. Direct methods use estimations derived from the known relationship between a variable attributed to the particular illness and the illness in question. For example, Jellinek (1966) used the relationship between liver cirrhosis (commonly associated with alcoholism) and deaths from cirrhosis and alcoholism to estimate the rate of alcoholism in a given population. In certain fields (as in alcoholism), this method has proved to be unexpectedly reliable, if it is remembered that the relationship between the variable and the illness can vary.

Mortality from overdose in heroin "addicts" is much higher than in the general population in similar age groups. Baden (1968) has used this relationship in estimating prevalence rates of heroin use ("addiction") in a given community.

Coming back to direct methods, it is being increasingly recognized that population surveys are more reliable than statistics derived from legal and health agencies. One of the main reasons, other than those already referred to, is that these agencies cannot have access to all the "addicts" in the given population. They encounter "addicts" in special circumstances, such as when in conflict with the law, when ill, or in need of social help. Not all "addicts" or users necessarily find themselves in these situations. In addition, many "addicts" may avoid seeking help because they do not believe that they need help or that the help available will be effective, or they are afraid that disclosure of use may lead to prosecution. At times, even when "addicts" reach these agencies, it may be for problems connected with "addiction" (for example, suicide attempt or theft) but not "addiction" itself, and it is therefore not surprising that these agencies frequently fail to identify cases.

To illustrate, Moss and Beresford-Davies (1967), in a community survey on alcoholism, found that 59.5 percent of the 527 alcoholics discovered did not consult their medical practitioners. In a field survey on heroin use in a new town (de Alarcon and Rathod, 1968), we found that 40 percent of our patients had not sought medical advice. In the survey on alcoholism just referred to (Moss and Beresford-Davies, 1967) it was found that 15 percent of the patients consulted their doctors, not directly for alcoholism, but for disorders that could be attributed to it. Similarly Dupont (1971), in a study of prisoners in the District of Columbia jail, found that 63 percent of the prisoners identified as heroin "addicts" were not known to the Bureau of Narcotics and Dangerous Drugs.

Noble, Hart, and Nathan (1972) also found that only 24 of the 74 narcotic users (that is, just over a third) in a remand home in England were known to the Home Office. We (de Alarcon and Rathod, 1968) found that 42 of the 50 (that is, 84 percent) confirmed heroin users in a new town were not known to the Home Office.

By virtue of the fact that field surveys have access to the whole population in the community (be it in the general community or in an institution, such as colleges and schools) that contains both the identified as well as the hitherto unidentified cases and users as well as nonusers of a substance, they are better suited to provide more reliable and greater information. The field survey (Moss and Beresford-Davies, 1967) on alcoholism sought information from thirteen different sources likely to encounter an alcoholic or his family in one way or another. They discovered 527 cases in all; and of these, 189 were known to the doctor; 51 to the police and probation officers; 54 to the Salvation Army and the Church Army; and 14 to such other voluntary bodies as a marriage guidance bureau, the Samaritans, and Alcoholics Anonymous. The de Alarcon and Rathod (1968) survey on heroin abuse discovered more confirmed users through information from heroin users (seventeen cases) and through health surveys of jaundice and attendance at casualty departments (seventeen cases), than through all other sources, which included police, probation officers, and doctors. The per thousand prevalence rates, according to this survey, was 8.50 against 1.4, as indicated by the Home Office figures for this town.

Dupont (1971) observes that according to the Bureau of Narcotics and Dangerous Drugs, there were 1,162 "addicts" in Washington, D.C., in 1968. A survey of prison population disclosed many more cases and the total number of "addicts" had to be raised 3.7 times to 4,300. When death rates were used as an independent screening technique, the figure arrived at was 4,200. By 1971, using various independent instruments, he estimated that there were 16,800 addicts in Washington, D.C. The disparity between his estimates and those registered by the Bureau cannot be due to new cases.

Field surveys also assist us in identifying the changing patterns of drug use and decrease or increase in the number of total users and new users over a period of time, and thereby help assessment of needs for, and the efficiency or otherwise of, policies on health and control. To illustrate, Whitehead (1971) repeated a survey of drug use among students in grades 7 to 12 in Halifax, a year after the original survey in 1969. The same questionnaire (anonymous and self-reporting) and sampling method (random selection) were used. In 1969, 1,606 students participated in the study and in 1970, 1,526 students. He found that there was a significant increase in the use of eight of ten types of drugs. The greatest proportionate increase was for LSD and other hallucinogens (73 to 209 individuals), glue sniffing (50 to 108 individuals), and marijuana (106 to 223 individuals), although tobacco, alcohol, and marijuana remained the most preferred drugs. In terms of rank order, tranquilizers and stimulants dropped from fifth to sixth and from fourth to seventh, respectively. Buickhuisen and Timmerman (1972) carried out a similar exercise in the Netherlands in 1969 and 1971.

Among the 11,659 students surveyed (80 percent of the schools in the Netherlands were covered), 11.5 percent had used at least one drug in 1969 and the proportion almost doubled in 1971, both in the ever-used group and in the used-more-than-twenty-times group (2.5 to 6.5 percent). Cannabis remained the most popular drug (88 to 95.9 percent) of the users. Amphetamines came second. An interesting feature was the tendency for persons to stop using illicit drugs as they grew older, especially after the age of twenty-one. In the case of the use of opiates (principally heroin), heroin use was monitored in the town just referred to (de Alarcon and Rathod, 1968) for three consecutive years (Rathod, 1972), and it was found that the number of new cases decreased from 32 in 1967 to 11 in 1968. The drop in cases was also reflected in incidence of jaundice, casualty attendance, and police arrests, suggesting that the reliability of survey methods was not affected. On the other hand, in another English town a first survey conducted in 1967 (Kosviner, Mitcheson, and others, 1968) and then a second in 1968 (Zacune, Mitcheson, and Malone, 1969) showed an increase in the number of cases of heroin users from 37 in 1967 to 51 (Camps, 1970) in 1968. Both groups of workers used the same methodology. Accounts of heroin use in a Negro community (Hughes, Barker, and others, 1972) provide another illustration of the value of follow-up studies.

The value of field surveys is being increasingly acknowledged by official agencies that are using the information to forecast estimates of drug use (Commission on Narcotic Drugs, 1971). Some such examples have already been referred to in the previous section.

Identification of groups specially at risk or vulnerable is one of the functions of epidemiology. Vulnerability and the criteria by which it is to be determined must be defined. This is *relatively* easy to achieve if vulnerability is defined as dependency but not if it is also desired to consider degrees of drug use that fall short of dependency. The chosen sample should also be unbiased for drug use—to use known drug users implies a bias. Prediction of vulnerability can best be achieved by prospective studies, but these studies are expensive and difficult because of the need to follow the subjects through years. Retrospective studies or comparison of users and nonusers at a point in time are more practicable if less reliable. Needless to say, these are the most popular methods used. One can choose as many predictive variables as one likes as long as the sample is homogeneous. Robins and Murphy's (1967) work is a good illustration of such studies. Their hypothesis (based on previous studies of known addicts) was that Negro youths from cities in the United States are especially vulnerable to the use of illicit drugs (including heroin). From the records of St. Louis public elementary schools for the years from 1930 to 1934, 235 subjects were selected. The subjects were male, of normal IQ, who were born and were still living in this Midwestern city. At the time of research all were aged thirty to thirty-five. Degree of adult adjustment was assessed on the basis of various records and personal interviews (221 subjects). Evidence of illicit drug use was found in 109 (49 percent) of those interviewed—103 had used cannabis, and 1 in every 10 of the subjects was assessed as "'addicted" to heroin. On an analysis of eight different variables, it was concluded that a combination of absent father, delinquency, and dropping out of high school characterized the group of boys most vulnerable to addiction.

Among other indicators of groups at risk may be mentioned sex, parental use of drugs, child-rearing methods, and the psychological state of the subjects. It has been shown that opiate use is generally three- to five-fold more common among men than women, while tranquilizers and hypnotics are used more by women than men. Smart and Fejer in Canada (1971) and Rathod (1970) in the United Kingdom have found that there is a positive relationship between the use of socially accepted drugs (for example, alcohol, tranquilizers, stimulants) among parents on the one hand and use of illicit drugs (for example, heroin, marijuana) among their adolescent offspring. Abraham, Armstrong, and others (1970) have shown that in Australia dependency on barbiturates was more common among those receiving attention for psychiatric disorders than among those attending medical services for other reasons. In the United Kingdom, Parish (1971) has found that psychiatric patients remain longer on hypnotics than others. The uniformity of findings across cultures is revealing. Route of administration can also make certain groups more vulnerable to develop an illness than others (for example, infections amongst those who inject intravenously). This is discussed below. Information on groups at special risk is of importance for preventive measures. It is apparently necessary to pay equal, if not more, attention to the parental use of drugs and parental child-rearing values and methods in prevention of drug use among adolescents.

We have seen that the study of vulnerable groups provides us with useful information on assessing the probability that an individual will develop a certain condition. This, however, means a study of a large and relevant group of individuals within a community. Some examples of risks to the individual are given below.

Risks to individual health through excessive use and use of multiple drugs, involving additive effects, have already been referred to. Other effects arise from the mode of administration employed and are seen at their worst in those who inject drugs intravenously ("fixing"). Sharing of syringes and needles, lack of concern for sterile syringes, and use of unsterile water involve risks of infection that at times can be fatal. Marks and Chaple (1967), for instance, found degrees of liver dysfunction in 80 percent of the 89 injectors attending psychiatric services in England. Litt, Cohen, and others (1972) monitored 23,028 presumably healthy adolescents who were admitted to a detention center in New York City over a forty-two-month period. Physical examination and urine analysis identified 7,272 as drug users. Liver dysfunction—often persistent—was found in 2,689, that is, 37 percent. As to death due to accidental overdose among opiate users, Gardner (1970) found that this was the major single cause of death in 59 of 170 cases collected from all over the United Kingdom, and in 12 of these, drugs other than opiates were implicated as the cause. Sixteen patients died of infective complications. Mortality rates from these figures cannot be calculated because the total number of opiate users in the United Kingdom is not known. However, James (1967) has calculated the death rate for known "heroin addicts" as 22 per 1000 per year—about twenty times that expected in the general population of comparable age but about three times more than observed among narcotic users in New York (Cherubin, McCusker, and others, 1972). Both in the United Kingdom and in the United States, the opiate user seems to be dying at an ever earlier age. Accidents endangering one's own life or those of others are also commonest among alcoholics and those dependent on narcotics (Godber, 1969; Kessel and Grossman, 1961). High mortality from smoking tobacco has also received attention (Russell, 1972). Another kind of risk is that of social dysfunction in the nature of poor work record, crimes of theft, and social uprooting. These have been repeatedly documented for alcoholics (Edwards, Kellog-Fisher, and others, 1967; Edwards, Hensman, and others, 1971) and for those using "narcotics" (Stimson and Ogborne, 1970; Chein, Gerard, and others, 1964; Willis, 1964). Such evidence throws light on the relationship between social and health morbidity on the one hand and drug abuse on the other hand. Unfortunately, data on use of prescribed drugs and their effects on social functioning seem to be lacking. On the other hand, it is pertinent to mention that the health and social hazards of drugs, like cannabis, have been exaggerated (Commission of Enquiry, 1970; World Health Organization Technical Report #478, 1971).

Despite lack of evidence or even evidence to the contrary, the belief persists that single exposure to injection of opiates leads to "dependence" or that the use of certain drugs (cannabis or amphetamines) inevitably leads to use of opiates by intravenous method (the so-called escalation from "soft" to "hard" drugs). Chein, Gerard, and others (1964) report an experiment on 150 male volunteers who were given an injection of morphine. Only three were willing to have another injection. Attention has already been drawn to the fact that many users stop use of illicit drugs as they grow older (Buickhuisen and Timmerman, 1972; Beese, 1968), and similar findings are reported for cannabis in the United States. Other workers—for example, Blum and his colleagues in the United States (Blum, 1964), H. Cohen in the Netherlands (1972), and Noble and Basnes (1970) in the United Kingdom—come to similar conclusions. Uniformity of such cumulative evidence across cultures should help to bury the myth of the escalation theory. On the other hand, it is very probable that those who use illicit drugs frequently and *in combinations* are more prone to continue this practice or to resort to drugs by the intravenous route.

It is possible that the risk of dependence is greater with some drugs (for example, heroin) than with others (cannabis), but in the absence of studies following the same untreated users over the years it is difficult to forecast the proportion of users who will eventually become dependent. Such data are very necessary to assess the dependence risk of drugs known to have a high dependency potential.

Epidemiological studies may draw attention to new health problems and thus expose an unfulfilled need for services. This is well illustrated by what happened in the United Kingdom in the middle 1960s. Between 1964 and early 1968, attention was repeatedly drawn to the new trends in illicit use of drugs, especially amphetamines and heroin (Bewley, 1965; Connell, 1965a; de Alarcon and Rathod, 1968; Kosviner, Mitcheson, and others, 1968; Stimson and Ogborne, 1970). The new trends began to be reflected in the Home Office statistics, and in the middle of 1968 formal treatment facilities were instituted and restrictions on prescribing came into force. Clinicians also began to impress on users the need for hygiene (sterile water, sterile needles, and clean skin) when injecting. Concurrently patients were encouraged to switch over to use of narcotics orally in preference to injecting (Stimson and Ogborne, 1970; Bewley, Fames, and Mahon, 1972; Chaple, Somekh, and Taylor, 1972).

COMPLETING THE CLINICAL PICTURE

Morris (1964) says "only an inclusive community study can hope to supply a clinical picture of the condition in proportion and as a whole." This is because drug abuse does not follow a uniform and predictable course nor is it likely that any clinic or institution will have access to the whole spectrum of cases, for example, some drug users may die, others manage to abstain, and still others continue the drug use and survive. Casualty departments are likely to meet drug users only in crisis situations (for example, accidents or overdose), but the psychiatric clinics or rehabilitation centers are likely to meet those who for one reason or another profess to have the "cures"; on the other hand, prisons come across only those who are convicted. There are others who may suffer their abscesses or jaundice quietly and seek no help at all; and still others who do not suffer any adverse effects, seek no help, and remain undetected. These are some examples of how the drug users differ; and if one wants to learn about the various aspects of drug use, what other better method than community (including hospitals and prisons) detection and monitoring? As far as the author is aware such a broad-based and in-depth approach has not been attempted but should be, if we want to learn the complete clinical picture of their behavior or illness—call it what you may.

As D. C. Cameron (1970) puts it, "Far too little is known about the natural history of various types of drug dependence in a given culture, let alone the variations in patterns to be found in differing cultures." This is partly due to lack of long-term follow-up studies of drug users (treated and untreated). Reference has already been made, for example, to evidence suggesting that with age many users stop using illicit drugs and to lack of substance in the escalation hypothesis. That initiation into use of heroin is a convivially communicable phenomenon is demonstrated by de Alarcon (1969) in the new town survey referred to earlier (de Alarcon and Rathod, 1968). As far as identification of syndromes is concerned, the contribution of epidemiology is still too meager to comment upon.

Epidemiology, through identifying differences in incidence in different groups, assists in elucidating causes of ill health. The search for causes has not been very fruitful, but certain common denominators have been identified. These are combination of availability, access, and expectation (mental set) from the drug in question. Social acceptance or rejection is also an important factor, a rejecting social setting discouraging overt use. This may explain why users of "illicit" drugs have to form clandestine groups that accept such usage and thus promote the expected effects. The very act of the use of illicit drugs is deviant behavior, but possibly no more deviant than that of exceeding the speed limit. Such single or very occasional users of illicit drugs or other drugs have not been proved to be any more abnormal in their background or personality than other citizens in a community. On the other hand, it has been shown that alcoholics, opiate dependents, and frequent users of illicit drugs, come from "broken homes" more often than would be expected (Robins and Murphy, 1967; Willis, 1964). Given the data of the Gluecks (1960) and other criminologists as to deficient or absent parental discipline and affection among other deviant groups (for example, delinquents) one may wish to postulate that an unsatisfactory home background is a common denominator of deviancy generally and some form of drug use (for example, "addiction") is an expression of general delinquency-proneness. Attention has also been drawn to the evidence that the frequent users of illicit drugs, including alcohol, are reared in a drug-accepting and drug-using adult environment. It is, therefore, tempting to postulate that adults provide learning models for seeking pleasurable experience through drugs. Both these propositions need to be put to test through studies of various at risk groups in a given community.

CONCLUDING COMMENT

Scientists, as D. C. Cameron (1970) puts it, recognize that "propositions and assumptions are, and of course must be, developed and utilized as a basis for the provision of essential services when objectively validated data are not available. Unfortunately, when such operating assumptions are utilized, for some time they may come to be accepted as proven facts rather than regarded as the unproven hypotheses they continue to be. Operating assumptions should be queried at frequent intervals." If society promotes consumption or use of other commodities why not drugs, and, also, why do we emphasize such heavy legal restrictions? If the criminal sanctions fail, what next?

The Addiction Research Foundation of Ontario holds that "after all possible information has been acquired and verified scientifically, the final steps in the formulation of legislation or government policy will be based upon value judgements" (Le Dain, 1970, p. 21). At the same time one should expect advisers and legislators to find it "intolerable that the process of subjective evaluation should take place in ignorance of the objective facts" (Commission of Enquiry, 1970). As criminal sanctions do show their limits, one expects other values plus scientific evidence to lead to new policy formulations.

Laboratory and Field Investigation

Jared Tinklenberg

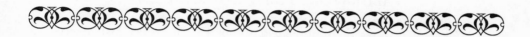

XII

Other chapters of this book discuss laboratory and clinical research, both of which provide maximal opportunity to control and systematically change the forces affecting the phenomena under investigation. The researcher is able to methodically control drug composition and dosage, the method of administration, the state of health and nutrition of subjects, and certain physical, psychological, and environmental aspects of the experiment. Sensitive measures and sophisticated equipment can be used to record and analyze precisely the events under investigation. In contrast, the field or "real life" researcher studies people as and where they are, adjusting measures accordingly. In some settings, such as prisons or custodial hospitals, a degree of control is possible, and some events can be systematically altered; but in most field work—for instance, in observations of drug dealers at work—the forces influencing the object of study cannot be controlled. Consequently, one may expect a greater margin of error in field studies. At the same time, however, one has the advantage of observing phenomena with the full range of complexity in view and with all contributing influences operative. By comparison, laboratory work, although more precise, is usually more limited.

The differential advantages of laboratory versus field study often facilitate a complementary two-way interaction. Findings from rigorously structured laboratory investigation can be tested in the field to measure their importance in natural settings. Conversely, information obtained from the field may be reanalyzed in the laboratory for elucidation of certain specific processes or elements.

Field and laboratory interactions are described in the following sections as well as the comparative advantages of each approach for drug classification.

In this chapter, a wide range of research activities is arbitrarily dichotomized into the two categories of laboratory and field. The reader should remain aware that these overgeneralized terms refer to the extremes of the research method continuum; many investigations occupy the middle range and have characteristics of both laboratory and field approaches to scientific investigation.

LABORATORY-FIELD INTERACTIONS

General features of drug-related phenomena are often first observed in field settings and subsequently reanalyzed in the laboratory where variables are systematically altered so that critical dimensions of the phenomena in question can be more precisely ascertained. Connell's classic field observations linked the self-administration of amphetamines by housewives and businessmen with the development of paranoid reactions characterized by unfounded suspiciousness, hostility, and persecutory delusions (Connell, 1958). However, in natural settings, it was impossible to determine precisely which variables of amphetamine ingestion contributed to the psychotic reactions. Were factors of self-selection operative, so that individuals who used amphetamines were likely to become psychotic without any use of drugs? Since amphetamines markedly disturb sleep patterns, could sleep deprivation have precipitated the psychotic reactions? Observations in natural settings could not adequately answer these and other important questions; it was necessary to perform laboratory experiments with subjects carefully selected to exclude people vulnerable to psychosis and in which the amount of sleep as well as other variables could be accurately recorded. Griffith and others conducted such controlled laboratory investigations and documented that paranoid reactions can be attributed to amphetamine effects per se and do not result merely from predisposing personality characteristics or sleep deprivation (Griffith, Cavanaugh, and others, 1970, 1972; Angrist and Gershon, 1970). Thus, the laboratory provided the setting where possible contributions to a given phenomenon could be controlled so that the relative influence of the various forces could be more precisely identified.

Another example of crucial information gathered in understructured field settings and subsequently refined by controlled laboratory research is that of the life-threatening interactions between antidepressant monoamine oxidase inhibitors and certain kinds of cheese (Blackwell, 1970). Over a period of several months, an astute physician observed, in uncontrolled settings, several patients who suffered headaches and other symptoms of hypertensive crises while being treated with monoamine oxidase inhibitors. The physician correctly linked these crises with the ingestion of cheese; subsequently, he and others reproduced the results in structured settings and established that markedly elevated blood pressure resulted from the interaction of the antidepressant medication with amino acids from certain brands of cheese. Without the field observations, it is exceedingly unlikely that any researcher would have conducted the relevant laboratory studies. On the other hand, if follow-through in the laboratory had not been undertaken, the field observations might have been dismissed as coincidental, and the culpable amino acid, contained not only in cheese but also in other foods, would not have been identified.

Information acquired from field studies may be refined in the laboratory through the use of sophisticated and sensitive measuring techniques. Recently, epidemiological data and clinical observations suggested that illicit drug use among adolescents increased the possibility of cerebral vascular accidents. Subsequent laboratory investigations utilizing advanced radiographic techniques have documented that some young drug users do have vascular changes not usually found in their age group that would make them prematurely vulnerable to strokes (Citron, Halpern, and others, 1970; Rumbaugh, Bergeron, and others, 1971). Another illustration of the movement from global real-life impressions to more refined laboratory measurements comes from work done by McGlothlin, Cohen, and McGlothlin (1966). Their naturalistic observations of people using LSD socially had suggested that these were introverted and artistically inclined people. Using a group of student volunteers for an unspecified experiment, McGlothlin and his colleagues first assessed their interest in taking LSD in the laboratory, and then gave psychological tests measuring introversion, artistic interests, and a variety of other characteristics. The refined laboratory measures confirmed the initial impressions from field observations; subjects with higher scores on scales measuring introversion were more interested in taking LSD.

The rigorous, controlled setting of laboratory investigations may also provide opportunities to dispel myths and misinformation derived from the street use of illicit drugs. Dimethoxymethyl-amphetamine (DOM), widely used in northern California during the 1960s and dubbed STP by street users for its properties of inducing serenity, tranquility, and peace, had the reputation of inducing altered perceptions for several days or weeks. Subsequent laboratory investigations in controlled settings indicated the effects of the drug dissipated in less than two days (Snyder, Faillace, and Hollister, 1967). Other drugs, such as the belladonna alkaloids, were probably responsible for the field observations of alterations in behavior that persisted beyond a day or two. Similarly, one large group of American street users had come to praise mescaline (a "hallucinogen") for its ability to produce "insight," sensory changes, mystical experiences, and the like. An analysis of tablets thought by users to be mescaline showed that the tablets contained various drugs, mostly amphetamines diluted with a variety of materials.

Information about drug-related behavior also flows from laboratory to field; laboratory findings are often elaborated in naturalistic settings. The field trial of a drug first tested in the laboratory is a common example. If after examination in controlled settings, a drug appears to have clinically useful properties, it is studied in field investigations with a more inclusive group of patient-subjects in order to determine the extent of its usefulness, as well as the types and incidence of side effects.

Another example of information transfer from the laboratory to naturalistic settings is the utilization of laboratory-determined personality factors in field work. For example, Kogan and Wallach (1964) have shown in laboratory studies that sex, age, self-confidence, and anxiety are associated with risk-taking. From this study, one would predict that those individuals most willing to take the highest risks in drug use—willingness to take drugs with a high probability of dangerous side effects concomitant with a possible high "yield" of euphoria and anxiety reduction—will be younger males, low in self-esteem, high in anxiety, high in defensiveness, and particularly sensitive to the pressures and opinions of their peers. Field work confirms some of these expectations derived from laboratory investigation; epidemiological studies have identified some of these characteristics among heroin users (Chein, Gerard, and others, 1964).

The above examples illustrate the reciprocal interactions between laboratory and field investigations. In some instances, information can be more easily obtained in unstructured settings and then extensively refined in the laboratory. In other situations, the flow of information is in the opposite direction—from laboratory to natural settings. The following sections describe some of the relative advantages of these different settings for acquiring information necessary for drug classification.

ADVANTAGES OF LABORATORY INVESTIGATIONS

An important research advantage of the laboratory setting is the opportunity to carefully select many of the variables in the experiment such as the precise composition of the drugs to be tested, the exact dosages, and the subjects to be used. The ability to choose the components of investigation in the laboratory is especially important in determining the basic pharmacological characteristics of a drug. The investigator can select the exact drug to be used—the crude natural product, the refined extract, or a pure preparation of the chemical presumed to exert most of the pharmacological activity of the drug. Drug composition has important implications for the results of the experiment, since mechanisms of drug action may be more precisely defined when synthetic or refined preparations are used.

The advantages of defining the components of an experiment in the laboratory are also important in the determination of the usual short-term effects of a drug. Virtually all of the acute drug effects seen in natural environments can be replicated in the controlled settings of the laboratory. The determination of the usual short-term effects of drugs in laboratory investigations permits the researcher to provisionally place the drug into pharmacological categories based on a prediction of consequences if the drug were to be used in natural settings. For example, if a new drug is found in the laboratory to produce primarily analgesia (pain relief) and mild euphoria in some subjects, the researcher can expect with a reasonable amount of certainty that some individuals in natural settings will misuse the drug by increasing the dosage until tolerance and dependency develop (see Chapter Eight). On the other hand, if controlled laboratory studies show that the acute effects of a drug include the unpleasant side effects of extrapyramidal stimulation with uncomfortable muscular rigidity and "chemical straightjacketing," as is the case with the antipsychotic phenothiazine drugs, the scientist can reasonably predict that the drug will not be misused even if used extensively in field settings.

The controlled conditions of the laboratory also permit precise determination of the differing effects of various drug doses—the dose-response function, another pharmacological characteristic important for drug classification. As discussed in other chapters of this book, the dose-response function indicates that any given drug is likely to have different effects depending on dosage levels. Although one may observe drug effects from one dosage and then infer that higher doses will induce more of that response and lower doses less, such inferences may be inaccurate. Alcohol provides a salient example; moderate doses usually enhance social interaction and assertiveness, whereas higher doses do not further increase these tendencies, but instead induce stupor and sometimes coma.

Accurate determinations of dose-response functions are important in the identification of significant nonpharmacological contributions to the observed "drug effect." Nonpharmacological variables such as set (the user's expectations) and setting (the total environment of drug use), are generally most influential at low doses and become less important at higher drug doses. Behavior during drug intoxication may be wrongly attributed to pharmacological effects, particularly at low doses. Observers unsophisticated in drug pharmacology may observe different "drug effects," dispute the properties of the drug, and differ on the classification of the drug for social control. The current dispute over classification of marijuana exemplifies this process and probably stems from the observations of varied nonpharmacological influences operative at the low doses commonly used in illicit settings.

Laboratory research is essential in the determination of *time-action characteristics* of drug effects—changes in drug effects during the time course of drug action. The initial phases of marijuana intoxication often include subjective sensations of increased sensory awareness and euphoria, whereas subsequent effects may be primarily characterized by sedation and lessened sensitivity to environmental stimulation. Observers who focus on the initial effects of marijuana will insist that marijuana should be classified with the drugs that exert central nervous system stimulation; others who concentrate their attention on the later phases of marijuana effects will classify the drug with the central nervous system sedatives; people who consider the entire time-action characteristics of marijuana will equivocate.

Another dimension of short-term drug use that may not be obvious from field studies and hence may benefit from elucidation in laboratory research is the role of false expectations in the perpetuation of drug use. Carefully conducted laboratory work suggests that individuals who habitually abuse alcohol experience increased dysphoria and hostility with sustained drinking rather than decreased anxiety, their stated expectation (McNamee, Mello, and Mendelson, 1968). These alcoholics finally stop drinking, not because their anxiety has been reduced to a tolerable level, but because intoxication has become so unpleasant. This finding suggests that episodic, binge drinking may stem partially from false expectations about the positive benefits that would accrue from drinking.

Part of the discrepancy between the alcoholic's persistent expectation of positive effects from alcohol and the actual negative effect he repeatedly experiences may be maintained by state-dependent learning, the phenomenon that information learned in a given physiological and psychological state is most efficiently recalled in that state, or conversely, less efficiently recalled in different states (Goodwin, Powell, and others, 1969; Weingartner and Faillace, 1971). In practical application, state dependency means that experiences occurring while an individual is intoxicated with a drug may not be remembered during sobriety, even though they can be recalled while the person is again intoxicated. With certain drugs, such as LSD, there can be selective recall; subjects remember the more positive aspects of the experience, and unpleasant effects are forgotten (Hollister, 1968). Since information obtained from individuals after drug effects have subsided may not be accurate, cross-validation with empirical observations during the drug experience is often essential (Cohen, 1969; Wikler, 1970). The necessary cross-validation would be difficult to do in field settings, and again laboratory investigation is useful.

Subjects in natural settings are unlikely to be truthful about drug-taking for a variety of reasons, both intentional and unintentional. In field research, people will often underreport both the extent of their drug use and the impact of drug-taking on their lives, although in other instances, the effects of drug use will be grossly exaggerated. The users of LSD and other potent psychotomimetics often tout their drug as enhancing creativity, resolving neurotic conflicts, reducing alcoholism, and so forth. Carefully conducted laboratory studies with precise measuring techniques have failed to substantiate any of these claims (Hollister, 1968). These findings illustrate a recurrent theme of this book—it is better for policy-makers to operate on the basis of systematically derived information than on unsupported subjective impressions and myths.

The availability of sensitive and precise measuring techniques in laboratory studies may also provide a differential advantage over field investigation. Sophisticated laboratory electroencephalographic (EEG) techniques can be used to measure brain processes that reflect basic psychological variables such as attention and the initial stages of information processing. Drug-induced alterations in these fundamental operations may have direct implications for a wide range of more complex human behavior. If EEG measurements of selective attention in the laboratory setting show definite impairment under the influence of a given drug, one might predict that complex behavior requiring intact attentional processes, such as driving an automobile or operating complicated machinery, could be vulnerable to impairment. Appropriate field studies could then be conducted to determine if these laboratory-based predictions are also valid in naturalistic settings. In this fashion, laboratory studies can facilitate predictions about the effects of drugs in natural settings and can focus field investigations into appropriate areas.

Some sophisticated laboratory measures (for example, some EEG tests) require no active participation or cooperation from the subject. These techniques, therefore, have advantages for drug studies since the subject's level of motivation or his ability and desire to cooperate is often affected by the drug taken. In addition, certain sensitive laboratory measures, especially those of a biochemical or physiological nature, reflect central nervous system processes that are independent of language and other social variables. These techniques permit testing of individuals who are unable to give accurate verbal or written reports of their drug experiences; in addition, these fundamental data can often be generalized to drug users from differing linguistic, socioeconomic and racial backgrounds. If a given drug exerts brain-wave patterns indicative of impaired tissue functioning, that drug dosage is likely to impair brain functions of individuals in a wide range of natural settings, regardless of psychological and social factors.

In most instances, laboratory studies can be economically and efficiently repeated with either identical conditions or with slightly altered variables. Thus, experimental replication, which is emphasized in Chapter Nine as a crucial but seldom performed operation, is much more easily accomplished with laboratory investigations than with field studies. Laboratory studies are also more likely to apply principles of converging techniques, that is, the simultaneous measurement of the same phenomenon at two different levels of biological organization. An example is the measuring of effects on brain function by concurrently recording electrophysiological and behavioral changes. The simultaneous application of two different measures will provide information that cannot be obtained by utilizing each measure separately (Platt, 1964; Stoyva and Kamiya, 1968).

Although laboratory investigations provide data fundamental to drug classification, the limitations of such data should be kept in mind. One must be particularly aware of the inevitable sampling limitations, the inherent constraints on considering long-term effects, and the inadvertent omission of important psychological, sociological, or environmental variables in experimental design or data analysis. Drug classification systems based solely on laboratory studies may be seriously deficient when applied to the "real world." Although the pressures of immediate circumstances may at times require the enactment of public policy before the completion of relevant field studies, such policies should be explicitly provisional and formulated to accommodate automatic revision as new information becomes available. Some of the advantages of naturalistic investigations are discussed in the following sections.

ADVANTAGES OF FIELD INVESTIGATIONS

A major advantage of field investigation is that all the forces influencing the phenomenon under study are operative. In drug studies, these factors include not only the obvious pharmacological variables, but also important psychological, social, and environmental variables, which, although not obvious, may be of critical importance in terms of social consequences. In some situations, these nonpharmacological variables are complex and difficult or impossible to replicate in laboratory experiments and can easily be inadvertently omitted from the experimental design or data analysis. Consider, for instance, the effects of moderate doses of alcohol in two different settings, both in late evening. In one setting, the alcohol user is at a lively party with boisterous, competitive acquaintances. In such a setting, the individual might become animated, assertive and possibly aggressive. On another occasion, the same alcohol user is alone watching a dull television show. Even though the pharmacological factors are identical and the same individual is involved, the behavioral response may be diametrical—drowsiness and sedation.

In our field investigations of drug-use patterns among California delinquents, complex nonpharmacological variables such as psychological expectation seemed to be an important determinant of aggressive behavior associated with short-action barbiturates, especially secobarbital (Tinklenberg and Woodrow, in press). These youthful offenders did not become sleepy from sedative-hypnotic barbiturates as one might reasonably predict from laboratory experimentation, but instead fulfilled the expectations of the current cliché, "Reds make you rowdy" by demonstrating various forms of violence.[*]

Psychological and social variables, difficult to replicate in laboratory studies, are especially important determinants of "drug effects" when low doses of the drug are involved. Indeed, factors of set (the individual's expectations of what the drug will exert) and setting (the sum total of environmental factors) partially explain the placebo effect—why many people respond to an inert substance if they expect it will have potent effects.

As previously stated, many apparent contradictions about drug effects and hence controversies over drug classification arise because low doses of the drug in question are used in settings where powerful psychological influences are operative. The totality of the resultant effects is erroneously attributed to the drug. However, with increasing drug doses, psychological and social factors become progressively less important contributors to the total drug response.

In many situations involving drugs, there is not only a multiplicity of psychological and social forces but also the possibility of more than one psychoactive agent exerting important effects on the phenomenon in question. When purified

_____

[*] The term *reds* is derived from the distinctive red capsule of Seconal ®, one of the most common trade brands of secobarbital. Illicit distributors sometimes market a variety of other drugs in similarly colored capsules in order to capitalize on the reputation of Seconal.

drugs are used for laboratory investigation, some active ingredients in the natural product may be inadvertently or intentionally eliminated, and the information for drug classification may be erroneous. Nicotine per se produces many of the effects of tobacco smoking, but not all the consequences that occur with the repetitive use of cigarettes, notably those which stem from the condensates in tobacco smoke, the so-called tars. Hence, human investigation with nicotine in lieu of natural tobacco will not provide complete information about the hazards of cigarette smoking. Conversely, the combustion of organic materials with low concentrations of nicotine does not precisely mimic the effects of tobacco because important nicotinic influences are reduced. Field investigations become pertinent.

In today's society, many individuals consume a wide range of psychoactive agents, another situation that renders field investigation preferable to laboratory studies. During the past thirty years many potent new psychoactive agents have been developed, partially as a result of technological advances. LSD is a dramatic example of a powerful new synthetic chemical that has recently entered the illicit drug-taking scene. Tranquilizers and mood elevators are but two of the many types of drugs now medically available. In addition, modern transportation has made it possible to obtain drugs that were formerly inaccessible. Until recently, hashish and cocaine could be procured only where they were geographically indigenous or in certain circumscribed urban centers. Now, in many parts of the world, these two drugs are widely available through illegal channels. One consequence of the increased variety of drugs presently in use is the greatly enhanced possibility of deleterious consequences of drug-drug interactions that result from the simultaneous or sequential use of two or more chemicals. In general, adverse effects resulting from drug interactions increase in proportion to the number of drugs given and the duration of administration. These important interactions may occur in several different ways, but unfortunately they cannot be simply predicted from the known laboratory effects of each drug used separately (Bressler, 1968). Attempts to predict these phenomena in laboratory investigations are difficult because of the tremendous number of possible combinations. Usually, drug interactions are observed in field settings, and subsequent laboratory experimentation is performed to clarify mechanisms.

The scientific consideration of sampling may also limit laboratory studies and necessitate field investigation. As described in Chapter Nine of this book, the research sample should represent all features of the phenomenon to be studied in concentrations appropriate to the total population itself. The ideal situation is seldom obtained and is particularly difficult to achieve in laboratory settings, in which subjects are rarely representative of the total population of drug users or, perhaps more importantly, of the relatively small number of individuals for whom social control of drugs is mandatory. The primary determinant of subject selection for laboratory research is usually availability; subjects most often consist of students, school or research staff personnel, prisoners, or other individuals easily recruited and whose behavior can be controlled. Laboratory researchers who are not investigating specific pathological conditions attempt to avoid using debilitated or psychologically disturbed subjects even though natural settings include these people who seem predisposed toward unusual psychiatric reactions as well as the abuse of drugs. In fact, the individuals for whom drug classification is most important seem to come predominantly from the ranks of the socially deviant and psychologically disturbed (Freedman, 1972). Experienced observers claim that unstable individuals are especially susceptible to unusual drug reactions and hence are most likely to demonstrate aberrant behavior under the influence of a drug (D. E. Smith, 1968; Weil, 1970). These same individuals are likely to demonstrate deviant behavior patterns in many other ways. Since most laboratory investigations are not deliberately conducted with unstable subjects, field studies are necessary to obtain the range of reactions representative of the population at large.

In addition to the sampling considerations of subject selection, sampling requirements of the phenomenon to be studied may necessitate naturalistic observations. Some rare but socially important phenomena, such as idiosyncratic drug reactions, occur so infrequently that they are unlikely to take place in a laboratory setting. Also, an inordinate number of subjects would have to be studied until a statistically significant number of episodes of the clinical entity, for example, pathological intoxication, could be observed.

Field investigations may also be required to establish scientific validity (discussed in Chapter Nine of this book). For instance, there are no laboratory measures that accurately predict drug-induced propensities toward assaultiveness in natural settings. Since laboratory measures of human aggression do not seem to be pertinent to aggression in natural settings, field studies are required. A similar problem is the prediction of a drug's *abuse potential,* a global term referring to the propensity of people in different settings to use the drug in such a way as to inflict deleterious consequences on themselves or others in their society. Since laboratory measures have been of limited validity in making these predictions, which are obviously of crucial importance for drug classification, field studies are necessary.

Field investigations are required for determining some of the long-term characteristics of drug use in social settings. For example, since the development of severe alcoholism usually takes place over a period of five to fifteen years, studies of the process require naturalistic methods. Similarly, since life-long patterns of drug use are usually established in adolescence, youths who today begin the repeated use of psychoactive agents are likely to continue to use drugs, at least intermittently, throughout much of their lives. The consequences of this repetitive use will not become apparent for decades. The practical importance of field investigations for obtaining information about drugs after they have been used for several years in naturalistic settings is illustrated by the experiences of the pharmaceutical industry. Despite elaborate animal and human laboratory experimentation, the full extent of both risk and benefit of a new therapeutic drug is usually not learned until it has been extensively used for at least two or three years in actual practice (Modell, 1963).

On a shorter time scale, subchronic studies of the effects of repetitive drug use that extend over several days or weeks often necessitate natural settings as well, because research subjects are simply unwilling to undergo the tedium and confinement required if these studies are conducted in a laboratory setting. For instance, studies have shown that individuals offered marijuana cigarettes *ad libitum* decrease their smoking over time. Does this indicate that lower doses induce the desired effect, suggesting "reverse tolerance," or merely that the subjects were bored using marijuana in a controlled experimental setting? This question, of importance to the classification of marijuana, cannot be answered in a laboratory. Either a long-term domestic study or appropriate cross-cultural investigations are required.

In addition to the practical and scientific advantages of field investigation, field studies may be required because of ethical considerations. In most laboratory studies, medical ethics require that the investigator inform the subject about the nature of the experiment, the possible effects of the drug, and so forth. This requirement may irreparably bias the results. By contrast, in most naturalistic investigations, the subject is using drugs on his own volition, and he is obviously not influenced by the process of obtaining informed consent. Also, the laboratory researcher is often unwilling to perform the type of experimentation that occurs naturally in field settings because of hazards to the subject. For example, despite the fact that much drug abuse occurs with adolescents who, because of psychological and physiological immaturity may be more susceptible to certain toxic effects of drugs than mature adults, most laboratory studies on drug effects utilize only subjects who are over the age of eighteen. The researcher does not want to risk exposing the teen-ager to drugs that might be especially injurious.

Laboratory experiments may be precluded by pharmacological hazards intrinsic to certain kinds of drug abuse such as the intravenous injection of large amounts of methamphetamine or the use of chemicals that have toxic impurities (R. Smith, 1969). Similarly, the drug abuser in natural settings may use drugs despite intercurrent infections, pronounced malnutrition, and other conditions that can specifically alter the effects of drugs and, in most instances, increase the risk of adverse effects. Hazards of investigation with regard to teratogenicity, mutagenicity and carcinogenicity may be less likely but may nevertheless preclude laboratory experiments and necessitate field studies. For example, women who could possibly be pregnant are excluded from most laboratory investigations.

Field investigations are also required to assess the impact of environmental influences intrinsic to our increasingly crowded, interrelated, technological, urban environment on the consequences of drug use. The importance of drug-environment interaction is suggested in well-done field studies of alcohol and driving (Dale, 1964; Zylman, 1968). Even very low concentrations of alcohol (0.01 to 0.04 percent) increase the chances of accidents during times of peak traffic density—6 to 9 A.M. and 3 to 6 P.M. However, during other times of the day drivers with these low blood alcohol concentrations were underrepresented in automobile accidents. The researchers suggest that many people driving in light traffic can compensate for moderate alcohol influences, but as traffic density increases, the need for intact attentional processes (quick reactions, and appropriate judgment) also increases; hence in heavy traffic, drivers who have any alcohol in their blood are more likely to experience an accident than if they had none (Zylman, 1968). The data also show that the chance of being involved in an accident after drinking is inversely related to the number of drivers who have been drinking. Thus, the findings are not confined to just the increased probability that intoxicated drivers are running into each other, but indicate that drug impairment renders the individual increasingly unable to cope with the complexity of his environment. The complex stimuli impinging on the contemporary individual in an urban setting are obviously greater than those experienced only a few decades ago when many people lived in predominantly agrarian or small-town communities.

Modern life entails a wide range of environmental factors that may have important but difficult-to-predict influences on the consequences of drug use; therefore, environmental factors may have implications for drug classification. The consequences of repetitive drug use may be significantly influenced by exposure to air pollution, radiation, pesticides, food additives, and other chemicals prevalent in modern life. Although definite data are not available, there are suggestions that cigarette smoking is more hazardous for inhabitants of smoggy urban centers than for people living in pristine rural settings. Since these and other environmental factors influencing the effects of drug use are in constant flux, and because important consequences of drug use often do not become apparent until after years of drug use—for example, cigarettes and lung cancer—ongoing field surveillance of the consequences of drug use offers inherent advantages for appropriately modifying drug classifications.

Epidemiological monitoring of changing effects of drug use would be analogous to continuous surveillance of airborne chemicals and toxins, a process that is now operative on a national and international basis (Stokinger, 1972). Continuous field surveillance has also been advocated as one of the most efficient and practical methods of protecting the public from teratogenic and mutagenic hazards of both legal and illicit drugs (Brent, 1972). Monitoring of the consequences of drug use may focus on different parameters according to the values and priorities of the country. Some countries might stress direct economic costs of certain drug-use patterns, while others might emphasize public health or morals. The important point is that critical information for drug classification necessarily changes as drugs are used in real-life settings, and in some instances can be determined only after a drug has been extensively used in real life. Ongoing field monitoring would aid in the detection of these changing trends. The principle of uncertainty, a recurrent theme of this book, is again underlined.

As discussed more extensively in Chapter Nine of this book, field investigations are also required to ascertain the ramifications of attempts to control the distribution and use of drugs. These ramifications are invariably complex and difficult to evaluate. For example, the prohibition of alcohol in the United States was effective along certain public health dimensions: the number of people dying from alcohol-related accidents decreased, and the number of admissions to hospitals for alcohol-related diseases declined in some states. But along other parameters—widespread law-breaking, corruption of law enforcement and judicial systems—efforts at eliminating alcohol were less successful. The important point is that ramifications of prohibition or other attempts to curtail the use of drugs are complex, difficult to predict, potentially far-reaching, and obviously necessitate field investigations.

At times, attempts to control the distribution and use of drugs rapidly alter important influences on patterns of drug use and create a naturalistic setting in which certain drug use variables can be efficiently investigated. When Operation Intercept was invoked by the United States government to suppress drug trafficking across the Mexican-United States border, McGlothlin and associates determined that with reduced availability of certain illicit drugs, there was a definite shift in patterns of drug consumption (McGlothlin, Jamison, and Rosenblatt, 1970). These important data, suggesting that drug abusers will readily transfer from the use of one drug to another, cannot be obtained readily in a laboratory setting and usually could not be acquired in field studies.

SUMMARY

Both laboratory and field investigations have inherent advantages and limitations in providing information about drugs. The reader, when pondering a question of drug classification, might well ask himself the question "What mode of investigation—laboratory or field—is most applicable?" The differential advantages of these modes of scientific inquiry are such that there necessarily is a complementary two-way flow of information between them. Laboratory research allows the investigator maximal opportunity to control and systematically change the forces affecting the phenomenon he is studying and increases the opportunity of precisely identifying which of the many influences impinging on the drug user are relatively more potent and which are less. The sensitive measures and sophisticated equipment available in laboratory studies are ideal for the precise identification of usual short-term drug effects, including the relative contributions of the various drug components, the dose-response function, and time-action characteristics. Laboratory measures of short-term effects may also aid in predicting tissue toxicity and other consequences of repetitive drug use in natural settings. These predictions may be based on the assumptions that bodily functions most markedly altered during acute intoxication are the functions most likely to be impaired chronically or permanently when biologically susceptible individuals use the drug repeatedly.

Field investigation offers the major advantage of providing an opportunity to observe all factors influencing the phenomenon under study. These factors in drug research include not only pharmacological variables but also psychological, social, and environmental influences which, although not obvious, may be important in drug classification. Field studies thus reduce the risks of inadvertent omission of important variables from consideration and permit testing situational factors that are impossible to replicate in a laboratory. Field investigations may also be necessitated because of scientific requirements such as appropriate subject selection and adequate sampling. Ethical considerations for the safety of the subject and practical difficulties such as studying the effects of drug use over long periods of time may also preclude laboratory research and require field investigation. Since the multiple factors that influence the effects of drugs are changing in today's increasingly urbanized and technological world, on-going epidemiological field surveillance is especially useful in monitoring consequences of drug use.

Studies on
Natural Groups

Richard H. Blum

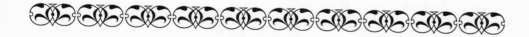

XIII

Work on real-life or natural populations is useful in classification for several reasons. One reason is that such work describes what drug effects are under conditions of actual use, be that for private, social, religious, or self-administered medical reasons. Just as one finds there is no perfect correspondence between drug action on a particular brain center and accompanying gross behavior, just as there is but limited predictability from results in animals to results in man, the findings from real-life studies show that laboratory results from the use of drugs on humans have but limited generalizability to conditions of actual use. Real-life studies show the range of behavior associated with drug use and effects and can specify some of the factors that account for these different behaviors and effects.

A second value in natural studies is that one can learn the consequences of control systems. Recalling that drug classification schemes with practical purposes are linked to control recommendations, it is certainly valuable to know what happens as a result. A related value is found when in a given population, even if no scientific or legal classification scheme is its base, there are customs and attitudes governing drug use. Information about how communities have adjusted to the availability of given substances can suggest conditions under which certain kinds of control mechanisms might work, or fail to work, elsewhere. Knowledge of how various societies have responded to drugs and styles of drug use also gives policy-makers an idea of the alternatives that can exist in public action.

A third merit derived from studies on natural populations is the opportunity to gain perspective on value judgments about drug use and problems. Just

225

as effects differ depending on the circumstances of use and population characteristics, just as outcomes of control systems differ depending on the conditions
under which they are operating, so too judgments about drugs, drug effects, drug
users, and control systems also vary, for drug judgments are related to other
values and life styles that are part of a group or culture. One can also learn
about judgments of particular interest, for example, those made by legislators or
the police or pharmacologists. One can see their judgments in the perspective of
the family, religious, and political background of individuals and groups.

A fourth value in research that employs natural populations is that even
though the investigations are on some aspect of drug use, the results are very
likely to be instructive about matters that bear, not only on drugs, but also on
fundamental features that help to account for the particular drug effects, styles
of use, or opinions held about drugs or drug users. These fundamental features
are, in turn, likely to be seen in such a way that one comes to discoveries about
people themselves, the way they live, and their institutions. For scientists, such
discoveries are exciting in themselves. For the policy-maker or politician, these
discoveries can reveal previously unknown things about the public he serves or
particular groups with which he is dealing. Why does one group favor punitive
controls or why is another group unlikely ever to suffer any ill effects from drugs?
How is it that a third group opposes a particular form of public action? Answers
to such questions can be very useful if one wants to know what public needs are
or how to plan some particular public action best to tailor it to fit given communities or where to look for support for particular programs.

Since the actions of scientists, legislators, and administrators working in
the drug field are themselves examples of natural groups at work, one set of inquiries addresses itself to what they do and how they came to do it. These may be
studies of politics in action, of the process of information-gathering and legislation
by decision-makers, of the allocation of resources in a community for various
drug programs, of a stage of scientific work as an expression of cultural assumptions or the diffusion of knowledge, and the like. One can immediately see that
this shift in research, moving from, for instance, pharmacological studies of drug
action to operational research on those persons acting on drug classification and
legislation, opens new vistas for the understanding of public policy. Insofar as
those engaged in action—or those publics they serve—learn something new about
their own assumptions, efficiency, interests, or goals, then such work can contribute directly to creative developments that arise from the opportunity to reflect on
how things are done and how, by using different assumptions, they might be
differently done. These organizational, operational, or systems studies represent
a fifth meritorious reason for work with natural populations.

PRINCIPLES FOR NATURAL STUDIES

No doubt readers can think of additional benefits—and possibly of some
risks too—entailed in such studies. The point to be made is that such investigations, whether conducted by psychiatrists, epidemiologists, psychologists, anthro-

pologists, sociologists, criminologists, economists, systems analysis experts, historians, political scientists, scientifically trained lawyers, or others, all take as their first principle that it is well to know what happens in the real world. The better to understand what happens, one asks under what conditions does it happen; for example, who is involved, what beliefs guide them, what drugs are available, where did they learn to do as they do, how do their personalities shape their actions, what institutional environments do the actions of interests occur in, and the like.

Another principle is that to find out what is happening one had best be as accurate and objective as possible. That means giving up the pleasure of basing judgments on one's own personal experience, opinions, or self-interest. Instead, one substitutes objective methods that reduce bias and error, as, for example, statistically sound sampling methods; the use of instruments or measures of proven worth; the use of controls or other comparative devices; data analyses methods employing statistical tests of inference; and, in coming to conclusions, adherence to canons of scientific logic. Each of these is applied in such a way that other investigators can readily check one's conclusions by conducting (replicating) the same study. This possibility of replication is basic to scientific studies.

Policy-makers who have not been trained in scientific method can be misled by arguments based on information that is itself inadequate. Although even good scientific work cannot claim to be sure to have provided adequate information, at least the method of the scientist seeks to reduce the possibilities for erroneous observation, inference, and reporting. Central to much activity of investigators who do study natural groups are efforts to assure the reliability of their instruments (that is, making sure the same result is obtained if the instrument is used—other conditions being equal—on different occasions or by different persons), the validity of their instruments (being sure they measure what they are said to measure), the clarity of their definitions of what is being measured, and the reasonableness of their inferences from the results they do obtain. This latter is usually a matter of statistical operations and is discussed in Chapter Nine. Also central to most studies that are experimental in nature is the notion of controls. One wants to be sure that the events or changes being observed and commented upon are correctly ascribable to particular preceding or associated events. This leads the scientist to seek to control the conditions affecting the outcome of his observations. A typical procedure in human studies is to employ comparisons by having control and experimental groups, as, for example, seeing how people behave when taking amphetamines and how the same (or like) people behave under quite the same circumstances when not taking the drug. To "control" for the possible suggestion effect of the smoking itself or the person's belief that it is an active he is using, the observer may give a placebo instead, that is, another pill that the person thinks is amphetamine but that is not. One of the most important things for the policy-maker to keep in mind is the frequency with which these methodological principles and controls are ignored when claims are put forth about the causes of what people do.

Causality is also an important concept to which scientific thinking may make a contribution that protects policy makers from overquick conclusions. Discussions of causality as such are both empirical and philosophical in nature, and one cannot claim that current scientific perspectives are final truths. Nevertheless most scientific workers these days who concern themselves with biological and social disciplines believe that nature—including human nature—is complex, and that whatever is the subject of inquiry is affected by multiple other conditions both antecedent and concurrent. This notion of multicausality implies that even if A is shown to determine X (that is, when A occurs then and only then does X occur), it does so only when the other determining conditions B, C, and so forth are constant, so that in fact X is determined by A, B, C, D, and so forth (and each requires control if a valid and proper experiment is being conducted). In most human investigations, the behavior of interest, X, is rarely linked solely to one identified event, A; but rather A is found to account for a portion of X and other events account for the rest. Furthermore, the extent to which A does determine X is likely to vary from one observation to another, even if B, C, and D are controlled, suggesting uncertainty, possible unreliability and error in measurement, the need to think in terms of probabilities, and the likelihood that unknown events F through Y are also important.

The practical import is to suggest that one be skeptical of single-cause arguments invoked to account for human conduct, especially if the arguments are couched in terms that exclude possible contributing roles of other factors. Indeed, some social scientists prefer not to talk of "causes," preferring instead to refer to probable relationships.

One must be on guard, for example, when a speaker claims "Heroin causes crime," instead of saying "There is evidence (of the following kind . . .) showing that heroin users (of the following sort . . .) engage in crimes (of the following type . . .) and that upon treatment (by which modality . . .) their crimes (measured in the following way . . .) are reduced by (giving the statistics and inferences based on probability theory)." Even the latter type of statement, qualified as it is, is likely to mislead unless one can also show comparative information on the crime rate by these same heroin users before their heroin use, and when using drugs other than heroin. It is also instructive to compare these heroin users with a control group of persons not on heroin, but of the same age, sex, ethnic status, and the like, who live in the same neighborhood (as, for example, their siblings or peers), to learn what the control group's crime rate is and what other factors besides heroin—or other drugs—are associated with either higher or lower crime rates among the controls.

Such qualifications seem tedious to those who want simple answers. Yet if there is anything that policy-makers and behavioral scientists are likely to agree on it is that people are not simple. It is the job of both groups to understand their complexity.

There are, of course, many other principles that constitute the scientific method. Each partakes of the basic assumption that there is reality, that men's observations can describe that reality in steps that increase accuracy, as inferred from replication, from building theories that allow predictions that upon test prove to be at least more accurate than a chance guess, and from the development in those sciences with practical potentials of a body of working knowledge that can be put to use and that works in daily life. It is never assumed that the knowledge that is developed is a description of "truth," but only that one has achieved an ability to make statements (or conduct experiments, make applications in practice, and the like) that are more or less probable and that give working approximations as to what is going on in the world, including the relationships among processes, events, and phenomena. Work in those disciplines that deal with humans in real-life settings rarely comes up with findings that show single causes or that are highly accurate. More often, such work shows some of the complexity of human behavior (including that which involves drugs), demonstrates that what one is observing is simultaneously affected by many factors operating at many levels (chemical, physiological, psychological, social) and that one can by study expect only to increase one's understanding but not to be able fully to identify all the events that occur to bring about that specific conduct (event, process, or whatever) or that regularly occur in connection with it. Therefore, it is best to have cautious goals for what research can do. At the same time, the success of behavioral studies in the drug arena has been great enough to give confidence that one is better off (if one wants to know facts) by doing and reading research than by making guesses, relying on personal sentiments, or otherwise using unscientific techniques. This is not to depreciate the wisdom that is independent of scientific training or experience; indeed, great insights come from wise observers and practitioners. One test of the implications and applications of that wisdom and those insights is, however, practically achieved through empirical research.

FIELD-LABORATORY EXCHANGE

The laboratory is an environment that allows the investigator maximum opportunity to control the events that affect the phenomenon he is investigating and to measure most carefully. He can, for instance, control dose, amount, and manner of administration of a drug; the genetic strain of the animal subjects and their state of health and nutrition; and the environment (temperature, number of animals together, noise). He can also make delicate measurements, utilizing elaborate electronic equipment and computers. The worker doing field studies takes people as they are and where they are, adjusting his measurements to field conditions. In some settings—for example, institutions such as hospitals or prisons —a degree of control is possible, but in others—as, for example, observations made on drug dealers at work or on the activity levels of commune hippies while on or off cannabis—flexible procedures are required. In consequence, one expects more error in field studies; on the other hand, the advantage is that one observes things as they are with the full range of complexity visible. The differential advantages and disadvantages of laboratory compared with field studies are such that there is a two-way street between the two. Findings made in the laboratory can be tested in field situations to see if factors found important in an experiment can also be detected in real life. Conversely, discoveries of factors operating in real life can be taken to the laboratory so that better understanding can be gained as to how the newly discovered processes or elements operate.[*]

An illustration of the movement from real life to the laboratory comes from work done by McGlothlin, Cohen, and McGlothlin (1966). Their observations on persons who used LSD socially had suggested that these were an introverted and artistically inclined group. Using a group of student volunteers for an unspecified experiment, McGlothlin and his colleagues first assessed their interest in taking LSD in the laboratory, gave psychological tests measuring introversion and artistic interests (and a variety of other characteristics), and then assessed the intensity of individual reactions to LSD. Findings were in the direction predicted.

Laboratory findings can also be put to the test in field settings. Aside from the typical case of the field trial of any drug first tested in the laboratory, for example, Kogan and Wallach (1964) have shown in laboratory studies that sex, age, self-confidence, and anxiety are associated with risk-taking. From their work one anticipates that those who are willing to take the highest risks in drug use, defined as willingness to take a drug with a high probability of dangerous side effects but also a possible "yield" of high euphoria and reduction in anxiety, will be younger males who are low in self-esteem, high in anxiety, high in defensiveness, and particularly sensitive to the pressures and opinions of their peers. Turning to epidemiological work, one finds that these are indeed some of the characteristics of heroin users as described by Chein, Gerard, and others (1964).

Another example comes from street experimentation. English youth, in their postwar experimenting with social and private drug use, combined sedatives and stimulants simultaneously. Instead of these drugs cancelling each other, as might have been expected, many users experienced pleasure, indeed more pleasure than from either drug by itself. Clinicians and other observers noting this, reported it to laboratory workers who then confirmed and defined such effects in controlled settings (Legge and Steinberg, 1962). In another instance, Connell (1958) observed the insidious development of paranoid reactions (unfounded suspiciousness, hostility, and persecutory delusions) among housewives and businessmen who were self-administering amphetamines. These reactions were confirmed by Griffith, Cavanaugh and others (1970) in carefully controlled laboratory studies (see also O. Kalant, 1966). Social and private settings served—and are still serving—as natural laboratories for the discovery of drug effects. In the laboratory, LSD had been thought to be a psychotomimetic, that is, a drug that produced or mimicked schizophrenic-type psychoses. It was hoped that the drug

[*] Some of the material in this chapter is taken (directly or slightly revised) from Richard H. Blum, "Social and Epidemiological Aspects of Psychopharmacology," in C. R. B. Joyce (Ed.), *Psychopharmacology: Dimensions and Perspectives*, Philadelphia, Lippincott, 1968, pp. 243–282.

could be used medically to study and to learn about mental illness. When some of the experimenters themselves began to use LSD for personal rather than scientific reasons, it became clear that experimental schizophrenia was not the drug effect. Even so, that early laboratory misimpression remains with us in the term *hallucinogen* (implying hallucination-producing), which is still used to characterize LSD and other drugs, even though reports from and observations on LSD users show that hallucinations may not occur at all (although sensory changes are likely) or, if they do, are but one of many outcomes (Hollister, 1968; Blum and Associates, 1964). A different example stems from street, not laboratory, error. One large group of American street users have come to praise mescaline (a "hallucinogen") for its ability to produce "insight," sensory changes, mystical experiences, and the like. Yet upon analyzing through one time period tablets thought by users to be mescaline, it has been determined that they were buying various mixtures, mostly amphetamines or LSD diluted with other materials (R. Smith, 1971).

FIELD STUDY METHODOLOGY

The systematization of knowledge necessary to the better understanding of drug effects, control effects, and people effects rests on the adequacy of the methods and logic used. Insofar as methods or logic is weak, the resulting information will distort rather than clarify our understanding of the conditions under which drugs or control measures produce undesired outcomes. The policy-maker or concerned citizen interested in drug classifications for control must himself be reasonably sophisticated so as to be able to judge the adequacy of the research findings that are presented to him as a basis for recommending one or another classification-and-control scheme. Since adequacy depends on the goodness of the methodology, the drug decision-maker must know something of research methodology. The trend of our times is in the opposite direction, for specialization of knowledge leads to increasing narrowness of scope and the widespread lack of understanding among policy-makers and citizens of the technological operations that affect their lives. In the case of drug-effects data, such a lack of understanding puts the policy-maker at the mercy of "experts." If, relying on professionals who are not in fact careful research workers and thinkers, the policy-maker is led to inaugurate or perpetuate laws and programs that are based on error, nations and the international community are in jeopardy. That is why we ask nonscientist readers, or scientists working in the drug field with data from disciplines other than their own, to undertake the hard work of learning new concepts and appreciating complex procedures and logic and to strive for a level of wisdom that makes them less vulnerable to misinformation and poor logic.

Ordinary Observers

The earliest field studies involving drugs were made by nonscientist observers. An observer, frequently a traveler, ventured forth among the people of a tribe or nation foreign to him and described what he saw, relying only on his mind, his eyes and ears, and the willingness of the people being observed to respond to his questions and to let him witness their conduct. In these early reports, whether they were of alcohol use in ancient Greece, hashish intoxication in the Middle East, opium traffic in China, or coca-chewing among the Incas, behavior involving mind-altering drugs is usually incidental to the general observations recorded. More recent works, on the other hand, focus on drug use and may extract from the accounts of early observers to build up a picture that is more comprehensive and more abstract. Such work—for example, Mortimer and Golden's (1901) analysis of coca-chewing by Incas—may well describe relationships between drug behavior and social variables (status, sex-linked roles, ritual, and the like) that can be investigated in other field studies or in the laboratory.

Group Studies

The next step (to impose an artificial order of progress) is taken when an observer sets out with the study of a group as his primary goal. He may aim at a general description of the group, as do many anthropological or sociological studies, or he may wish to focus particularly on drug use or drug responses in relationship to some one or several cultural or social variables. At this point the observer becomes an investigator: he plans his study, sets up the standards he will use to identify the group of interest to him, develops the concepts and hypotheses to be used in seeking out information about the group and its members, and brings along with him tools that will enable him to gather the information he needs. For the most part, the tools used by anthropologists and sociologists have been no different from those of early observers from Herodotus on: their eyes to watch with and their ears to listen. Insofar as they begin to ask questions of group members—whether these are tribesmen or patients in a hospital—the investigators must also employ some kind of sampling procedure to determine who is to be interviewed. They must also have questions to ask. These questions constitute an interview schedule. Asking the same questions or making observations of different people under similar circumstances, as, for example, under drug influence, is evidence of systematization in field work.

Systematic Sampling

An important next step, one that increases the likelihood that generalizations made about a group will be accurate, occurs when the observer moves from casual to systematic sampling. Sampling takes place whenever one has to select certain individuals (or objects) out of a larger partially inaccessible universe of individuals. It is usually impossible even to study the total population of interest.

One wants to learn enough from the sample to be able to make accurate statements about the larger population from which it was drawn and therefore needs to sample so as to achieve a representative distribution. There are a number of ways of accomplishing this in human populations, among them techniques of sampling at random (that is, so that every individual has an equal chance of being included in the sample), by systematic (every Nth case) devices, or by matching, one example of which is to construct a sample having the same proportional representation of relevant characteristics as those in the total population, as is done in quota sampling. By such methods as choice of target population, as in stratification, and of statistical techniques for describing the distribution of characteristics and for drawing inferences about their relationship to the larger population, one can achieve quite respectable generalizations on the basis of studies of relatively small samples. The size of the samples needed varies with the degree of accuracy required, the distribution of the traits in question, and the size of the total population.

Reliable Instruments

It is inefficient to draw a careful sample, or to observe a total population if its numbers are small enough, and then to use a poor instrument for fact-finding. One wants instruments, as far as possible, to be sources of knowledge rather than error. That leads the investigator to select for data-gathering instruments that are reliable and valid. A reliable instrument is one that yields consistent results upon different applications (to the same objects of study), in the hands of different people, and that is internally consistent as well (that is, various measures of internal correlation reach acceptable levels). A valid instrument measures what it purports to measure. The instrument, whether it is an interview, a rating scale, a psychological test, a sociometric device, a physiological stress indicator, or something else, must be prepared in advance so that its reliability and validity are demonstrated and its range of inherent error known. As with any tool, an instrument requires the personnel who are to use it to be trained. For example, an interview, which may appear deceptively simple, is subject to large errors depending upon a variety of intruding factors only some of which can be controlled by careful development and investigator training. The bias of the interviewer (an intruding variable familiar to laboratory workers when described as the experimenter effect, or the demand quality) is one of the most pervasive intrusions. The relationship between interviewer and subject is another, for it colors perceptions that mediate and control subject responses. One present trend designed to increase the accuracy as well as the scope of interviews is to supplement a basic interview schedule with standardized tests (that is, with published norms that show the range and distribution of scores for stated populations). Questionnaires and behavior-rating scales are also widely employed. Each of these devices has its limitations; any tool for delineating phenomena and facilitating observation loses as well as gains information—for example, as a microscope by magnifying gives greater detail, it loses the broader scene.

Special Samples

It often happens that an investigator has a special interest that cannot be met by describing behavior in a naturally occurring group. This may be the case even when the naturally occurring group is selected because it is known to contain individuals of special interest, as, for example, a sample of outpatients taking antidepressives, of jail inmates with a wide experience in illicit drug use, or of students volunteering for drug experiments. Quite often the investigator wishes to concentrate on persons who cannot be identified as members of some real group to which access is easy. In that situation, he will develop means for case-finding and further means for case identification (see Blum, 1962). Some device is required that allows one to scan a population among whose members the cases of interest are expected to occur, and then a refined device to identify those who have the experience or trait that the investigator seeks. One may scan the population by means of survey sampling, by a review of agency or institutional records, or by enlisting the cooperation of physicians or police or other knowledgeable persons who see special populations. Case identification requires some standard by which to judge persons, on the basis of their experience. Here one might use medical or psychiatric examinations, psychological tests, health inventories, response to nalorphine test injections, possession of marijuana, use of drug jargon, or any other "proof" that the subject is or has done what one is interested in. If the trait being sought is elusive not because of known rarity but because of unclear or poor definition as can be the case for cases of drug "dependency" or "abuse," then proper sampling begins first with proper definitions (Smart, 1973; Edwards and Hawks, 1972; Christie and Bruun, 1969).

Prospective Studies

Techniques that involve case histories (see MacMahon, Pugh, and Ipsen 1960), are retrospective methods. In prospective studies, on the other hand, one follows a population forward in time. For example, persons exposed to some event are contrasted with those not so exposed, the population having been selected on existing knowledge of the frequency with which the interesting event occurs: the inquiry is directed to its possible sequels. The subjects may be chosen before the occurrence of the event, as in a typical laboratory procedure; in the field one must rely on the event occurring and, further, on some being exposed to it and some not. An alternative is to select a population at random, or perhaps for convenience, then to follow such outcomes as the development of alcoholism, and finally to return to the data gathered over the years to see what variables were the "events" associated with later heavy alcohol use. Ordinarily, but not invariably, public health scientists refer to the prospective comparison of exposed and unexposed populations as a cohort study; the study watching and waiting for outcomes of interest is described as "longitudinal."

SPECIAL GOALS AND METHODS

The goals of the investigator, of course, determine his methods and his populations for study. He may be interested, as Morris (1957) puts it, in "community diagnosis." For example, he may seek to identify groups of persons vulnerable to heroin addiction; he may want to know what the distribution of and trends in tranquilizer use are. He may be interested in community change; for example, the spread of marijuana use to middle- and upper-class youngsters. He may be interested in individual changes; for example, paranoid psychoses associated with amphetamine use, positing that the personal and environmental factors relating to amphetamine exposure and the psychotic experience are both of importance. An investigator may also wish to focus on the provision or evaluation of services (that is, public action, controls); for example, asking what the characteristics are of citizens who come for treatment of their heroin addiction and receive methadone compared to those who do not volunteer for care or who come but receive psychotherapy instead of methadone.

Let us say an investigator wants to know, through program evaluation, if drug-use prevention programs conducted in public schools are working. That investigation is a complicated one, for he must learn what kind of drug use the schools are hoping to prevent and to what extent. He must also identify what is going on in that educational effort so that, if there is any result, one knows what form the intervention really took. That is a form of process analysis. He might, in his design, try to persuade the schools to try three different approaches, one a control in which no education on drugs was formally given, another in which ordinary classroom instruction by means of books, movies, and outside lectures was used, and a third in which group leaders led the children in discussions not only about drug information but also about the emotional and social significance of various kinds of drug use and related conduct. Simultaneously the investigator might be studying the children themselves to see what different patterns of drug use they had as a function of their age, choice of friends, family background, neighborhood, type of school attended, personality as measured by tests, and the like. Were he to follow the students for several years, a follow-up (prospective) method, measuring their drug exposure, experience, and intentions regularly while they were receiving education, the investigator would be in a position to say what kind of drug education had what kind of an effect over time (increasing, shifting, decreasing, no change) on what type of child. Such a study, sponsored by the U.S. National Institute of Mental Health, is in fact under way (R. H. Blum, principal investigator, 1972–1975).

A different method would be applied if the investigator were interested in identifying new patterns of use—types of people or syndromes of people-plus-drugs—based on self-reported outcomes of use linked to styles of social and private use. He might begin with a given environment or social role; for example, students in a university, heroin users buying on the same street corner, drug dealers working in one city, or street youth living in the same neighborhood. In each situation, he would observe what drugs they were using and how (supplementing observations and reports with laboratory analyses to be sure what the drug really was, since users of street drugs often do not know what or how much of a drug they are getting) and would then seek data on outcomes. He could do this by having each user keep a daily diary, by having members as informants in each social group report their observations, by having an independent observer record behavior, and by having systematic special observations—as, for example, occasional medical examinations or tests of psychological performance. Behavior could be tied to expectations of outcome by having participants say what they knew about drug effects and express themselves as to whether or not such effects were compatible with their desires for themselves or their social roles. Were one interested in predicting the future drug behavior of people in the various categories being developed, one could ask nonusers of a particular drug to name peers whom they admired and aspired to be like, a sociometric procedure. If investigation revealed those persons were users, the prediction would be that the nonuser would become a user. Or, if one were interested in predicting volunteering for treatment or response to arrest one might ask users about their dissatisfaction with current social status and their drug effects. One could also address their interest in and ability to engage in more conventional work and living, not only by interviews but by checking with employers or using other institutional data sources. Those who were dissatisfied with the drug life and had conventional capabilities would be predicted to be more likely to enter treatment or to respond to a drug arrest by terminating illicit use. In point of fact, all the foregoing methods and findings have been reported: Hughes, Barker, Crawford, and Jaffe (1972); Feldman (1968); and others by Blum and his colleagues (Blum and Associates, 1969a, 1969b, 1972b).

Sociological and social psychological studies, as well as some anthropological ones, rely on techniques that may or may not be termed epidemiological. A typical sociological approach is the method of participant observation, which is much the same as the direct observation method of the early traveler. It differs only in that the observer works harder to become part of the group while at the same time using his scientific conceptual framework to identify factors in the group that account for what is being observed. The participant observer may have the opportunity to conduct informal tests of emerging hypotheses by actually altering group structures or relationships, doing this without departing from his own role in the group. He may also have the opportunity to systematize his observations by means of sociometric devices (asking members, for example, to rank each other in terms of their prestige, or to choose those they would prefer to be with when taking a drug). Attitude scales can also be employed, these being quantifiable tests designed to measure the sets or expectations of people (for example, measures of trust in persons offering or prescribing drugs, measures of rating the efficacy of one or another means for handling nervousness, or measures of willingness to have new experiences). A sociological participant observer might well set out with these devices to live on a hospital ward and to predict in advance of medication which patients would show the greatest response to a strong tranquilizer, perhaps basing his predictions on observations of ward dynamics, for instance, power conflicts among doctors, nurses, and the agitated patients. Or he might live in a family with an alcoholic father and show that increased drinking occurs when the wife subtly encourages it even though ostensibly opposed.

An investigator who attends to the nuances of interpersonal behavior, the interaction of families, or the operation of unconscious factors in the personality is going beyond conventional sociological methods, which limit themselves to either visible events or inferences related to elements of group composition, for example, role, status, reference groups, and the like. The investigator who is interested in psychodynamics is more likely to be a psychiatrist or psychologist.

Assume that a research worker has heard from drug users descriptions of their relations with their families that differ markedly from those offered by non-users of the same socioeconomic level. Among the middle class for instance, youthful users of illicit drugs describe their relations with parents as more disagreeable, affectionless, and distant; and they see themselves as more different from their parents in their beliefs and goals. The investigator can accept that this is the way the youthful user feels—or represents the adoption by the user of a point of view that is fashionable in his circle—but it cannot be taken as evidence of actual familial difference. To test these assertions, one would have to compare families under direct observation. One could use interviews, ratings, tests, and the like. One method would be to take a random sample of all families in a given neighborhood with same-age children with illicit drug-taking opportunities. These families could be scored depending on the average kind and amount of drug use by their children. Then the families would be seen by an interviewer-rater who would not know the children's drug use so as to avoid prejudicing the findings. Then, to be sure of independent agreement, a second rater might see the family. Since the interviews in the home are less controlled than is desirable for a psychodynamic appraisal, the most extreme families (highest and lowest on children's illicit drug use) could be invited to participate in special sessions, for instance a programmed discussion of child-rearing with the entire family present. These discussions could be filmed and the results independently rated by two clinicians so that reliability of judgment could be assured.

The foregoing describes another piece of actual research (Blum and Associates, 1972a). In this study, in which some statistical methods were used for weighing family characteristics, the results were such that children with high-risk drug use could be predicted with considerable accuracy on the basis of what their families were like. Analysis also revealed that what was defined as risk-taking use of illicit drugs correlated very highly with excessive cigarette smoking and dangerous outcomes from alcohol use. It was also learned that the likelihood of using drugs in dangerous ways was associated with individual factors as well, for example, a history of feeding problems in infancy, misbehavior in school, and a lack of personal confidence. Given these combined features, it is possible to classify and thence to predict with high accuracy which youth are at risk of suffering ill drug effects associated with excessive tobacco smoking, or heavy drinking, or will use LSD, amphetamines, and opioids with attendant risks of arrest, ill health toxic reactions, and the like.

The psychologically oriented investigator may also apply psychomotor or physiological measures to determine base lines, correlates, or outcomes, as, for example, in the study of the impact of treatment programs on heroin use. In a study on the U.S. Army in Vietnam, in which chromatographic techniques were used for urine analysis, it was found that over an eight-month period the prevalence of heroin use declined markedly (Jaffe, 1972). By examining the social and environmental characteristics of persons whose urine is positive for heroin, it becomes possible to pinpoint potential heroin users before they are exposed to their use of that drug during Army service and to experiment with special educational or environmental control programs for them.

A number of fruitful investigations have focused on psychodynamic and other features of personality. When using naturally occurring groups, as distinct from laboratory or clinical subjects, such studies ask the following sorts of questions: What personality changes occur over time as part of being in the drug life or being exposed to heavy use of one or another drug? Do personality features differ for persons who use the same drug in different ways or who have different kinds of reactions to the same or drug-setting experience? How do psychodynamic features interact with attitudes and expectations about drugs to help account for the kinds of drug experiences that individuals seek or report? Are there personality features that predispose persons to become interested in the drug life; vulnerable to drug involvement or addiction; or, contrariwise, relatively immune to disapproved or disabling use or effects? How is the distribution of drug-related conduct in a population linked to the presence of environmental (or genetic) circumstances (for example, stress, absent parents, and the like) that are expected to create personality difficulties that are in turn expressed by problem drug use? What means for treatment or prevention can be suggested, tried, and tested—based on awareness of the personality features of groups with special drug problems? In the course of testing or treatment using drugs, what range of reactions occur that are specific to given personality structures or states (including psychopathological ones)? How does the study and enumeration of these special drug effects become useful in constructing drug classification schemes helpful in research or clinical treatment? (See Chapter One.)

The range of studies that address these or related questions is great, ranging from comparative investigations such as Louhivoori's (1971) in Finland and Stevenson (1956) in Canada to analyses such as Pichot and Buchsenschutz (1972) in France, the longitudinal work as Jones (1967), and the English epidemiologically related work of De Alarcon (1969). Clinical and theoretical work on personality and the addictions has been emphasized among psychoanalytic workers, among whom, following Freud, the names of Glover (England), Kielholz (Switzerland), Meninger and Knight (United States), Simmel (Germany), and Tahka (Finland) may be mentioned.

From such work one concludes that personality features—and of course the environmental and genetic features productive of them—as well as possibly correlated neurophysiological states play an important role in determining drug-setting predispositions and reactions, as well as responses to preventive or correctional intervention. Although general principles are not easily formulated, given the diversity and subtlety of drug-setting–personality interactions, the following may be set forth. (1) One should not confuse that which is disapproved (that is, people using drugs illicitly) with that which is psychopathological (psychiatric illness). (2) When drugs are taken within the normal range of dosage, one should not attribute everything that subsequently occurs to the chemistry of the drug, overlooking that personality expressions are also on view. (3) Destructive and disabling forms of drug-related behavior do not just happen, but likely are the consequence of preexisting developmental trends. (4) Drug classification systems that are based on observations of diverse effects specific to personality features should be so constructed that they do not exclude those personality features or ignore the range and variability of such drug-person interactions. (5) Drug control and intervention systems, when being planned or tested, also should assume differences in impact dependent upon personality and its correlates.

SCIENTISTS' ORIENTATION

A primary tool of methodology exists, not in the hands, but rather in the head of the research worker. His concepts direct his attention, define his focus of interest, influence his choice of instruments and designs, and modify the method by which he processes data. Concepts also influence his interpretation of his results. In field work, as in the laboratory, the conceptual framework will be borrowed from the primary disciplines in which the investigator has been trained. His terms and referents will be part of a body of empirical data and of theory. However, his scientific approach will also be subject to influence from the larger culture and smaller social groups of which he is a member, and from his own idiosyncratic experiences. An historian of science is more likely to identify the nature and limitations of an investigator's world than the worker himself. For example, a non-Communist who reads Sigg's (1963) fine studies of hashish use in Morocco may be struck by Sigg's Marxist interpretation of determinants of drug use. One who reads the discussion by Chein, Gerard, and others (1964) of the etiology and control of opioid addiction may be struck by the authors' humanistic, antipunitive, and possibly even antipolice position. One who reviews congressional or medical or Food and Drug Administration expert testimony regarding the "abuse" of amphetamines, tranquilizers, and barbiturates may find remarkable the reliance on anecdotal material in support of conclusions that contain a set of value judgments strongly condemning dependency or euphoria as such. Similarly, physician prescribers or pharmaceutical industry sellers of tranquilizers may be strong in support of the beneficent effects of such substances on mental illness, for example, attributing to such drugs all recent reductions in the number of hospitalized mentally ill (as in the United States) without mentioning concurrent changes in community and hospital psychiatric practice—humans find satisfaction in thinking that they know what they are doing and that what they are doing produces the good effects observed and humans do tend to oversimplify or justify that which they do for ease or self-interest (that is, prescribing a tranquilizer without having made a diagnosis or selling tranquilizers without establishing specific efficacy).

Unless methodology is sound, there can be no protection against the intrusion of bias in judgments of drugs, drug users, and drug intervention programs. Even with sound methodology, biasing factors occur. Only alertness to their omnipresence and an open-minded interest in bias as determinant in human affairs can help scientists, policy-makers, and citizens to at least appreciate how easy it is to err and to encourage all of us to temper certainty with statements of probability instead.

HISTORICAL STUDIES

In reviewing fieldwork itself, one begins with the library, for much in the way of earlier observations has been put to good use by historians, anthropologists, and occasionally ethnologists and epidemiologists. The emphasis in the early observations, and necessarily on current work utilizing such sources, has been on mind-altering drugs that either had or were thought to have so marked an effect on behavior or so strong a therapeutic potential that people on the scene were moved to write down what they saw happening. The use of such substances has been consistent, for they have usually been employed at first for medical (including folk medical) and/or religious purposes and have afterward become "social" drugs in the sense that their use has become less ceremonial, more secular, and perhaps more individual or private. The frequency with which drugs known from early times are described varies of course with the literacy of the period and the adequacy of records, with the availability of the drug itself, and the size of and the impact upon populations employing it. Much has been written on alcohol, opium, tobacco, coca, and cannabis. A few historical studies have attended to coffee, khat, mandrake, and the natural hallucinogens. For the most part, synthetic drugs have been so recent that their study becomes part of direct scientific observation rather than the subject of historical review; exceptions are Grimlund (1963) on analgesic use in a Swedish factory town and Connell's (1965b) brilliant description of the epidemic of ether drinking in Ulster in the late eighteenth century. To mention but a few among other historical studies there are De Monfried (1935) on the hashish trade; Laufer, Hambly, and Linton (1930), Corti (1932), and Laufer (1942a, b) on the diffusion of tobacco;

Youngken (1957) on *Rauwolfia serpentina;* Lubbock (1933) and Owen (1934) on the opium trade; the erudite Burton (1910) on coffee; Loeb (1943) on intoxicants in relationship to agricultural technology; and, among the most insightful of hundreds of travelers' reports, there is Wissman's description (Wissman, von Wolf, and von Mueller, 1883) of the political and military aspects of the introduction of cannabis to the Congo Baluba. Blum and Associates (1969a) have described the events most commonly associated with the diffusion and acceptance of, and the resistance to, social drugs. Historical analysis, both of the distant and recent past, suggests to some investigators the nature of present trends in drug use and offers a basis for predicting what kinds of use will be most common in the near future. One thing that historical analysis reveals is that abuse as such is a recent concern.

It seems possible that the relative recency of emphasis on abuse is a function of increased secular as opposed to ceremonial use of drugs (this in association with the industrial revolution and with colonization). The volume of descriptive writing about drugs has been much greater in recent times, and rising humanism and sophisticated notions of interdependent community welfare have led concurrently to the definition of social problems as such. In any event, the use of historical documents can lead to descriptions of relationships between drug behavior and other social variables that can be put to the test in contemporary observation.

Connell's work on Irish ether-drinking may be used as an example of the historical-epidemiological approach (Connell, 1965b). He describes the increased availability of ether when manufacturers in England produced it as an industrial solvent. At the same time as the price of ether was falling, alcohol itself was the subject of increasing criticism by temperance campaigners, and it was becoming more expensive. As legislation and agrarian advance reduced illicit alcohol distillation, Irishmen accustomed to homebrew were looking for a substitute. Imported ether soon came to be distributed to doctors, druggists, hawkers, bakers, and others, although tavern keepers themselves were reluctant to handle it because its low cost brought little profit. The Ulster area, where ether use became most prevalent, had been the object of heavy temperance campaigns, mitigated by the willingness of a leading temperance worker to take reformed drinkers to physicians who would sell ether to the thirsty. The area was also the home of repatriates from Glasgow, who had learned there the reputation of ether as preventive and remedy against cholera. They taught its general use as a folk remedy. Connell concludes that epidemic use of ether was a consequence of its availability, of its prior acceptable use (in folk remedies and by prestigeful persons), of its appeal to manliness (a hot and volatile drink), and of the strong need felt for an intoxicant by those thousands suffering a homebrew loss. Following this epidemic use, there was a reaction against its use at all; church and government cried, "Abuse!" and proclaimed that terrible things were happening, although physicians did not report many actual untoward consequences. The alarmists carried the day: and within a few years legislation, priestly denunciation, government control of commerce, and the rising fortunes of the local folk who could once again afford a tastier brew combined to suppress ether-drinking.

CONTEMPORARY STUDIES

Connell relied on historical documents: but an investigator interested in use of drugs by a contemporary group can look at that group directly. Typically, the behavioral scientist or epidemiologist with such an interest defines his population either in terms of a particular drug or in terms of a particular group. If a drug, he must engage in case-finding and case identification and construct his sample from the results of his search. The search itself may rely on cases already identified by physicians, other medical agencies, and the like; it can employ survey methods in populations suspected of harboring cases; or it can move down a chain of cases following either lines of introduction ("infection" by analogy with parasitic illness) or lines of acquaintance ("exposure"). If studying a group that is using drugs, rather than identifying cases of a particular drug's use, the investigator does not need to identify cases from a larger population, thereby constructing a special sample of interest. Instead he must identify a naturally occurring group whose members engage in the behavior in which he is interested.

POPULATIONS USING SPECIFIC DRUGS

An excellent example of the case-finding approach is the work of Chein, Gerard, and colleagues (1964), who sought out New York City youngsters who were using heroin and compared them with delinquents who were not using heroin and with nondelinquents, all groups being drawn from the same area. Work on a smaller scale with special populations defined and sampled on the basis of their use of a particular drug has been done on nitrous-oxide sniffers (Danto, 1964), glue and gasoline sniffers (Sterling, 1964; Ackerly and Gibson, 1964), amphetamine users (Brown, 1963), hallucinogen users (Ludwig and Levine, 1965), and numerous other groups. Perhaps the cases most often studied are alcoholics. The work of Knupfer and Room (1964) is an example. With the advent of popular marijuana use, a number of studies have sought out young marijuana users in the United States and Canada (Commission of Enquiry into the Non-medical Use of Drugs, 1970; National Commission on Marijuana and Drug Abuse, Washington, D.C., 1972). These studies are probably second in number to alcohol case findings. In Scandanavia, the focus has been on stimulant users (Martens, Netz, and Sundwall, 1967, Narkotikaforskning, 1970; Ahrens, Kihlbom, and Nas, 1969).

To illustrate the development of samples drawn from a population of drug users, the splendid work of McArthur, Waldron, and Dickinson (1958), comparing smokers and nonsmokers, and of Stevenson (1956), comparing criminal narcotic addicts with several other groups, will be briefly described. McArthur and his colleagues followed Harvard undergraduates who had been carefully studied for a number of years. They identified those who, as adults, were non-smokers, those who were smokers, and those who were heavy smokers. They also identified those who reduced smoking after having used cigarettes. This longitudinal study was able to compare childhood-rearing practices, family background, socioeconomic circumstances, student interests and personality, and student drug habits (alcohol and tobacco) with later smoking habits, the latter gathered through follow-up procedures.

There were many important findings: for example, family and subcultural background was closely related to later smoking behavior, as were sociability and personality. Anxious men became heavy smokers, but only if the habit was established under pressure of other influence: anxiety itself did not initiate smoking. Those who smoked tended to be more sociable; heavy smokers had more personality disorder. Sociability was not related to cessation of smoking; personality and the amount smoked were. Alcohol use and smoking habits were related. In this study, it was found that social and personality factors associated with the initiation of drug use differed from those associated with the later intensity of individual use or with those associated with likelihood of continuing or stopping. That is not an unusual finding. Factors associated with exposure to, let us say, illness can be different from those associated with susceptibility or with the course of individual symptomatology, and these in turn can be different from those defining the treatment methods to be employed or the response of the illness to treatment. It is well to keep in mind that behavior data and time-sequence data must be carefully ordered in social psychopharmacology; that is, one must be careful to identify clearly what phase of drug behavior is being related to other variables.

A study in British Columbia matched addicts with nonaddicts on background, sex, age, race, intelligence, and education (Stevenson, 1956). Techniques used included historical document analysis, psychological tests, psychiatric interview, observation, institutional records, and so forth. In addition to comparing addicts with abstinent former users, with medical addicts, with nondelinquent siblings of addicts, and with nonaddicted delinquents, the investigators used regional and personal historical materials to trace the development of narcotic use in British Columbia and to outline drugs transmission routes. Among many important findings were those reporting that addicts had been criminals before use and that their initiation into heroin use had been part of a close relationship with an older user. In contrast, nonusers had less exposure to the drug and had more information about bad effects. Heroin use was more intensely associated with the kinds of association made by the group than with personality defects, although hedonism, aimlessness, heavier alcohol use, and promiscuity more often characterized users before drug initiation. Even though the addicts tended to use heroin as a "total solution" to personal difficulties, 24 percent of the addicts had spontaneously abstained from use for a year or more, primarily because of difficulty in obtaining drugs. The investigators relate individual narcotics use in British

Columbia to the facilitating cultural setting, calling attention to earlier Chinese opium-smoking, the existence of the frontier ethos, and immigration by unstable adventurous males. The work pattern of seasonal labor as well as those attracted to such work was believed to lead to unemployment and then crime and that in turn to prison and acquaintance with older criminal addicts who taught new-comers both heroin use and the criminal activities necessary to engage in the habit. The authors note that the heroin problem is a minor one in contrast to alcohol abuse—an important point made by others, but often overlooked when assigning priorities to drug research and social legislation.

DRUG-USE CORRELATES IN NORMAL POPULATIONS

Samples selected from populations of special interest need not be limited to drug-dependent persons or their nondependent cohorts. One may be interested in the drug behavior, or in correlates of such behavior, in a normal population. If so, sampling follows typical survey research designs. Jeffreys, Brotherston, and Cartwright (1960) studied drug consumption in an English housing development. They found that two out of three persons took nonprescribed medication, that women did so more than men, that those self-prescribing more frequently also used their physician more often, that first-born and children in small rather than large families received more medication, that mothers who were themselves high-frequency self-medicators gave more to their children, and that "nervous" mothers (self-described) were more frequent self-medicators.

Ahrens, Kihlbom, and Nas (1969) found that parents of children who were using or were predisposed to using cannabis self-medicated more. Smart (1971) in Canada has similar data. As Kihlbom notes (personal communication, 1973), as an alternative to the inference of parental teaching or children's learning, copying, or identifying, it may be that the "nervousness" feature was common to both parents and children predisposing both to self-medication whether through licit or illicit channels.

In the United States and Canada, arising from concern over youthful drug abuse, there has been a spate of descriptive studies of the drug use and correlates among high school and college students (Berg, 1970; Smart, 1971; Blum and Associates, 1969b). These find, in general, that more common forms of use are correlated with family income and education, with liberal political stance, with liberal arts rather than physical science academic majors, with less rather than more club or organizational membership, with less conventional career goals, and the like. Ill effects from such drug use are found to be unusual (whether illness or arrest), and the distribution of use follows a log normal curve (there is no clear-cut division of the population into users and abusers). Existing laws are ineffective as deterrents (among users) and users do not view their conduct as criminal.

Drug use tends to be multiple; that is, users of one illicit drug have greater likelihood of trying another one than nonusers; furthermore, the use of approved social and medical substances correlates with the use of disapproved (illicit) substances. Most 1972 data show an increase for regular illicit use of marijuana with continued spread downward by age and across social classes.

A pilot population study (Blum and Associates, 1969a) later confirmed by the more adequate sampling of Manheimer, Mellinger, and Balter (1969) examined patterns of mind-altering drug use in a quota sample drawn in two California cities. The study attempts to link frequency of drug experience, variety of drugs used, and variety of purposes for which they are employed to personal and social factors. Findings suggest that illicit or exotic drug use is closely related to greater-than-ordinary experience with licit drugs, that the most unusual pattern of drug experience is abstinence from all centrally active drugs (including alcohol and analgesics), and, as in other studies, that in spite of relatively high incidence rates for illicit use, there is no evidence for the "inevitable link" between marijuana and heroin. (Most heroin users do try marijuana first; few marijuana users try heroin.) Other relationships suggested by this small sample survey are that there is greater childhood exposure to medication, more gratification from being sick as a child, more repressive and discordant childhood handling of emotion by parents, more childhood eating problems—and more adult ones—among the sample with more drug experience. In addition, people with high drug experience reported more cravings for ordinary food and drinks, more fear of becoming dependent, more fear of being exploited because of drug use, and more feelings of guilt and social vulnerability about drug-use habits. Frequent drug experiences as such appear to be associated with curiosity, sensitivity to peer-group pressure and encouragement, self-exploration, and suicide risk. In terms of background, frequency of drug experience was associated with youth, religious uncertainty, and higher educational levels.

INSTITUTIONAL POPULATIONS AND INSTITUTIONAL STUDIES

Special populations have also been subjects for research: they include medical and psychiatric patients (Downing and Rickels, 1962; Satloff, 1964); volunteers for experiments (Lasagna and von Felsinger, 1954); institutionalized addicts (Wikler, 1953; Kolb, 1962); institutionalized criminals (Fabing, 1957); and so on. These populations are sampled during routine contact, at which time the psychopharmacologist may wish to relate either their past or present natural drug use or their subsequent behavior to some social, personal, or physiological variable by means of natural observations, interviews, tests, and the like.

He may wish to exploit the client's presence by engaging in controlled observations of social phenomena, as, for example, during clinical trials (Cahn, 1953; Uhlenhuth, Canter, and others, 1959; Marks, 1963; Joyce and Swallow, 1964). Raskin's (1961) study of medication-taking behavior is an example. Patients in psychotherapy were described in terms of whether or not they took all, some, or none of the psychoactive drugs prescribed for them. The attitudes of "resisters" were then studied. These patients were also found to be resistant to psychotherapy as well as drugs, to be better educated, more knowledgeable about psychiatry, to have less favorable views of their physician, and—in the eyes of raters—to be less likable. The patients perhaps agreed, describing themselves as hostile. The study shows how drug-taking as well as drug reaction is an important area for investigation, and it links response to attitudes, relationship, and personality. In doing so it obtains results consonant with others on patient cooperativeness (E. M. Blum, 1958).

For a more complete picture of the sequence of actions that lead to taking a drug, it is also necessary to study the man who prescribes the drug and the institution in which he works, for both institutional and personal characteristics have been shown to influence prescribing behavior (Klerman, 1960; Pearlin, 1962).

Considering what goes on in medical practice as an institutional study, in this sociological sense, one finds that prescribing varies with physician speciality, age, and point in time of training (Cooperstock, 1971), with the nature of the relationship between doctor and patient (Balint, Hunt, and others, 1970), on the doctor's nervousness and inexperience (Appleton, 1965; Mendel, 1967), and on the sex and age of the patient (unrelated to illness) (Levine, 1969; Shepherd, Cooper, and others, 1966). The doctor's own licit drug use and belief in the efficacy of pharmaceuticals also is associated with the rate of both prescribing and recommending over-the-counter drugs (Blum and Wolfe, 1972) and doctors' heavy use of drugs is in turn predicted by their psychological health as youths (Vaillant, Brighton, and McArthur, 1970).

These findings suggest that the rates at which physicians prescribe psychoactive drugs vary considerably. Insofar as one might wish to introduce greater rationality into the distribution of drugs that are under control, that is, making the control that is implicit in classification schemes more systematic within medical practice, it is evident that much work with physicians and patients remains to be done.

Investigation of an institution and its staff, in order to learn more about prescribing habits, attitudes communicated to patients by physicians to alter drug impact, and the role of psychoactive drugs in affecting patient behavior in an institution, represents a slightly different type of study. Instead of sampling from a flow of clients over time, or every Nth person in an institution, one begins to look at whole groups or institutions as such. This method, which is that of the study of social systems or natural groups, is used by social psychiatrists, social psychologists, anthropologists, and epidemiologists. Each of these disciplines has contributed to psychopharmacological knowledge. Such studies are illustrated here.

Klerman (1960) investigated staff attitudes, decision-making, and the use of drug therapy in a mental health center. He found that older physicians, especially those with administrative duties, favored drug therapy, whereas younger doctors were opposed to it. Attendants and practical (qualified) nurses were in favor because drugs reduced disturbed or trouble-making behavior. Staff workers with psychotherapeutic orientations were most resistant to the use of somatic treatments, including drugs; physicians in this group felt guilty when giving drugs. Psychologists and social workers were opposed to drugs, partly because of their own inability to prescribe them (Klerman says they were in competition with the psychiatrist for status) and partly because of psychotherapeutic leanings. The people who were most in favor of drugs also had the least tolerance for disturbed behavior—and were those whose jobs required them to have the most contact with the patients least like themselves, saving the younger, brighter, and better-educated patients for psychotherapy.

The latter finding is much in keeping with one from a major study of differences in treatment given by psychiatrists to persons of differing economic status; Hollingshead and Redlich (1958) found that psychotherapy was primarily given to higher-status patients, somatic therapies to lower-status ones. An additional variable affecting choice of therapies was the background of the psychiatrist himself; those favoring somatic and directive treatments were more often from Old American families, made more money, married women from backgrounds like their own, and so forth, whereas psychiatrists preferring analytic and psychological treatments were much more often from relatively recent immigrant (Jewish) backgrounds, made less money, had mixed marriages, and so forth. Pearlin (1962) reaches conclusions similar to those of Klerman; personnel emphasizing control and docility of patients were in favor of drugs; those interested in interpersonal relationships were against. One staff faction might be said to have seen tranquilizers as reducing their own work problems, those of managing patients; the others as reducing their work pleasures in alert personal exchanges.

CASE HISTORY AND SOCIAL CONTEXT OBSERVATIONS

The chain of events that leads to a drug effect in a patient does not begin with the hospital itself; it may be said to begin with the events that lead a person into one or another channel for care. The natural history of distress, its alleviation, and the subsequent drug experience become the object of interest. Some patients will seek medical help; others will prescribe for themselves; still others will ignore their symptoms. Given the evidence that symptom exacerbation or decisions to seek medical care are associated with stressful interpersonal environmental events, and not only with pathological changes in tissue (Hinkle and Wolff, 1957; Caplan, 1961; Zola, 1964), the scholar interested in tracing the full sequence of symptom-defining, role-assuming, care-receiving, drug-taking, and drug-impact events finds himself looking at the individual in the whole community in work, family, and peer-group settings. In company with community psychiatrists, public health workers, sociologists, and others, the perambulating psychopharmacologist will want to know what makes people hurt, what they do about it, and what happens as a result. He may very well wish to undertake studies of the use of drugs in these nonmedical environments; studying, for example, home remedies, or the diffusion of prescription drugs through nonprescription channels.

GROUP LIFE

Many revealing studies of natural groups have provided insight into how drug use and effects are imbedded in and consonant with other features of life, be that life in a primitive tribe, an Indian subcontinental village, a friendship group of American marijuana smokers, or a neighborhood group of heroin users. Alcohol use by Indians of the Guatemalan highland has been observed by Bunzel (1940). In Chichicastenango for example, drunkenness partakes of the sacred and it is through drunkenness that the Indian communes with respected ancestors. The visitor to that village on a feast day may judge "abuse" as he sees inebriated Indians lying on the street, whereas the drinker is fulfilling a familial and religious duty. Alcohol use studied in three Greek villages (Blum and Blum, 1970) shows that food intake patterns were associated with variations in drinking, that notions of manly self-respect and womanly reputation protected against excessive use, that effects contributing to sociability were sought on festival occasions, and that alcoholism itself was rare, given the strength of village and family life. A number of peyote-using tribes have been described (La Barre, 1938; Slotkin, 1956) with an exhaustive study of the Navajo conducted by Aberle (1966). Its findings have been referred to in Chapter Twelve of this book. They show how peyote-cultist drug judgments of effects differ markedly from those of anticult Navajos and that outsiders are in turn divided in assessments. Carstairs (1954) studied two Indian subcontinent villages for differential use of cannabis and alcohol. He discovered that persons committed to active aggressive work and values by virtue of their caste and occupation preferred alcohol and those with contemplative or religious lives preferred bhang. Both specific and nonspecific drug effects were harmonized with group and cultural values.

Drug-using subcultures or groups have been studied in Western society. Preble and Casey (1969) have observed the life of street heroin users in New York City. They find that little of what goes on can be attributed to heroin effects per se since drugs ingested are often dilute and, further, cannot account for the complex "hustle" of these addicts whose involvement "in the life" provides meaning, excitement, work-avoidance, income, and a variety of experiences all of which are drug-related, even drug-centered, but certainly are not due to specific drug effects. Longitudinal study of users is also required for understanding of sequential events, for example, physically dependent heroin users may stop using (drying out) not necessarily because drug effects felt are undesirable but because they are, when there is tolerance, insufficient or because, after drying out one can get the desired effect more cheaply.

Among other group life studies, one must remember one of the first that was simultaneously political, sociological, and psychiatric; that of New York marijuana use in the late 1930s (conducted by Bowman and Jellinek, 1942) for the Mayor's Commission. The commissioned scientific studies on behalf of the U.S. National Commission on Marijuana and Drug Abuse (1972–1973) and the Canadian Commission of Enquiry on the Non-medical Use of Drugs (1970–1972) expand that fine tradition. Some centers of drug use have attracted particular attention, the Haight-Ashbury District in San Francisco being foremost. Dozens of investigations were conducted there in its heyday, from 1966 through 1972, among which are anthropological observations (Weakland, in Blum and Associates, 1969a), psychological examinations (Kendall and Pittell, 1970), psychiatric-neurophysiological research (Blacker, Jones, and others, 1968), survey research (Manheimer, Mellinger, and Balter, 1969), and neurological-psychological child and family studies (Blum and De Tobal, 1972). Canadians have the Yorkville study by Smart and Jackson (1969) and, within a treatment setting, Yablonsky's (1962) observation on Synanon. From these and other investigations one must draw the conclusion that drug involvement is a way of life that is replete with values, styles, and symbols and that is not wisely reduced to metabolic processes or drug effects as such. In such settings, the study of physiological processes can be partly isolated, as Blacker, Jones, and their colleagues (1968) accomplished with such distinction in their laboratory, but what emerges impressively are the relationships among various levels of functioning, from neurophysiological to aesthetic. If there is a message for drug classifiers to be derived from the richness of such group enquiries, it is to be aware of reductionism or notions of single causes or uniform reactions.

H. S. Becker's (1953) early studies of musician marijuana users emphasized the importance of learning over time how to use marijuana in order for any effects to occur, that learning process consisting of the communication not only of smoking techniques but also of an interpretation of experiences and a language of sensation. Becoming "clean" can also be a symbolic exercise to demonstrate self-control and to deny dependency. (That can be seen in alcoholics and tobacco smokers as well.) Resumption is justified on the grounds that "it is so easy to quit." Longitudinal study also provides understanding for sequences that alternate drugs with differing specific effects, for example, persons "strung out" on stimulants (uppers) will begin taking barbiturates or opioids (downers) to achieve rest or sleep (R. Smith, 1971; Bentel and Smith, 1971), thereby beginning a cycle of up-and-down drugs.

It is not to be assumed that anticipation of drug effects accounts for all typical sequences of use over time. As Becker and others have noted, the reasons for beginning use are different from those for continued use. Furthermore the reasons for resuming use after discontinuation may involve still other elements. For example, a study of LSD users (Blum and Associates, 1964) showed how initiation into use was precipitated by an association with prestigeful persons who were already using, by positive information about drug effects, the existence of anxieties and depression for which the person thought himself responsible (and thus personally correctable by drug ingestion), and the presence of introspective trends. How people responded to initial use depended not only on dosage but on the setting. Institutional administration, as in medical experimentation, rarely led to euphoria, mystical experiences, or insights; administration in a religious setting was likely to lead to (being interpreted as) religious experiences, whereas use in a social-party setting more often was experienced as aesthetic and pleasure-giving. Those who continued to use the drug felt they were performing well or becoming better people, although their families or employers were likely to render a less optimistic evaluation of effects. Those who discontinued did not like loss of control or were responding to pressures from families or employers. Of particular interest in terms of subjective effects was that those who continued LSD did not claim it eliminated their emotional distress but that they felt it almost or nearly did (what the investigators term *presque vu*)—a sensation close to that reported by humans with electrodes implanted for self-stimulation of the brain who stimulated themselves not because they were fully satisfied but because the sensation was one of a promise of fulfillment.

A recent work focuses on professionals and academicians who use marijuana (Goode, 1970). The emphasis here is on the recreational potential of that drug, a pleasant aside in life but not a dominating interest. That recreational use is what Zinberg and Robertson (1972) speak of when they note that being a user is not a dominating characteristic for users themselves but may be for observers; that is, what the user does incidentally is considered by those who know of his use as the main characteristic for judging him. The user enjoys a pleasant but peripheral experience, like a cocktail hour, but the disapproving nonuser stereotypes the user as a "pothead," and may believe him to be criminal or disabled. As Becker observed, both user and nonuser seek justification and support by joining with others who share their views; and both sides, ethnocentrically, view themselves as wise and right and think others are engaging in dangerous behavior or prejudiced thinking.

OCCUPATIONAL GROUPS

Studies of drug effects and use by students are observations on people holding particular social roles. It can be particularly helpful to look at what holders of particular roles believe, do, and experience when that occupation is of special importance in drug distribution or control. Illustrations of such occupational studies may be found in investigations that focus on the drug distribution practices of physicians in relationship to their own drug use and beliefs as to the power of pharmaceutical preparations (Blum and Wolfe, 1972), in studies of narcotics law enforcement officers (Skolnick, 1966; Blum and Munson, 1972; Blum and Wahl, 1964), in observations on pharmacists (Blum and Smith, 1972), on legislators responsible for drug laws (Blum and Balbaky, 1969), and on illicit drug traffickers (Blum and Associates, 1972b). Studies of educators' views on drugs and features immunizing them from illicit trafficking are available (Blum and Wahl, 1964; Martinez, Ross, and others, 1972), as are some bearing on the recommendations of community leaders vis-à-vis drug policies (Blum and Associates, 1972a).

In the study of physicians, it was found that their prescription practices, own self-medication, narcotics records control in their offices, beliefs as to public drug control, and views on the efficacy of pharmaceuticals were interrelated. In this sample, in which 16 percent admitted to self-administration of narcotics and 28 percent had tried marijuana, it was found that an overall measure of drug effects, that is, the belief that pharmaceuticals were powerful forces for harm or health, correlated with the strictness of controls recommended, including restraint in prescribing. Physicians who believed that drugs did not have, in general, much potency tended to recommend their use and not be concerned about nonmedical (unsupervised) social and private use. Control-oriented doctors believed in the power of drugs, believed in the power of physicians to control drugs, and believed that society's power ought to be employed in controls beyond medical practice. Were these findings to be replicated, one could suggest that there is a fundamental position vis-à-vis the power in drugs that is associated with a fundamental position regarding the desirability of controls and the central role of the physician in that control. If that be so, then physicians at least have a general view of pharmaceutical efficacy that underlies much of their implicit—if not explicit—evaluation of drug-effect data and of classification and control schemes.

Findings (Blum and Associates, 1972b) from a very different occupational group, California drug traffickers, also yield data on drug effects. For example, most of this sample had used most of the illicit drugs available, but the one that had first worried them the most as to their own inability to control their use or reactions was alcohol. Although most had used heroin and other opioids, only a minority felt they might be dependent on it. (This is compatible with other findings to the effect that street heroin use does not inevitably lead to dependency on it.) Although most were aware of ill effects experienced by customers and colleagues as a consequence of drug use, few quit using or selling for that reason; and, overall, the majority held that drugs did more than damaging things for those who employed them illicitly. There were differential evaluations of course; marijuana was rarely indicted as dangerous whereas heroin was often so indicted.

Dealer studies also yield information on the impact of the criminal law. Although the risk of arrest to a regular drug dealer in California is quite small in any one year, those who continue in the life are likely to be arrested, especially if they come from lower-class backgrounds and use/sell opioids. Arrest does deter some from dealing, although deterrence is not permanent. Many of those in jail intend to deal upon release. On the other hand, among those who were dealing, there was often unhappiness with their lives, which led many to at least contemplate quitting. Fear of arrest and the criminal milieu were major contributing factors. Those who were dealing most successfully, or were in the relatively invulnerable group of middle-class marijuana and hallucinogen dealers, seemed least likely to want to quit because of the fear of arrest and imprisonment. Some of these dealers, however, could be expected to quit spontaneously as they became older and as family and group middle-class values argued against their continuing an illicit career.

CONTROL IMPACT

Studies of the impact of existing or planned public action programs can guide policy-makers. The foregoing work with dealers shows that the criminal law is but partially effective in control; studies of nondealers show that conventional morality and being part of a law-abiding environment give most support to internal controls over drug-taking, not the fear of the law. Indeed, studies on how police departments operate (Blum, Gordon, and Egan, 1973) make it evident that even when there is strong public pressure for enforcement, only a minority of users and dealers may be at risk of arrest. Review of their cases shows that, in spite of statutes calling for stiff penalties, few dealers will ever serve long terms in prison. If they do go to prison—or juvenile detention centers—some may continue dealing behind prison walls. Inside the prison, drug traffic takes on special significance as a symbol of opposition to and autonomy from the authorities. In that way, prisoners are recruited to use and traffic. Kaplan's (1971) is the most extensive analysis of the consequences of the criminal law. His work, limited to marijuana laws in the United States, concludes that the costs of that law far exceed the benefits, given current conditions of widespread use and the inability of enforcement endeavors to punish more than a very few offenders. Although many crimes other than marijuana offenses are characterized by a very low ratio of arrests to violations, Kaplan argues that the marijuana laws have the added costs of affecting in socially undesirable ways the distribution system for the drug.

Intervention by treatment is another favored control procedure, whether offered voluntarily or required involuntarily. There are extensive studies of alcohol treatment programs. In general, if treatment goals are limited to improvement rather than total "cure," such treatments do succeed in the majority of cases. In spite of strong advocacy of one or another school or style of alcohol treatment, the evidence suggests that all are about equal in their effects. This applies to compulsory treatment as well; it appears as successful as voluntary treatment. Evaluations of treatment efficacy with drug users, mostly heroin addicts, since these are a group most likely embraced by the medical model of the ill person, are very limited. Analyses of posthospital careers of users released from the U.S. Public Health Service hospitals show that most return to drug use upon release. The rate of return varies greatly with the patient's previous history; the general rule is that those who were most conventional and mature before admission do best upon release. That rule applies to many forms of intervention, be these psychotherapy, prison, juvenile detention, or the like. More recent studies of the now popular methadone maintenance programs suggest a considerable degree of success for older addicts. (Spiegel and Sells, 1973). However, drug use cannot be a pure measure since methadone is itself an opioid that has dependency liability. As for illicit drug use, this does appear susceptible to reduction by methadone programs, apparently depending upon the age and class background of the patient. Fujii (1972), using economic criteria alone and accepting treatment evaluations as presently available, concludes that methadone maintenance is, in the United States, the best method for the price.

Such restricted economic analysis emphasizes immediate costs and gains including those of treatment, employability, and reduced criminality. It does not embrace some of the broader debates about methadone maintenance programs in which costs are linked to the duration of maintenance, the diversion of methadone into the illicit marketplace, and the possible suppression of recovery through maturation and abstinence generated by nondrug treatment. As with other new treatments with new kinds of patients or clients, evaluation is one step behind changing times, and its results undergo continual revision. Today one finds this empirical uncertainty reflects in arguments about methadone that necessarily occur when data are inadequate and when emotions run strong. One should not, under these conditions, despair of the use of evaluation research but, to the contrary, seek to make it more rapid, more systematic, more comprehensive, and obligatory.

In the United Kingdom, Hawks reports (1971) on heroin users there, including follow-up on their treatment under the British heroin maintenance system. Unlike the situation in the United States, crime is not a significant correlate of such use (although delinquent backgrounds may be). Since heroin maintenance does not aim for abstinence, the choice of measures of success and failure is limited. The data to date show that heroin users—even if maintained in a medical setting where ample care for other ills is available—have a death rate 28 times normal for their age. A follow-up showed that sepsis, overdose, and suicide were the most common causes of death. If the goal of treatment is to cherish life, it cannot be said that the heroin maintenance program is a success, although there is no control population to allow one to say that such a program is worse than alternatives. If the goal is to accede to the user's wishes, providing ample care if and when he wishes to use it, and to avoid the development of criminality and drug traffic in association with addiction, doing all of this at very low cost and with a minimum of public concern or governmental attention, the United Kingdom heroin treatment outcome may be considered a success. As with all other measures, outcome evaluation depends upon the criteria employed and the values and interests of those judging. Tinklenberg (1973) has provided a general review of the findings regarding both treatment (medical or social) and penal interventions with American drug users.

PREVENTION: INTEGRATED USE AND CONSUMPTION REDUCTION

In considering preventive efforts, one must be aware of a range of theoretical as well as practical alternatives. For example, a long history of work in the field of alcoholism has led scholars to conclude that alcohol consumption and its effects are, in essence, controlled by interpersonal factors that operate as part of the social institutions of the family, peer groups, the church, and the like. In consequence, the differences observed among ethnic groups, either in their homelands or as immigrants, show that some (for example, Jews, Italians, and Greeks), are less susceptible than others (for example, Irish-Americans) to alcohol problems. The observed differences have led to proposals that safety in drug use arises from teaching people the proper use of drugs and providing controlled settings for such use. Some postulate that the lack of authoritative teaching and models and the availability of uncontrolled settings (and, of course, thereby uncontrolled dosage and purity of drugs) lead to excess and to unpredictable and adverse outcomes. The implications of this approach, a containment model by means of informal social control, call for family teaching of safe drug use, integrated into mealtimes, festivals, and rituals with the extension that both education and legal controls aim to localize where, how, when and in whose company, and for what purposes drugs are consumed. How much is consumed is not the major issue. Some support for this view comes from geographical studies of alcohol consumption, which suggest that, when northern and southern climates are compared, what matters is not the amount but the circumstances of use and the kind of substance (wine compared with distilled spirits, consumption of which varies by region), for these in turn are associated with lesser or greater problem outcomes. The historical success of the English, detailed by Zacune and Hensman (1971), in reducing their several epidemics of adverse outcomes of spirit use through controlling the time and place of liquor sale and consumption can also be adduced in evidence. Taking such interpretations to heart, advocates of prevention programs for the modern drugs of abuse (in this instance, the illicit use) have argued for forms of legalization that include regulation of sales and education for safe use. The Amsterdam cannabis-sanctioning clubs are an instance in practice as Kaplan's book (1970) is an instance in argument from evidence and theory.

Recently a somewhat different point of view has been offered—Ledermann (1956) in Finland, De Lint and Schmidt (1968) and Smart and his colleagues in Canada (1969 to 1973). The thrust of the original Ledermann finding is that alcohol use follows a smooth curve with no clear distinction, statistically, among social drinkers, heavy drinkers, and problem drinkers. It is a logarithmic normal curve which shows many low-rate users, fewer middle-rate users, and few large-rate users. Data from Australia, Belgium, Canada, Finland, France, Holland, Sweden, and the United States, provide evidence that the distribution of alcohol consumption can be similar from place to place, that consumption is linked to bad outcomes (liver cirrhosis), and, by inference, that in order to reduce outcome problems one must reduce per capita consumption.

The earlier model, the integrated use or sociocultural viewpoint, does not concern itself with volume consumed. It may conceivably encourage increased consumption by giving education on how to use, liberalizing the law so as to provide reduced control over availability and encouraging particular forms of use (that is, wine over whiskey, cannabis over heroin). The two models are clearly in opposition. The essence of the consumption distribution model calls for overall reduction in the use of all psychoactives (because the data show high correlations in the use of one compared with another substance) and, prevention through education to restrain use and control over availability of all substances. Smart (1973) calls attention to the success of prohibition in the United States because liver cirrhosis death rates did go down (his definition of success is hardly that of Kaplan's or others who measure the increase of individual criminality, self-poisoning, and organized crime). Smart cites the Finnish experience (Makela, 1972) showing that an attempt to increase moderation by shifting consumption to wine and beer, facilitated by a 1969 change in the law to allow unrestricted beer sales as opposed to earlier sale only in state-controlled stores led to a 48 percent increase in the rate of beer consumption and no reduction in use of hard spirits. After 1969, the overall curve for consumption showed higher per capita consumption with an increasing proportion of drinkers now consuming enough to pose liver cirrhosis hazards (in excess of 10 centiliter per day). Smart concludes, "Liberalization merely encouraged people to add a new drinking habit to those already held, without getting them to relinquish any of the older ones."

The extension of the alcohol consumption model to the control of current illicit drugs rests on the assumption of the adequacy of the log normal curve as a descriptor of use, on the demonstration of high correlations among different rates of use, on the inability clinically to distinguish predisposing factors of problem users, on the refutation of cultural and geographical observations either showing or presuming equal volume consumption over time among groups suffering diverse effects, on the demonstrability of a variety of adverse effects as a function of consumption per se (regardless of how, how spaced, what form, and so forth), and, of course, on agreement as to what adverse effects are and when they emerge as a function of consumption over time. The implications for policy are quite different, although whether policy formulations can themselves be effective in doing anything more than channeling rather than opposing social trends is itself a question. Smart (1972, p. 12) observes, "What is known of the effectiveness of control by legal means inspires little confidence that planned prevention of drug use is possible." On the other hand, the success of England in controlling the gin epidemics, of China in reducing opium use, of the United States in controlling opium use in the early 1900s suggest that there are certain conditions under which legal controls, probably in combination with other social and economic trends, may be effective. The very fact that some of those same controls, for example, narcotics laws in the United States, did not prevent growing rates of use (during the 1960s and 1970s) although they may have set upper limits on these rates or their duration demonstrates the importance of comprehending the interaction between the criminal law and other features governing drug demand, social and individual conformity to law, and the operation of enforcement.

Given this diversity of opinion one can sympathize with the policy-makers who, listening to "experts" disagree, are impatient with "expert" disagreement and uncertainty. Yet there is no easy out, for the same problems, facts, and interpretations that face the scientist also face the policy-maker, and without that awareness of conradiction, one cannot determine the priorities for fact-finding nor may one, as Mao has written, be able to maximize constructive public action.

EDUCATION

A popular form of prevention is education in the schools. At the moment few studies are available, although thorough evaluations are under way. Swedish studies (Ahrens, Kihlbom, and Nas, 1969) do not indicate a strong impact of classroom teaching. Smart, reviewing other work, writes (personal communication, 1973) that education can affect alcohol consumption; and both Cohen (1973) and Soskin and Korchin (1972) can show that, using involvement not in school programs but in more comprehensive efforts, high levels of illicit use can be reduced. Stuart (1972) in Michigan reports that education in the classroom increased illicit drug use, a finding compatible with California survey work showing increasing illicit use during a period of increasing educational intervention. Woodcock (1973), in England, has analyzed the conditions under which education will be introduced, proposing that education of teachers should occur when illicit prevalence is low but increasing; but that direct education to children should occur only when illicit drug prevalence is very high. Additional work on the conditions associated with various educational outcomes is under way in several countries. In Holland and Australia, such evaluation, Woodcock reports, is wisely preceding the authorization of large-scale school programs. The conflict and uncertainty about education results must rest in part on the conflict among—or absence of goals for—school programs, as well as the failure to match educational methods to the susceptibilities of what are very diverse populations (measured by age, intelligence, anxiety levels, information, drug use habits, and the like) within classrooms. It may well be that greater clarity as to impact will emerge as we see which methods with which goals differentially affect which groups of young people.

CROSS-CULTURAL STUDIES

When someone wishes to compare several cultures with one another to see if certain common conditions are associated with like behavior in quite different settings, he will conduct a "cross-cultural study." The methods for studying each culture, whether it be a nonliterate tribe, a peasant society, or even a technological society, are those employed in any observational field study. The description "cross-cultural" implies that the results of several such studies are examined within a common framework.

There are several cross-cultural studies on alcohol use and alcoholism (Horton, 1943; Field, 1962; Child, Bacon, and Barry, 1965). Child and his colleagues utilized a library collection of descriptions of hundreds of nonliterate societies (The Human Relations Area Files). They first sought variations in alcohol use. Then they set up a classification of predominant kinds or styles and attributes of drinking in these cultures: integrated drinking, the best measure of which is ceremonial drinking; inebriety; hostility associated with drinking; and quantity of alcohol consumed. They hypothesized that the style of drinking would be related to personality in the culture and that personality in turn would depend upon child-rearing practices. Taking the descriptions of child-rearing from the field studies available for all the cultures in which alcohol-use patterns were described, they tested three specific expectations, each linked to the amount of drunkenness in cultures. They anticipated that drunkenness in adults would depend upon child-rearing practices associated with individual conflicts over being dependent, with individual desires for independence, and with the extent to which the individual indulged in unrealistic fantasies (dreams, wild hopes, and the like). They found, for example, that the fact that men are more likely than women to be alcoholics—which was true for *all* societies studied—depends upon these child-rearing variables. Where drunkenness among men is common, the culture emphasizes self-reliance and achievement (independence) and disallows the natural dependency (weakness, getting help from others) that a boy child or adolescent feels. On the other hand, in cultures where dependency needs are indulged in infancy and where nurturance is diffused among children and adults, they found low degrees either of drinking or of drunkenness.

Integrated (nonabusive or non-conflict-engendering) drinking occurs most often in societies with long histories of alcohol use; nonintegrated (individualistic, potentially trouble-making) drinking more often occurs in societies in which drinking has come only after contact with another more dominant culture. High amounts of integrated drinking occur most often in complex societies; high rates of consumption need not be so disruptive. Drunkenness, however frequent, does not necessarily mean that to the members of a society it presents a social problem or that there is drug abuse. It appears that the pattern of use, the values and social forms associated with it, and the attitudes of the group members (and *observers*) are related to what is called abuse. The cross-cultural studies tend to take the view that when individual inebriety or pathological drinking occurs it is related to personal conflict, anxiety, and frustration, which in turn depend at least partly on how children are reared and what special environmental stresses exist.

A different cross-cultural approach is shown in Zacune's (1971) study of the adjustment of Canadian heroin users, a few of whom migrated to England in order to take advantage of heroin clinics there. He found they enjoyed more normal lives there because of legal opioid availability; however, some missed the excitement of the addict hustle and not all followed a lawful life given the opportunity to do so.

Another cross-cutural investigation covers a range of psychoactive drugs, alcohol included (Blum and Associates, 1969a). It utilized the same library of anthropological observations as Child, Bacon, and Barry (1965) and, for nation-states, the reports of nations to the International Narcotics Control Board (INCB) in Geneva. For 247 nonliterate societies it was found that both native and foreign observers cite considerable abuse of alcohol, cannabis, tobacco, and opium. When there are differences between foreign and native observers these are over cannabis and tobacco; few of either foreign or native observers report excessive use of stimulants in tribal societies. Use is most common in tribal societies for social purposes—enhancing or smoothing interpersonal relationships; multiple functions are also common. Stimulants, alcohol, and tobacco are usually only social; hallucinogens are rarely social but often magically and/or religiously employed; opium is most often implicated for private (psychological) escapist purposes. Almost as many societies disapprove as approve psychoactive drug use; restraints are common on hallucinogen and stimulant use; outright opposition is most common for opium. Children are often denied hallucinogens and cannabis. Males primarily use alcohol, hallucinogens, and cannabis; both sexes use opium, stimulants, and tobacco. Persons of lower status more often use alcohol, cannabis, and opium. Levels of drug use are generally related to child-rearing methods, the nature of the environment, food production methods, kind of relationships, and social structure. These data show that abuse is most likely to be judged as present in situations of harsh environment and in which there is class stratification based on wealth and/or occupational status, military glory, and bellicosity.

Shifting to nations that rendered reports to the INCB during the 1960s (only opioid, coca, and cannabis are reported), one finds that reported abuse of those drugs is less where populations are Christian, where there is political activity by interest groups, and where newspaper circulation is high. In general, narcotic abuse, as measured by INCB data and culture characteristics, is associated with status in less rather than more technologically developed nations. If INCB data incorporated alcohol problems and recent data on the prevalence of marijuana, LSD and, amphetamine use in Western countries—given the propensity to equate "abuse" with illicit use—then these findings would dramatically alter.

Reference to the INCB data introduces the problem of the adequacy of existing statistics used in assessing drug use and problems. Almost always when data are gathered through official agencies, they suffer from distortion, for what government agencies count or receive by way of count or reports is likely to be different from statistics gathered from more intimate and/or confidential contact with people. In psychiatric epidemiology for example, the official cases that come to the attention of clinics and hospitals are always far fewer in number than cases of illness, defined by the same psychiatric criteria, that are found if one gets acquainted with each family in a community. Generally, there are consistent differences between those found and those not found, as, for example, in the severity of disorder, in age and sex, in ethnic background, and the like. Using criminological "dark number" studies one finds, as a further example, that more crimes go unreported than are reported and that more offenses are not followed by arrest than are so cleared. The rate varies with the offense—homicide reporting and clearances are considerably greater than for burglaries. If one is counting drug users and relies only on arrest or treatment statistics, one will miss those individuals who have avoided both.

Illustrative are Bruun's (1972) findings on official compared with unofficial alcohol consumption rates. Nonregistered consumption in Norway is estimated at about one-third more than the official estimates; in Finland, about one-fifth more. In rural Greece (Blum and Blum, 1965), official statistics may report no more than a fraction of actual consumption. In the United Kingdom, official counts of heroin users miss those persons who have not yet entered the registry and clinic system (De Alarcon and Rathod, 1968; De Alarcon, 1969). In the United States, even official estimates are at variance; Ball and Chambers (1970) estimate 200,000 heroin addicts, the Director of the Bureau of Narcotics and Dangerous Drugs estimates 500,000. Resting on population surveys of drug-life use rather than on current addict status, one may estimate many more persons with one or more incidents of heroin use. On the other hand, street users cannot be relied upon to report either how much of a drug they are using or even what drug they are taking. J. Smith (1973) shows how laboratory studies reveal that errors in illicit drug "labeling" run as high as 50 percent, especially with regard to contaminants and impurities. Gibbins' (1971) Canadian film documents that doses reported by amphetamine users are not those actually ingested. Such studies as these point to the need to supplement observers' reports with laboratory work when accuracy as to drug and dosage is required.

These diverse estimates and the problem they reflect in counting, when placed against INCB opioid-use information, which shows greater use in underdeveloped countries, can lead to the demonstration of the need for similar data-gathering methods applied internationally if international statistics are to have any utility at all. Internal studies like, for example, those on alcohol use within countries (Lolli, Serianni, and others, 1958; Sadoun, Lolli, and Silverman, 1965; Cahalan, 1970) can be useful in showing regional and biosocial differences. The consistency of variables such as age, sex, urban status, socioeconomic position, and the like, can then be tested cross-culturally (Mercer and Smart, 1972). To the extent that there are constants in drug use and problems across nations by groups sharing the same characteristics, then both the prediction of which groups are likely to take up particular forms of new drug use and which groups are most vulnerable to problem use is made more readily. Such estimates have direct value in planning public action.

COUNTRY STUDIES

Under the press of public concern over youthful drug use several nations have taken stock of their situations. Relying on a variety of data sources, being careful about methods employed, and extending their concern beyond assessment of use and its significance to an evaluation of their laws and the impact of intervention programs, these nations have set the stage for full-scale evaluation of where they stand and where their public policy should take them. Such nation-wide integrated endeavors are termed country studies. These are best illustrated in the United Kingdom by the work of Zacune and Hensman (1971) in the Addiction Research Unit under stimulation from the World Health Organization and with the support of the United Kingdom Medical Research Council. In Canada, the reports of the Commission of Enquiry into the Non-medical Use of Drugs (1970, 1972) are comprehensive. In Sweden the work of the Narcotics Commission and in Norway of the Ministry of Health are in a similar vein. In the United States, several governmental commissions have addressed themselves to drug use and policy, notably the President's Commission on Law Enforcement and the Administration of Justice, 1967, and the National Commission on Marijuana and Drug Abuse (1972). The United Nations Social Defense Research Institute (Rome) (UNSDRI) is encouraging other nations to engage in similar studies so that each nation may evaluate its problems and policies internationally and vis-à-vis international law and collaboration in the light of reality. At present, countries committed to the UNSDRI-sponsored program of self-study and rational policy-planning include Afghanistan, Brazil, Egypt, Indonesia, Iran, Italy, Japan, Lebanon, Mexico, Norway, Panama, Singapore, and Yugoslavia. For an illustration of an excellent extant country study, England, the reader is advised to obtain Zacune and Hensman (1971), supplementing it by Edwards (1971). The Edwards and Hawks WHO paper (1972) is an additional guide.

The inference from the country studies done so far is that societal reactions to drugs have at times been markedly out of touch with events, that certain policies applied to drug control have worked costly hazards rather than notable benefits, but that inspection will also reveal interventions that have succeeded in their goals. That nations have considerable choice in learning to live with drug use becomes very apparent. Such study also assists in the process of forming policy, not simply by providing facts but by introducing notions useful in measuring policies as they are applied, "applying accountancy to examination of drug legislation" as Edwards puts it, following the thrust of Kaplan's (1971) method. Such study also can give rise to reflection on the meaning of terms, the sources of action, the alternatives and the process of judgment. Zacune and Hensman along with Edwards introduce the path to reflection simply and cogently. Policy-makers would do well to attend to what they say and, should a country study be required, to consider their methods.

Benefit–Cost Approach to Evaluation of Programs

Robert C. Lind

XIV

Like many areas of public policy, drug regulation is characterized by the absence of any systematic framework or method for evaluating and choosing policies and programs. Policies are adopted and programs are initiated with only partial knowledge of the direct costs to the agencies with primary responsibility for their implementation and with no knowledge of the indirect costs imposed upon individuals, businesses, and other governmental agencies. Seldom are the basic objectives or purposes specified in operational terms, with the result that the effects of a policy or program cannot be measured and evaluated. Policy making and program selection in the field of drug control are analogous to buying unspecified goods at an unknown price and then not verifying what in fact was received and paid out.

There appear to be two reasons for this lack of professionalism. First, decisions pertaining to the control of drugs are made in a setting characterized by a high degree of uncertainty and widely varying, often conflicting, objectives for control. Because the sources of uncertainty and the motivations for the many competing objectives are not clearly described, it is difficult in debating policy to distinguish conflicts stemming from differences in individual assessments of the probable outcomes from conflicts resulting from differences in objectives or values.

This chapter has benefited greatly from the work of my research assistant, Perry D. Quick, and from the helpful comments of my colleagues in the International Research Group on Drug Legislation and Programs and in particular from the help of my friend and colleague Richard H. Blum.

The second reason for the present state of drug policy is that the tools of modern management science for structuring the analysis of complex decisions made under uncertainty have not been adequately applied. Only recently have economists and systems analysts begun to consider the problem of drug regulation. For the most part, drug use, drug abuse, and drug control have been analyzed from a legal, moral, medical, or sociological point of view rather than that of an economist concerned with the optimal allocation of scarce resources.

Economics and systems analysis can contribute to the evaluation and selection of drug-control policies in two ways: First, the benefit-cost framework of decision analysis can be used to structure the complex and uncertain decisions that face the policy-maker. Second, because many policies involve actions that have both direct and indirect economic effects, economic analysis can be applied to predict the impact and the effectiveness of various controls. The purpose of this paper is to set forth an analytical structure based on modern management science that applies to the field of drug policy and to demonstrate the power of economic reasoning in assessing the impact of various controls.

This framework combines the approaches of benefit-cost and cost-effectiveness analysis with an explicit treatment of uncertainty. It is designed to facilitate rational decision-making by providing a structure within which data, judgments, assumptions, and values can be systematically brought to bear on a decision. The reader should be cautioned that this framework can facilitate rational decision-making but cannot substitute for the decision-maker. It should also be stressed that while quantification plays an important role in the application of this technique, benefits and costs that cannot be quantified are brought specifically into this analysis as intangibles upon which value judgments are made. Therefore, if properly applied, this approach is not vulnerable to the usual criticism that it excludes qualitative and judgmental factors that are often the major determinants of a decision.

This paper is divided into two parts. The first develops a framework for decision-making as it pertains to the setting of drug-control policies and the selection of programs to implement them. This procedure addresses the problems of defining objectives and outputs, of measurement, of developing alternative programs to achieve given objectives, of predicting program performance, of evaluation, and finally of presenting a display of the results to the decision-maker in a way that facilitates his decision. The second uses this framework to establish the questions to be asked and the information required to evaluate the controls established by the Vienna Convention (United Nations Conference, 1971). The purpose of the second section is not to evaluate the Vienna Convention, but rather to show what such an evaluation should include.

SCARCITY AND DRUG CONTROL

The control of drugs requires the use of scarce resources and therefore is in conflict with other activities that compete for the use of these resources. Institutions and agencies with drug-control responsibility require personnel, capital equipment, and other factors of production just as do productive activities that produce housing, wine, transportation, and other good things. In 1970, one state in one country (California in the United States) spent more than $100 million enforcing its narcotics and dangerous drug laws (Etienne, 1970). The use of these resources in the control of drugs means that we must forego the production of others goods and services. Put in financial terms, the resources for drug regulation must be bought and paid for; and the amount spent can be raised only by spending less for something else.

The implication is that drug control must be considered like all other goods that compete for scarce resources, and this scarcity requires us to strike compromises between the amounts of food, shelter, education, drug regulation, and so forth, that we might ideally desire. Because productive resources are scarce and because the control of drugs requires their use, decisions pertaining to drug control cannot be evaluated in moral, legal, or medical terms alone. To do so would eliminate from consideration the constraints placed on society by the limits of technology and resource availability and the fundamental choices that these limitations force upon us.

Drug control, like other things, is not a matter of all or none, but a matter of degree. How much a community will choose to spend on drug control will depend on its wealth and how it values incremental improvements brought about by drug control compared with other goods and services. All other things being equal, the amount that a community will choose to spend on any public program will increase with the wealth of the community. In general, the wealthier we are the more we demand of most goods and services, including those that are publicly supplied. This basic economic premise has important implications for the design of international programs involving countries with widely disparate per capita incomes.

Resource allocation for the control of drugs can be subdivided into the analysis of three separate but mutually interdependent decisions: (1) How much of the resources of various societies should be devoted to the control of drugs, that is, how much money should be allocated to the institutions and agencies that perform this function. (2) How much of this total should go to each of these production units, for example, how much will be spent on treatment centers as opposed to law enforcement. (3) Within production units, how much should be allocated to various tasks, for example, should police attempt to stop the distribution of illegal drugs or to stop the production of such drugs or some combination of both.

The first decision involves contrasting the incremental benefits from increases in the control of drugs against the incremental social costs of obtaining the gains from higher levels of control. These social costs represent the foregone opportunities to produce other goods and services and can be measured in dollar terms. To arrive at the optimal expenditure on drug control, one should increase the amount spent on this activity to the point at which the incremental cost of obtaining an increase is just equal to the incremental benefits. If resources are allocated optimally, the last unit of expenditure in any activity will produce an increment of output the value of which will be the same for all activities.

This condition is fundamental to optimal resource allocation and can be demonstrated in terms of the allocation of resources to drug control. Suppose, for simplicity, that the purpose of a program to control a useful but potentially fatal drug were to reduce the number of deaths resulting from misuse. Further, suppose that by investing an additional $100,000 in the program one could reduce the number of fatalities from misuse by ten. Put differently, for each $10,000 spent, one life could be saved. To answer the question whether or not such an expenditure is justified one would have not only to weigh the $10,000 in cost against the value of a life, but in addition one would have to consider the alternative uses of these funds.

Suppose, for example, that if one spent the same amount on highway safety that twenty-five traffic fatalities could be prevented. This would mean that for each life saved the cost would be $4,000 rather than $10,000. Therefore, if saving lives were the only objective, it would be more cost-effective to invest in automobile safety than in drug control. This is true regardless of the value placed on life. Because at some point there are diminishing marginal returns from expenditure on any given activity, the number of lives saved from additional increments of expenditure would at some level of expenditure decrease to the point where another increment of expenditure for traffic safety would save no more lives than if it were spent on drug control. Only at that point should one consider the drug control program.

This example illustrates two points. First, if the incremental return from one activity is less than from another, resources are not allocated optimally because the total return can always be increased by transferring some resources from the activity with the lower return to the activity with the higher one, for example, in the above case from drug control to highway safety. Second, decisions about drug-control programs cannot be divorced from consideration of alternative expenditures that produce similar outputs or effects. In theory, one must consider all alternative possible uses of the resources in both the public and private sectors of the economy. However, as a practical matter it is often salutary to consider alternatives that are directed to similar ends, such as other public health or law enforcement programs.

Exactly the same points can be made with respect to the allocation of resources among agencies and the allocation of resources to tasks within a given agency, except that the range of feasible alternatives is limited by institutional constraints. Regardless of the return from money spent, an expenditure can be justified only if the return is at least as great as could be obtained by allocating those funds to some other agency or task. Put in economic terms, the opportunity cost of a given activity is the return foregone by not allocating those funds to the next best alternative. Optimal resource allocation requires that every expenditure be cost-effective in that the return from that expenditure is greater than its opportunity cost. This principle is basic to the evaluation of public expenditure decisions including expenditures for the control of drugs. The remainder of this paper develops and demonstrates an analytical procedure for implementing this principle.

BENEFIT-COST APPROACH

The basic tenet upon which the benefit-cost approach to decision-making rests is that in deciding upon any course of action one should consider all the consequences of that action and weigh the desirable consequences, the benefits, against the undesirable consequences, the costs. The basic criterion is that, if and only if the total benefits are greater than the total costs, should a given course of action be adopted. Further, if there is more than one alternative for which the benefits exceed the costs, then one should select that alternative for which the net benefits, benefits minus costs, are the greatest. This criterion is simple and has a strong intuitive appeal. For this reason, it is widely accepted and therefore forms a solid basis for a general approach to decision-making.

That one should weigh benefits against costs in evaluating decisions and choose a course of action that maximizes net benefits might appear trivial and one might expect that in fact existing drug policies and controls were based on such a calculus. While the principle that benefits should exceed costs is indeed simple, the implementation of this principle is, in practice, both difficult and complex. Further, in the field of drug regulation there is very little evidence that policy decisions are being based on a systematic analysis of all the possible consequences.

The application of the benefit-cost principle in the field of drug-control policy requires that policy-makers systematically and explicitly identify the consequences, direct and indirect, of each policy or program considered. Only then can the decision-makers weigh the various consequences against one another and reach an informed decision. While one cannot categorically state that this is never done, there is little evidence that such a procedure is the basis for establishing drug policy, and there is substantial evidence that it is not. The appalling lack of pertinent data and the fact that such data are not being collected for policy-making indicates the absence of systematic analysis. For example, consider the class of controls that make the production, distribution, and use of certain drugs a criminal offense. While the enforcement of these laws has wide-ranging effects, any accounting of the benefits and costs must at least include the direct enforcement costs to the criminal justice agencies, that is, how much was spent by the police, the courts, and the correctional system. Even these basic cost data, which could be collected at reasonable cost, are in most instances not available and are not being collected. A further indication that programs are not being systematically evaluated is that one seldom finds clearly defined policy or program objectives, hence the benefits and costs cannot be explicitly identified or adequately measured.

To make the benefit cost approach fully operational one must solve three classes of conceptual and practical problems: (1) the measurement of benefits and costs, (2) the treatment of uncertainty, and (3) the treatment of time. These problems are discussed in the following sections. In the course of addressing these issues an operational procedure is developed for the practical application of the benefit-cost framework to decisions pertaining to the control of drugs.

IDENTIFICATION OF OBJECTIVES

The first step toward the measurement of benefits and costs is to identify the consequences of a given policy or program that one would consider when evaluating it. Those consequences that one would value positively, and therefore want more of, are called benefits; those that one would value negatively, and therefore want less of, are called costs. This process of defining the criteria on which to base a decision is that of setting objectives.*

Objectives provide the basis for formulating and for evaluating alternative policies and programs. If the stated objectives are to be useful in the decision process they must represent those things that are valued for their own sake and not for how they might affect the achievement of some other objective. If one chooses an objective that is not valued for its direct effect, but is implicitly assumed to produce or be correlated with some other effect, then programs may be designed and evaluated on the basis of effects that in fact may not produce or be correlated with the real objective. A misstatement of the objectives can misdirect the entire process of formulating and evaluating alternatives for control.

This misdirection can be illustrated with an example. Suppose that one's objective were to reduce crime associated with drug use and that an increase in police manpower was one alternative being considered. To evaluate such an increase one would consider its effect on the level of drug-related crime. Suppose, however, on the basis of an implicit assumption that increased law enforcement would always reduce drug-related crime, the objective chosen was to increase the size of the drug unit. In this instance, the program that assigned the most men to the drug unit would, by definition, yield the greatest benefit regardless of its real effect on drug-related crime. By incorrectly specifying the objective, the decision-maker would exclude courses of action that do not involve an increase in police manpower. Not only would the assumption implicit in this definition preclude consideration of other courses of action, but in this case it could result in choosing a course of action that would increase drug-related crime. The reason for this will subsequently be discussed. The point here is that in defining objectives one should specify those effects that are valued for what they are and

---

* It should be noted that a cost can be considered a negative benefit and conversely. Similarly, a cost corresponds to the negative achievement of an objective so that the process of defining objectives includes the identification of all effects that are either benefits or costs.

not for what they are assumed to produce. In economic terms, objectives should correspond to final outputs and not to intermediate outputs that may be used to produce the final output.

Whenever possible, objectives should be stated in quantitative terms to achieve the degree of specificity required for systematic evaluation. If one is to evaluate a program or policy with respect to a given objective he must be able to determine whether the level of achievement of that objective has increased or decreased as a result of the program or policy, and by how much it has increased or decreased. This essentially requires that the objective be quantified. Clearly, evaluation and quantification are closely related.

Some objectives are easily quantified, for example, it is natural to state a change in the level of drug-related crime in terms of the number of crimes, the amount of property losses, or both. For other objectives it is more difficult. The general procedure for quantifying an objective that is not expressed directly in numerical terms, is to find a quantifiable indicator that is believed to be positively related to the achievement of that objective and to use this indicator to measure the level of achievement. While a complete discussion of the selection and use of indicators or measures of performance is beyond the scope of this paper, it is important to stress that in selecting an indicator one must think carefully about whether it is properly related to the objective.

Consider the problem of measuring the beneficial effects of tranquilizers. Immediately there come to mind a number of ways in which these drugs have made people feel better and lead more productive lives. However, many of these effects take the form of changes in emotional states that may be difficult to quantify. To the extent that these drugs are effective, the debilitating effects of mental or emotional disease will be reduced. In measuring this reduction, one might compute the change in the number of cases requiring hospitalization or the change in the number of patients who are productively reemployed as a result of the introduction of this class of drugs. On the other hand, if there were beneficial effects not highly correlated with these measures, then hospitalization or employment statistics would be inappropriate as indicators for these other effects, and the analyst must find other measures.

Indicators should be selected primarily on the basis of how well they correspond to the underlying objective they purport to measure. At the same time, there may be several indicators with the desired properties so that the analyst has some choice. In such situations, consideration of the availability of data will often determine which indicator is best suited. There are many situations in which the analyst may have to strike a compromise between the degree of correlation with the underlying objective and the availability of data.

Clearly, there may be some objectives for which, because of data limitations or because of inherent problems of quantification, it is not possible to construct a meaningful indicator. In this case the objective should be described qualitatively, making clear those qualitative factors that one values. It will be shown that given such a description, a decision-maker must explicitly or implicitly place a value on these qualitative factors in making a decision.

VALUATION OF BENEFITS AND COSTS

Suppose that the decision-maker has identified and stated the objectives in quantitative terms, with the exception of some objectives that are described qualitatively. In addition, suppose for the moment that the outcome of a control program or policy is known with certainty so that risk and uncertainty do not enter the problem. Then for any program or policy there will be a set of numbers representing its performance with respect to each of the objectives as measured by the appropriate indicator. The problem the decision-maker faces is that different consequences are measured in different units and, therefore, are not commensurable. The decision-maker could simply make a decision based on this display or he could attempt to convert the various consequences to a common unit of measurement, in most cases money, so that the benefits and costs can be compared in terms of this common unit. This task of assigning monetary values to various consequences constitutes the valuation problem. It should be noted before turning to the details of valuation that even if the analytical process were carried to the point of stating the objectives in operational terms, and no further, rational debate and decision-making would be greatly enhanced.

Obviously, if one is to subtract the benefits from the costs they must be measured in a common unit. While in theory any common unit would suffice, as a practical matter benefits and costs are generally stated in monetary units. One reason for this is that the resource costs of a program and some of the benefits may already be measured in terms of money. Second, individuals make a large number of market transactions in which money is the medium of exchange, and therefore they are comfortable in valuing most goods and services in money terms. For this reason it is natural to measure the consequences of a policy or program in the same terms that we value these other goods and services that compete for our scarce resources. For example, if someone were asked what value he would place on reducing the number of heroin addicts by half, and told to state his answer in terms of Mercedes-Benz cars, before answering he would almost certainly convert cars into money before arriving at an answer. Money is in this sense the natural unit of measurement for benefits and costs.

The procedure for valuing benefits and costs is as follows. Suppose a given consequence of a course of action were a benefit; the value of this benefit to an individual would be the maximum amount he would willingly pay for this consequence. If the consequence were a cost its value would equal the amount that individual would willingly pay to eliminate that consequence. For example, if organized crime were a consequence of a system of controls, the value of this cost to any individual would be the amount he would willingly pay to eliminate this crime.

If an individual is acting on his own behalf as a citizen and consumer, then the value he places on costs and benefits will depend on his wealth, his values, and the prices of competing goods and services. If, instead, he is acting in the capacity of a corporate executive or public official, the value he places on benefits and costs will reflect corporate or public objectives as interpreted by him, the resources available to the organization, and prices of other goods and services.

PROCEDURES FOR SELECTION

Once benefits and costs have been valued it is a simple procedure to apply the benefit-cost criterion. While this approach is conceptually sound, there remain some practical problems associated with its implementation. We now consider several different approaches to the application of the benefit-cost approach and evaluate the potential of each for contributing to rational decisions in the field of drug policy.

The first approach is that of *applied decision analysis*. In this procedure, once the problem has been specified, the decision-maker assigns values to the various consequences of each alternative according to his preferences, given the role he is performing. For example, a public official deciding whether to institute a given program would value its consequences according to his perception of public needs, political considerations, and the like. In the formal method of decision analysis, these values are explicitly stated by the decision-maker to the analyst, who then computes the net benefits of each alternative based on these stated values. On the basis of his calculations, the analyst presents to the decision-maker the decision that follows given the values he has set on each of the alternatives' outcomes. Therefore, in this procedure the decision-maker explicitly encodes his preferences into the decision process by stating the value that he attaches to the outcome of each alternative. He then chooses the course of action that maximizes the net benefits of the outcome based on the value he has imputed to each one.

For some decision-makers this is a very useful procedure, but many public officials are not willing to explicitly state the value they place on various consequences of a given course of action. There are a number of reasons for their reluctance. First, if such statements became public, the official would be extremely vulnerable to criticism. For example, an official who did not consider drug use to be a problem would not wish to be on record as placing no value on reducing such use if he knew a portion of the voters held a different view. Second, by stating the value on each consequence of a particular decision, the public official may become committed to a position that may later limit his options if he changes his mind or if he wishes to engage in political bargaining. Finally, any decision-maker might be unwilling to commit himself in advance to a decision based on values that he has put on each of a number of separate consequences of the decision. He may prefer to look at all the consequences simultaneously and then make a decision without going through this process of valuing the individual consequences. For these reasons, many decision-makers, particularly decision-makers in the public sector, are unwilling to go through the process of encoding the values they place on various outcomes and to make a decision based on these value statements.

The second procedure for applying the benefit-cost approach, developed from theoretical welfare economics, traditionally has been called *benefit-cost analysis*. Benefits and costs are not measured by the values of a single decision-maker, as they were in decision analysis, but rather by the sum of the values set by each individual affected by the decision. For example, to compute the benefits from a program that would reduce the number of heroin addicts, one would take the value to each citizen of such a reduction and then take the sum for all individuals.

Measuring benefits and costs in this way is appealing in that, since the members of a community have to pay for drug control or any other publicly financed program, presumably the program is for their benefit. The argument is that unless a public program benefits the citizens it serves more than it costs them, the program is not justified. It is important to note that costs of public programs that fall on private businesses are ultimately borne by the public either as consumers who pay higher prices for goods and services or as owners who share in reduced profits. Furthermore, these benefits and costs should be computed according to how they are valued by members of the community.

The problem that arises is how to estimate the sum of what individuals would willingly pay. In some instances this can be done, in others it cannot. Consider a program to reduce property crimes associated with drug use. The benefits are the reduction in property losses and can be valued in terms of the reduction in the value of stolen goods, on the assumption that society would willingly pay an amount up to the cost of crime to eliminate it. On the other hand, it may be impossible to measure, in terms of the community's total willingness to pay, the benefits from a program to reduce the harmful effects of drug abuse on the users themselves.

From a practical standpoint, classical benefit-cost analysis has two drawbacks. First, there are many situations in which it is not possible to estimate or infer the community's total willingness to pay. Second, even if benefits and costs could be measured perfectly in these terms, this procedure does not explicitly account for the role of the decision-maker. Seldom will the benefits and costs as seen by the decision-maker coincide with those measured according to classical benefit-cost analysis. In the United States, many well-documented benefit-cost studies have been shunted aside because their implications for program selection have been incompatible with the political interests of the decision-maker or decision-making group. Nevertheless, to the extent the benefits and costs can be measured in terms of the public's willingness to pay, these data can be important, if not decisive, input into the decision-making process.

Next we present the *cost-effectiveness approach,* which combines many of the features of both applied decision analysis and classical benefit-cost analysis.

The primary advantage of this approach is that it is methodologically less rigid and can be tailored to the specific needs and personality of the decision-maker while at the same time maintaining the advantages of both structure and quantification. The basic difference between the cost-effectiveness approach and both decision analysis and benefit-cost analysis is that all benefits and costs are not measured in dollar terms. Typically, resource costs and other costs and benefits that can be easily measured in monetary units will be stated in terms of money. However, other consequences of a program may be measured and displayed for the decision-maker in terms of other units, for example, the reduction of the number of crimes committed or the reduction of the number of addicts. Still other consequences may be stated in qualitative rather than quantitative terms, for example, decreased anxiety that one's child will use drugs. Furthermore, in computing the monetary value of costs and benefits, the decision-maker can use either the decision analysis approach, in which he assigns his own values to these benefits and costs, or he can use the classical benefit-cost analysis in which the benefits and costs are estimated in terms of the community's valuation.

With this approach, the decision-maker is presented a display of consequences for each alternative that includes a statement of resource costs measured in monetary units, a display of other benefits and costs that are measured in terms of nonmonetary units, and a display of qualitative descriptions of other relevant consequences. The decision-maker can then look at the various alternatives and weigh the relative advantages of each to arrive at a decision. It should be noted that if the number of objectives is large, the display before the decision-maker may be both large and complex. When uncertainty and timing problems are introduced, the complexity becomes even greater.

Consider a simple example in which a program of drug control has one objective, namely to decrease the number of drug users, and the decision-maker is considering alternative programs to accomplish this. Suppose the decision-maker has before him the resource costs and the effectiveness measures for each alternative. He must decide which, if any, of the programs should be undertaken, and if one should be undertaken, at what level. In deciding which program should be undertaken, he should choose the program that provides the greatest effectiveness per dollar spent, that is, is most cost-effective. He then must decide whether, in fact, the benefits from that program, in terms of the reduction of the number of users, exceeds its costs. If the decision is yes, then he must still decide on the optimal level of the program. This involves trading the incremental benefits against the incremental costs as described in the earlier section on resource allocation.

Next, consider a slightly more complex example in which the decision-maker is considering alternative programs for the treatment and rehabilitation of addicts. Here he must deal with the multiple objectives of reintegrating these individuals into the community, of reducing the number of users, and of reducing property crime associated with drug use. Further, suppose he chose to measure the reduction of property crime in terms of the reduction in dollar value of property loss and that the reduction in drug use was measured by the reduction in the number of users. The remaining objective of reintegrating former users into society is more complex and has many dimensions. One facet of such reintegration is that the individuals who were rehabilitated would become productive citizens and hold down jobs. Therefore, as a benefit from reintegration he could measure the productivity of rehabilitated users in terms of their earnings. In addition, other benefits from the reintegration of these individuals into the community might be quantified or described in qualitative terms. Finally, there will be the resource costs of each of the programs. Given these data on benefits and costs in both qualitative and quantitative terms, he could compute the net benefits associated with those benefits and costs that are measured in terms of money. For example, he could add the benefits from the increased productivity of the users and the decrease in crime and subtract the costs of the program. Suppose that the costs of the program exceeded the monetary benefits; then this net cost, resource costs minus the benefits from employment and reduced crime, would be the opportunity cost of obtaining the other objectives of rehabilitation. Suppose, on the other hand, that the monetary benefits exceeded the resource costs and that all other consequences of rehabilitation were benefits. Then the total benefits including intangible ones will certainly exceed the costs. The point is that even if some but not all of the benefits and costs can be stated in money terms, it is useful to do so. Such partial measurement can often illuminate the basic choices for the decision-maker.

Of the three techniques discussed, the cost-effectiveness approach described above is probably the best suited to the needs of policy-makers in the drug field. It incorporates the basic structure of the benefit-cost approach and makes use of quantification, but it avoids some of the pitfalls of applied decision analysis. It seems likely that at this stage in the development of drug-control policy, public officials with responsibility for decisions in this field will feel more comfortable with an approach that does not require placing an explicit monetary value on all possible consequences. Two recent studies (Fujii, 1972; McGlothlin, Tabbush, and others, 1972) are excellent examples of how this framework for analysis can be used in the evaluation of alternatives for the control of opiate addiction.

DIRECT AND INDIRECT COSTS

Any analysis for public policy decisions must consider the resource costs of that decision. These certainly include the direct costs required to implement that program. These are the costs to the agencies that have the primary responsibility for implementing a given policy or program. At the same time, there may be substantial costs to individuals, businesses, and other governmental units that result from the program. These indirect costs are as real and as important as the direct costs and should be taken into consideration in making any policy or program decision. This point is especially true in the drug field where various forms of control require that individuals and businesses follow certain procedures, for example, drugs must be prescribed by doctors and prescriptions must be filled by licensed pharmacists. Despite the fact that indirect costs are important to drug regulation decisions, these costs have often not been measured.

The results of any analysis using the benefit-cost framework will also depend upon what group is considered when benefits and costs are computed. Put differently, it will depend upon whose benefits and whose costs will be reflected in the decision. For example, the net benefits to a particular community may be positive if the costs are borne by the federal government, whereas, from a national point of view the net benefits would be negative. Similarly, communities may find programs to be desirable if they ignore the adverse spillover effects on surrounding communities. A law enforcement program in one community may only succeed in displacing crime, rather than preventing it. As a result, crime will rise in neighboring communities. At the international level, a program of controls may produce net benefits from the point of view of some countries and net costs for others. This point is exceptionally important in looking at the establishment and implementation of international cooperation with regard to drug control.

UNCERTAINTY

In the previous section we discussed the measurement of benefits and costs and the use of these measurements in the decision process on the assumption that these benefits and costs were known with certainty. This assumption was made to simplify the presentation. However, in real situations, a high degree of uncertainty surrounds policy-making and program-selecting. It is simply not possible to predict with certainty the outcome of any policy or program. Therefore, the benefits and costs are uncertain: any course of action may lead to a number of possible outcomes, each with a different degree of likelihood.

When uncertainty is introduced, decision-makers must consider all the possible outcomes of a given course of action, taking into account the relative likelihood of each one. The language that has been developed for precisely describing the relative likelihood of uncertain events is that of probability. The probability that one assigns to any outcome is a subjective judgment of the relative likelihood that that outcome will occur. In situations in which one can perform repeated and controlled experiments and in which, in a large number of repetitions, the relative frequency of a particular outcome is a constant percentage of the total number of trials, this percentage can be used as an estimate of the probability of occurrence. However, for most important decisions in life one cannot perform such experiments and must make a decision on the basis of little or no experimental evidence of this type. One must base such decisions on his own subjective judgment of the probability of various outcomes.

It is extremely important for the purposes of policy-making to realize the subjective nature of probability and to understand that no amount of data and no amount of experimentation will establish with certainty that a given outcome will occur or even the probability of it occurring. Such data simply tend to confirm or dispute that certain probability estimates are about right. This is particularly important for the way in which one looks at data. One begins with certain knowledge and beliefs about what a given policy will do. If he is then confronted with evidence that is consistent or inconsistent with his beliefs, this evidence should tend to confirm or modify his beliefs but should not replace all previous information. A decision-maker, therefore, will always be confronted with situations in which he must make decisions on the basis of his beliefs about possible outcomes and these beliefs will always be subjective. However, experience has shown that educated judgments based on knowledge and reason are better than wild guesses.

A comprehensive discussion of the procedures for introducing uncertainty into the formal evaluation procedure is beyond the scope of this paper; however, the basic points to be remembered are that the uncertainty needs to be described and that probability is the language for describing it (English, 1968; Howard, 1966, 1968; Raiffa, 1968). Therefore, decision-makers should accustom themselves to using this language. Second, probabilities for decision-making are the subjective judgments of the decision-maker. Nevertheless, these probability assessments are likely to be better if they are based on knowledge and reason. At the same time it should be recognized that knowledge and reason can reduce but never eliminate uncertainty.

TIME

A further complication is that the benefits and costs of any program are generally spread over time, and the question of timing is significant. Whether or not the benefits from a program are realized now or ten years from now is a matter for serious concern. Similarly, one is not indifferent as to when he must pay the costs. Therefore, the timing of benefits and costs is of some importance, and the question arises as to how to weigh costs and benefits at different points in time. The basic economics approach to this problem is to measure benefits and costs in terms of money and to discount them to their present value using a rate of discount chosen by the decision-maker. As a practical matter, it is often appropriate to use a rate of return on other investments as the rate of discount.

Because capital is productive, a dollar invested today will yield $1 + r$ dollars one year from now, where r is the rate of return that may be earned by any investment in the market. Similarly, if the $(1 + r)$ dollars is reinvested, one will have $(1 + r)^2$ dollars at the end of two years and $(1 + r)^n$ dollars at the end of n years. Therefore, to produce a dollar of income n years from now, one needs only to invest $1/(1 + r)^n$ dollars today. This amount is the present value of a dollar in year n. To compare benefits and costs at different points in time, the standard procedure is to first discount them to their present values and then to compare these discounted amounts.

While this procedure is common in business and finance, it may not be immediately obvious why it is appropriate in analyzing public policy decisions. There are two answers to this question. First, because public investments compete with other investments, it is reasonable to require that funds invested in the public sector yield a rate of return as high as investments yield in the private sector. Otherwise, that money would yield greater benefits if invested in the private sector rather than the public sector. This is, in essence, the comparison one is making when one discounts benefits and costs at the rate earned on other investments, which in free market economies is equal to the market rate of interest. The logic of classical benefit-cost analysis is that one should not collect taxes that could be invested in the private sector of the economy unless the return from the use of these taxes is as great as the return earned on alternatives in the private sector. For economies in which this distinction does not apply, the point is that money should not be invested in drug-control programs if the rate of return is less than the return that could be obtained, say, in steel. This is a straightforward extension of the concept of opportunity cost and the cost effectiveness principle to expenditures over time.

The second reason for discounting is that it provides a conceptually valid procedure for comparing things at different points in time. It should be noted, however, that unless benefits and cost are measured in terms of a common unit, for practical purposes money, discounting cannot be done in a straightforward way. A full discussion of discounting is beyond the scope of this paper, but we stress that as a practical matter benefits and costs that can be measured in dollar terms should be discounted and compared in terms of their present value (English, 1968; Lind, 1968; Krutilla, 1961). This requires at a very minimum that one predict when costs and benefits will occur. The timing of all benefits and costs is a factor that must be explicitly considered in evaluating alternatives.

APPLICATION TO DRUG POLICY

The first step in the rational design and evaluation of policies and programs for the control of drugs is to define the objectives. Without doing this, it simply is not possible to design and evaluate programs on a rational basis. It is difficult, if not impossible, to design effective programs without knowing what it is that one wants to achieve; and similarly, one cannot evaluate whether or not the programs will do what they are intended to do unless one knows the ultimate goals. This is what defining objectives is all about.

It should be noted at this point that the question of classification is closely related to the establishment of objectives. For the most part, we want to control the production, distribution, and use of certain drugs because of the effects that they are presumed to produce on individuals and on society. If our objective is to control the personal and social effects of given drugs, then for purposes of control we need classification schemes that group these drugs according to the known effects of these drugs on people and society as they occur in a real-world environment. For these reasons common classification schemes, like the chemical structure of drugs and the effects of these drugs under laboratory conditions, are of interest from a policy point of view only in so far as they relate to the human and social effects of drug use as it actually occurs, and in particular to the social and human effect that we wish to control.

Given a set of objectives, the next step is the design of alternative policies and programs for the achievement of these objectives. This step is particularly important because unless one develops the best possible alternative, one cannot select it regardless of how sophisticated the criteria for selection. There is a strong tendency in the development of policy alternatives in all fields of public policy for individuals to get locked into narrow approaches to the problem. For example, law enforcement officials are likely to consider programs that involve new legislation and new enforcement powers. Public health officials are likely to think in terms of treatment programs, and the like. It is important in the design phase that the widest range of courses of action are considered so as not to overlook promising alternatives. Even if there are political or resource constraints that make a particular alternative at first appear infeasible, this alternative should not be ruled out in the early stages of the design process. That is the task of evaluation.

Considering a wide range of designs and different approaches is advantageous because in many cases the optimal program design will consist of a combination of several basic approaches. It is, in fact, likely that in most countries a rational drug policy will contain enforcement, treatment, and other components. In designing policies or programs in the drug field one should look for combinations that exploit the complementarity and mitigate the weaknesses of various single approaches to the problem.

Suppose one were considering several alternative programs or policies. Before one can evaluate these policies, it is necessary to predict their outcomes. One way to do this would simply be to make an uninformed guess as to the various consequences of a given course of action. However, the accuracy of such guesses can often be improved by considering relevant data and by using models of economic and social phenomenon.

If one wished to predict the effects of drug education on drug use he should consider previous studies on this subject; and if none were available, he might wish to pay to have such a study performed. A second approach to prediction is to consider a policy in the context of an economic or social system and to make use of a model of this system. For example, if one were to enforce drug laws more effectively and thereby decrease the supply of a given drug, economic analysis can be used to predict that the effect of this policy will be to increase the price of the drug. As will subsequently be demonstrated, economic reasoning can be used in many cases to predict the effects of various programs and, in particular, to demonstrate that many have little chance of success.

The task of predicting the outcomes of various policies is not one that lends itself to a general solution. However, it is useful to discuss briefly some of the reasons why policies fail so that the decision-maker can identify situations in which a given policy may not produce the desired effect. There are two basic reasons for failure. The first is that the tasks set forth by a given program or policy are not carried out; and the second is that even though the tasks are carried out, the completion of the tasks does not achieve the desired objective.

Consider first the reasons why a given task might not be performed. First, the people responsible for performing that task simply may not do their job. This would be the case, for example, if law enforcement officials did not carry out their duties to enforce drug laws. Second, even if the personnel with responsibility for carrying out a given task were committed to doing the job it might be technically infeasible, given the budgeted resources. For example, it may be impossible to stop the flow of drugs across international borders by policing without employing thousands of border police. Another situation in which a program is not feasible arises when there are insufficient resources, at any price, to do the job. This is particularly likely to be the case in the short run where there is a shortage of trained personnel or leadership to carry out a particular task.

Suppose, however, that a task called for under a given policy or program was performed perfectly, it still might be the case that the performance of the task would not produce the desired effects. Three examples will illustrate this point. Consider first the enforcement of drug laws and the reduction of drug-related crime. It is often argued that increased enforcement of drug laws to reduce the illicit flow of drugs will result in a reduction of drug-related crime. Most economists writing on the subject of the economics of drug control have been quick to point out, however, that increased enforcement is likely to cause just the opposite effect, an increase in the amount of drug-related crime (Erickson, 1969; Holahan and Henningsen, 1972; Koch and Grupp, 1971; Little, 1967). The effect of increased enforcement is to decrease the supply of drugs available to the drug user. If the demand for drugs is inelastic, that is, an increase in price will lead to a relatively smaller decrease in the quantity purchased, then a reduction of supply will lead to an increase in the total amount expended on drugs. If, as is generally assumed, drug-related crime arises from the need to support the cost of drugs, then an increase in the total amount spent will very likely lead to an increase in crime to support this expenditure. If one wished to reduce drug-related crime, ideally, he would increase the supply of drugs and thereby lower the price to the user. One of the merits of the British policy of making heroin available to addicts is that it appears to have significantly less crime-related drug use.

This example becomes even more significant when we consider the results of a recent study that estimated the price elasticity of demand for heroin at less than 10 percent (Little, 1967). This implies, for instance, that if the supply of heroin is reduced sufficiently to cause a 10 percent decrease in the amount purchased, there will be a 100 percent increase in the price. This means that although the amount purchased will drop by 10 percent, the amount paid will increase by 180 percent. Now consider this in terms of some actual numbers. It has been estimated that the value of yearly heroin consumption in New York

City is about $500 million. Now suppose a 10 percent reduction in the quantity sold were effected through increased enforcement, then the total amount spent would increase by $400 million. If, in turn, it is true that addicts must steal goods valued at 5 times the amount they pay out in support of their habit, then depending on how much of this increase is financed by property crimes, such a policy could result in an increase in property crimes of as much as $2 billion annually.

Such estimates of demand elasticities and of amounts spent are always open to question because of data problems. However, the basic point illustrated by these numbers is valid even if the numbers were off by factors of 2 or 3. Enforcement of drug laws will significantly increase the amount spent on drugs as well as the crime to support this expenditure.

Consider now a second example. The United States is encouraging other countries to engage in programs of crop substitution. As an economic proposition, it is clear that farmers are going to cooperate with crop substitution only if it is profitable for them to do so. Therefore, in order for the program to be effective, subsidies must be paid on other crops, because if these other crops had been more profitable in the first place they would have been grown. Suppose, however, that as a resut of subsidies to other crops some farmers do switch to these crops. The result of this switch will be a reduction in the supply of the drug-related crop and a corresponding increase in its price. Therefore, an even higher subsidy will be required to produce further crop substitution, and this will be a self-defeating process. Therefore, economists looking at programs for drug control can see immediately the utter hopelessness of significantly reducing the importation to the United States through a program of worldwide crop substitution (Holahan and Henningsen, 1972).

Finally, consider a third example. Suppose that drug abuse resulted from the use of drugs legally produced for medical purposes but diverted to illegal markets. One might suppose that the way to stop such abuse would be to stop the flow of legally produced drugs into illegal markets. One must be very cautious in proceeding on such an assumption because if a market for such drugs for illegal use exists, and if it is sufficiently profitable for someone to supply these drugs, an illegal source of supply will develop when the flow of legally produced drugs has been stopped. This substitution is more likely if the technology of growing or producing a given drug is relatively simple. Therefore, by cutting off the flow of legally produced drugs into illegal markets one may simply create a market for the illegal production of these same drugs, with the result that these drugs will be sold at a slightly higher price but with a very small reduction of use. Furthermore, one may create other problems in that the illegally produced drugs will not meet the same standards as the legally produced ones, and there will be the problem of coping with the illegal industry. To some extent this describes the Swedish experience with respect to amphetamines (Goldberg, 1968).

The last two examples illustrate a basic economic premise that should not be overlooked. Where there is a demand and a profit to be made, a supply will develop. Further, when individuals are confronted with controls that inhibit the achievement of desired ends they make adjustments to minimize the impact of these controls. For example, when certain goods become more expensive or unavailable, people turn to substitutes. With drugs, this usually means using other drugs that are cheaper and more readily available. Such substitution resulting from increased enforcement was recently documented by McGlothlin, Tabbush, and others (1972) in connection with Operation Intercept. If one is to analyze the impact of controls, one must consider these responses. Most controls in the drug field can be analyzed in terms of their effect on the supply or the demand and therefore economic analysis provides a useful, but little used tool for predicting the outcome of various controls.

At this point, suppose that we are considering a number of alternatives and that we have predicted the possible outcomes of each, assigning to each one the probability of occurrence. We can then proceed to use the benefit-cost approach to choose among these alternatives. Alternatively, if one were to adopt the cost-effectiveness approach this would mean developing a display for the decision-maker of the costs and effects of each outcome associated with each alternative and a description of any intangible benefits and costs. The decision-maker would then have before him all the basic data required for the decision. The only problem might be that the number of possible outcomes would be so great that the complexity would be beyond comprehension. In this situation, he might wish to employ the techniques of formal decision analysis. As has been pointed out, the great virtue of quantifying everything in dollar terms is that it is a systematic and sound procedure for reducing a complex decision to a more simple one. Regardless of the exact application of the benefit-cost approach, this process of reasoning from means to ends and of considering the relevant tradeoffs can only enhance policy-making in the drug field.

VIENNA CONVENTION ON PSYCHOTROPIC SUBSTANCES

It is interesting to consider the Vienna Convention (United Nations Conference, 1971) in terms of the framework that has been established. It should be emphasized, again, that the purpose of this exercise is not to evaluate the Vienna Convention. That is far too large a task. It is rather to identify certain costs and benefits and raise certain questions that should be considered in any evaluation. It is also important to note that the proposed Convention is but one in a series of international measures to control illicit drug use. A complete analysis should apply the benefit-cost approach to the entire system of controls both to assess the cost-effectiveness of the system and to assess the burden borne by various countries as a result. Thus while this particular discussion focuses on the application of benefit-cost analysis to the Vienna Convention for purposes of illustration, it should be kept in mind that conclusions reached with regard to the Vienna Convention, when considered in isolation, may be modified if one were to consider the complete control system. This is especially likely in the case of the distribution of costs and benefits among nations.

This analysis must focus primarily on the cost side because the Convention does not state the objectives with sufficient precision to provide a basis for identifying the benefits. While the preamble of the Convention (p. 1) speaks of the "public health and social problems resulting from the use of certain psychotropic substances" and of a "determination to prevent and combat abuse," these statements are not specific enough to determine what, in fact, the ultimate objectives are. This is clear to anyone who has considered the meaning and the use of the term *abuse*.

It can be argued that this lack of specificity is appropriate insofar as the purpose of the Convention is to set up the machinery for international cooperation in the solution of problems related to drugs. Insofar as it serves this function the Convention is like a constitution specifying the rules and procedures by which the solution to specific problems will be agreed upon and implemented. However, it is important to note that the Convention goes far beyond the establishment of such machinery for international cooperation. It spells out in detail specific regulations. Where specific regulations are being considered, they should be considered with respect to their contribution to specific, well-defined objectives. Whether it is appropriate to specify objectives operationally in a document such as the Vienna Convention is a question that is beyond the scope of this paper. However, any individual or government that attempts to evaluate the Convention should do so with specific objectives in mind.

For the purposes of discussion we look at the Convention from the point of view of an individual country considering the question of ratification. Because circumstances in each country are different, it is likely that the objectives will differ from country to country. Rather than posit the objectives of a particular country, the discussion will focus on the cost side of the benefit-cost equation where various classes of costs can easily be identified. A full discussion of possible objectives and benefits itself constitutes a major paper (Lind and Lind, 1972). It should be emphasized that while we have not chosen to speculate about possible benefits, it should not be presumed that they do not exist or are not significant. They may well justify the costs. It should again be emphasized that this section does not presume to be an evaluation of the Convention, but is rather a set of comments directed to those who might perform such an evaluation.

The Convention sets up specific control and enforcement procedures that require action by the various participating governments. Therefore, the first cost that one would estimate is the cost to the government of carrying out and enforcing the provisions of the Convention, including support of personnel, capital equipment, information dissemination, and subsidy programs. It is important to note that, like the benefits, these costs will vary depending on the circumstances of the country. In particular, the costs are likely to be very high for countries that are producers of psychotropic substances. This would include both less developed countries, where drug-related crops are grown, and developed countries with sizable pharmaceutical industries. Therefore, it is clear from the outset that the costs will be distributed unevenly among nations.

The second set of costs are those imposed by the Convention on the manufacturers and distributors of drugs. These costs are primarily for increased drug security, record keeping and other basic transaction costs. For the most part it can be expected that these costs will be borne by the consumers of drugs, although it is possible that some of the costs will be borne by the pharmaceutical industry in terms of reduced profits. This point is extremely important, because in the case of pharmaceuticals it means that the increased costs of production will be borne by the citizens of the consuming country rather than the producing country. To compute the total cost borne by consumers, one must take into account both the increase in the price of pharmaceuticals and the quantity of pharmaceuticals used.

A third source of costs arises from the fact that the terms of the Convention call for the governments of some countries to shut down the production and exportation of certain commodities. To the extent that the resources used to produce these commodities can be reemployed only at lower levels of productivity, there is a cost involved to that country. Where there are no good substitute activities and where labor and capital are relatively immobile, for whatever reason, these costs may be substantial. Where the exportation of a drug-related substance is a major source of foreign exchange, these costs may be extremely severe in that they represent not only a loss of productivity but a loss of foreign exchange as well. This may have serious implications for the country's balance of payments. Related to this is the fact that in developing countries a shortage of foreign exchange often has serious implications for a country's ability to carry out development programs. These factors are, therefore, likely to be more important for certain countries in the underdeveloped world and, to a lesser extent, important for developed countries with large pharmaceutical industries.

There may be a number of intangible political costs as well. The provisions of Article 22 require that countries make their national laws with regard to drug control and drug abuse correspond with the provisions established in the Treaty (United Nations Conference, 1971, pp. 21–22). Therefore, one's national policy becomes tied to the international control mechanism, considered by some to constitute a surrender of national sovereignty.

It should also be noted that the costs are highly uncertain and that by signing the treaty a country is committing itself to possible unspecified future costs. For example, under Article 13 (p. 15), a country may incur substantial increase in enforcement costs if it is notified that it must stop the export of a given substance. This can occur as a result of an initiative of another party with no corresponding expense to the countries that make such demands.

It is clear from the foregoing discussion that the costs to a given nation may be substantial and that these costs will be very different depending on the position of the country involved. It would be extremely interesting to ascertain if any of the countries that have signed or ratified the treaty have done so with any knowledge of its implicit costs.

While we cannot actually define the benefits to a particular country, because the objectives stated in the Convention are too vague, we can comment on factors affecting the success or failure of its provisions by considering the resources of the countries involved and their incentives to participate. Earlier, we noted that a program or policy may fail either because the tasks set forth are not carried out due to technological infeasibility, insufficient resources, or lack of incentives or because completion of the stated tasks does not achieve the desired objective. Now consider how the Convention measures up in these areas.

The articles of the Convention deal mostly with licensing, inspection, prescriptions, record keeping, and export/import controls. Given sufficient resources, all these activities are technologically feasible; but, without a substantial commitment of resources, it may be impossible to enforce laws prohibiting the production and export of certain psychotropic substances. The resources required for, say, effective surveillance of a country's borders might be beyond the limits of either its ability or willingness to pay for this activity.

It is not likely that such a commitment will totally deplete a country's treasury; but, rather, the resources required may not, in the participant's view, yield a commensurate level of benefits. Since there are no provisions for equitable distribution of benefits through compensation among countries, it would be politically unwise for a public official to execute an activity that does not yield positive net benefits internally. Thus, it is clear that only if the benefits exceed the costs to a particular country will there be an incentive to fully implement the provisions of the treaty. Therefore, in evaluating the success of a drug-control program involving many countries, international cooperation hinges on the design of policy instruments through which the benefits to each participant exceed the costs. This point is not new to diplomats; however, determining whether given countries will find it in their interest to in fact implement the terms of the treaty requires the kind of benefit-cost computation advocated here.

This problem of incentives could be handled by a system of compensation in which countries that obtain net benefits would compensate countries that incur net costs. Another approach would be to establish sanctions for noncompliance that would impose on noncomplying nations costs that would be greater than the net costs of implementing the provisions of the treaty. Put differently, a participating country will have an incentive to comply only to the extent that the net cost of the marginal resources they commit to compliance are less than or equal to the marginal costs of noncompliance. It therefore follows that to evaluate the effectiveness of the sanctions for enforcing the treaty one needs to know both the net costs to various countries of abiding by the treaty and the net costs of incurring sanctions set up by the treaty. Further, countries that find that the costs exceed the benefits of the treaty may avoid these costs and the sanctions as well by investing minimal amounts in token enforcement of the provisions of the treaty.

Given the uneven distribution of costs and benefits and the differences in the wealth of various nations, it is highly likely that some countries will find it in their interest not to participate or to engage in token enforcement. If this is the case, will it affect the overall effectiveness of the system of controls for the remaining countries that do participate? The answer is clearly, yes, because the Convention basically attempts to control the supply of various drugs to medical and illegal markets. In most instances, the supply required by illicit markets is relatively small in terms of the world's potential capacity for producing these drugs. For example, the total United States market for heroin may be supported by 3,000 to 7,000 acres of opium poppies, while in 1969, more than 100,000 acres were planted in India and Turkey alone (Holahan and Henningsen, 1972). Therefore, industries could be developed in a few nonparticipating countries to supply the world's illicit markets. In fact, there is a strong incentive for some countries not to participate and to enjoy the high returns from supplying the illegal markets.

Stated more generally, even if controls were effective at controlling existing supplies, an incentive is created for developing new sources of supply. The incentive is likely to be particularly strong where the controlled drug has an inelastic demand because illegal suppliers can charge a very high price without significantly reducing the amount demanded. To the extent that one supplier controls a given market or segment of the market he can also obtain high monopolistic profits. These new sources are likely to be more difficult to control because they will be designed to circumvent control. Furthermore, these sources will provide drugs at a higher cost and perhaps of less good quality. This, as we have seen, is likely to result in a greater expenditure on illegal drugs throughout the world, at least in the short run. Thus, possible, but not necessarily inevitable, side effects of programs aimed at control of suppliers include an increase in drug-supporting robberies, prostitution and vice, the spread of traffic of impure substances, and the development of organized crime.

While these are problems that one should consider when proposing to control the supply of drugs, it should not be assumed either that they are insurmountable or that they are inconsequential. This judgment should be based on an analysis supported by data as well as on intuition.

It should be clear that many critical questions remain unanswered. Some of these questions have not even been asked. While it would take sizable effort to properly evaluate the treaty, it is clear that even the rudimentary first steps have not been taken. The message and plea of this paper is that future decisions involving important issues of national and international policy be based on a more systematic analysis of benefits and costs and be addressed using the basic tools of modern management science.

Classification for Legal Control

John Kaplan

XV

Earlier chapters have discussed the manifold problems encountered in attempting to classify drugs as biochemical, pharmacological, and behavior-altering substances. The difficulties become far greater, however, when we attempt to classify drugs for the purposes of legal control. Then, we must concern ourselves not only with the variables that, in some sense, are inherent in the drug itself, but also with the host of variables involving the legal, social, and political system of the society attempting the classification. Moreover, since these latter elements, within the realm of social science, are less understood than the questions in the domain of pharmacology, biochemistry, and even psychiatry, the problems are not only more complex but also less conductive to certainty.

Moreover, we are not engaged in an abstract philosophical, or even scientific, endeavor. Here, we are classifying drugs for the pragmatic purpose of making concrete decisions about their legal treatment—whether the drug should be prohibited entirely, used and sold freely, made available to citizens only through doctor's prescription, subject to rationing, or any one of a variety of other legal controls.

LEGAL TREATMENT OF COMMON DRUGS

However, before we go on to discuss in a somewhat more systematic way the variables that impinge upon the proper classification of a drug for legal purposes, it is helpful to examine the general kinds of legal treatment accorded to several of the most common drugs in Western societies.

Coffee

Coffee may be sold and used in all nations, although, at times, its use has been punishable by imprisonment or death. Although in many countries coffee bears a tax that is disproportionate to the taxes on other imported foodstuffs, this is generally not regarded as an effort aimed at discouraging its use. Rather, coffee is taxed highly for revenue purposes—a high tax being justified on the grounds that it is a "luxury" or that it is "unnecessary." In either case, the judgment does seem to reflect the fact that coffee is felt to do its user no "real" good. The fact that it is a drug that, moreover, can injure at least some of its users seems to be reflected solely in nonlegal, social controls. For example, the sight of an eight-year-old having a cup of coffee is sufficiently remarkable to be remembered for some while.

Tobacco

The regulations on tabocco are not a great deal more onerous than those on coffee, despite its far greater danger to the public health. In some nations, manufacture and sale of tobacco products is a state monopoly; and, in most of the rest, this drug is taxed far more heavily than most other consumables—thus reflecting, as does coffee, the demands of public finance. However, the high prices charged by the government monopoly and the high taxes where the products are privately manufactured and sold is a public health element. Demand for tobacco, though not completely inelastic, is inelastic enough in the usual ranges to provide greater revenue while still, at the margins, the taxes discourage consumption. Other regulations are attempts at guarding the public health, specifically designed to reduce consumption. Thus, in many nations, tobacco advertising is restricted, and its sale to minors is purportedly forbidden—though often no real attention is paid to this last restriction.

Moreover, cigarette manufacturers in the United States have recently been required to put a notice on their packages saying that "The Surgeon General Has Determined That Cigarette Smoking Is Dangerous To Your Health." And although, in the United States, some money is spent to convince users of the harmfulness of this drug, the amounts spent do not remotely approach either that taken in through taxes on tobacco or that expended by the tobacco industry to promote sales.

Alcohol

To describe completely the present controls on alcohol would take a sizable volume. It is a drug that causes enormous social havoc and is dangerous to a sizable proportion of those who use it. The United States and several other Western countries have, for brief periods, attempted to prevent its use through a prohibition that made the manufacture, the sale, and, in some places, the use of alcoholic beverages a crime. This type of control, however, has generally been abandoned and is used today only in certain Moslem countries where it is supported by strong religious sanctions.

Present methods of control are less ambitious but are generally regarded as more successful: the drug may be sold through either a government monopoly or by those licensed and often carefully regulated; it is heavily taxed, and there can be strong controls on its sale to those under the age of eighteen or twenty-one, depending on the jurisdiction. Moreover, its advertising is often restricted and sale is commonly forbidden close to schools or churches or at late hours of the night.

Furthermore, many jurisdictions have specific legal arrangements directed at the alcohol abuser. Thus, some have "posting" laws whereby a public official can determine that an individual is abusing alcohol and thereby make it illegal for anyone to give or sell the drug to him; others can civilly commit the alcoholic for compulsory treatment; and many jurisdictions attempt to provide social services to alcoholics and otherwise reduce their number through the enforcement of purportedly criminal laws against public drunkenness. Moreover, since, in motorized Western nations, the alcoholic is more and more likely to be driving an automobile, the enforcement of drunken-driving laws, aided by technological developments such as the breathalyzer, brings a sizable number of alcohol abusers into the criminal system for treatment.

Finally, although in many nations little is spent to warn the public against the dangers of alcoholism, this method of control is not unknown. France, for example, which has perhaps the world's most acute alcoholism problem, devotes considerable effort to public information on the dangers of excessive use of alcohol.

Cyclamates

The control of cyclamates in the United States exemplifies the next model of drug regulation—though this type of regulation is also commonly applied to conduct other than that associated with supply and use of drugs. This type of legal regulation is called the vice model because it is best known for its application to vices such as gambling and prostitution. Although it carries in its name "vice," connotations of immorality, there is no necessary connection and it can be applied to commodities or services that are felt to injure their user. The name is simply a historical accident, since the model was first named in a discussion of "morals" offenses. Under the vice model, the seller and manufacturer are made guilty, but not the buyer or user. The theory behind this distinction is that sufficient control may be exercised over a product by using the criminal law to try to deter suppliers, without attempting to apply the criminal sanction to the far larger number of users. Sometimes too this model is justified in moral terms, on the theory that the user is merely a victim of his own weakness and is more to be pitied than censured, while the seller who profits from the weakness of others is morally reprehensible.

In any event, the vice model is extremely common. It has been used, as mentioned before, to protect drinkers from the dangers of alcoholism by criminalizing the sellers of such products; it has been used to protect motorists and passengrs from traumatic injury caused by automobiles that lack seat belts or padded dashboards by criminalizing sellers and manufacturers of these dangerous instrumentalities; and at present, in some nations, it protects people from the danger of cancer of the bladder caused by dietetic soft drinks containing cyclamates (at least if those people turn out to have metabolisms like those of rats and would drink enormous quantities of such drinks). Probably the most interesting thing about the control of cyclamates is that in the United States it has worked to keep cyclamates off the market—when essentially the same method of control was applied to alcohol from the end of World War I to 1933, the "noble experiment" was a fiasco.

Medical Drugs

The next type of drug control is that used for medical drugs, in some jurisdictions antibiotics, in others major tranquilizers, insulin, and a host of others. We will call this method of regulation the medical model. This model seems to be the preferred one for drugs that meet three conditions—drugs that have medical uses, that are capable of harming their user, and that are not especially sought by illegal users. Under the medical model, the medical profession is given control of the right to obtain the drug. The ordinary citizen can purchase it if, and only if, he has the permission of a physician who is given almost uncontrolled discretion in this matter. If the physician approves, he will give the drug user a prescription that will allow a licensed pharmacist to sell the prescribed quantity. If the user does not have a prescription, but can still get someone to sell him the drug, he will commit no crime, but the seller will be guilty of a criminal offense— or, more significantly, if a pharmacist, he may lose his license. In short, the cyclamate or "vice" model, punishing the seller, but not the user, is applied to medical drugs used without a prescription. Moreover, there are many variations in the medical model to further limit the supply of a drug. Prescriptions for that drug can be made nonrefillable, limited in amount prescribed at any one time, subject to governmental inspection, or even restricted, as are amphetamines in Sweden and morphine in the United States and other countries, to the treatment of less than the full range of conditions to which it medically might be appropriate.

Amphetamines and Barbiturates

The amphetamines and barbiturates resemble most medical drugs in that they both have legitimate medical uses and can harm a certain percentage of their users. They differ, however, from most such drugs in that they are in substantial demand for nonmedical, or recreational, purposes. Although jurisdictions differ in how they treat this nonmedical use, the modern trend has been to decide that the vice model is not sufficient. As a result, several nations have attempted to deter the nonmedical users of these drugs through the threat of criminal penalties.

Marijuana and Heroin

Finally, there are drugs such as marijuana and heroin that, in most countries, are subject to complete prohibition, of use as well as sale. Since these drugs have no "recognized" medical use (at least in those countries), the medical model cannot be applied; and, because they are considered too dangerous, the vice model and cyclamate models are also unavailable. As a result, both sale and use of these drugs are criminal—without the safety valve provided by the amphetamine and barbiturate model in which medical practice channels a sizable percentage of the drug use into legal channels.

Within the category of criminal treatment there is, of course, a wide variety of possible social responses. Not only do these range in different nations from relatively low to extremely severe penalties for drug users but also, in several nations, users have the option of submitting to medical treatment in lieu of criminal punishment. Such treatment is nonetheless classified here under criminal measures for two major reasons. First, the treatment is involuntary, being compelled under threat of criminal punishment; second, the conditions of treatment, inpatient with no option to withdraw, usually approximate those of penal incarceration.

OTHER MODELS

Several things should be noted about the models of legal treatment applied to these various drugs. First, although the differing treatments cover an enormous range, additional legal models could be devised. It has been suggested for example, by some advocates of marijuana legalization who fear commercialization, that the "flower children" model should be adopted. By this model, all taint of commercialization would be removed by a law that permitted anyone to grow the drug for himself, and use (or even give away) as much as he wished. The only act that would be forbidden would be sale. Interestingly enough, this model bears some relation to the treatment of prostitution in some nations. These hold, apparently, that there are certain things that can be given away but should not be sold—or, in some fewer nations, bought. On the other hand, the fact that the legal treatment of prostitution has not been what could be called one of the law's greater successes, may be a good reason to be cautious about adopting the "flower children" model.

Another possible model that has not been considered here is a rationing system. Such a system might attempt to control either any one drug or a combination of drugs by allowing each consumer a certain number of defined "psychoactive equivalents." Such a system has been seriously proposed and may be a fertile avenue for exploration. Indeed, there are even the beginnings of such a system discernable in a number of jurisdictions.

However, although a society might choose among a wide range of drug-control models, these models, as a practical matter, are limited in number; and there are genuine constraints imposed, as it were, by the logic of the social system. For instance, though nothing inconsistent in the vice model forbids sale or production of a drug but not possession of small amounts, a legal system that attempted to do the reverse—permit sale or production of the drug but forbid the possession of small amounts would have given inconsistent directions, insofar as it is impossible to sell the drug without exerting some kind of possession over it. Such a law would either be unenforced, as far as the forbidding of possession is concerned; or else it would amount to a redundant and quixotic exercise of criminal power in purporting to permit sales that were in fact forbidden.

Similarly, a legal system such as that of the Netherlands or of Lebanon, which essentially allows the growing of the cannabis plant but not the possession of the dried leaves or resin, cannot be very serious about prohibiting the drug. That is not to say that if, for instance, the plant that produced a drug had useful by-products (as in the case with Turkish opium where the cuisine of an area is based on the use of a poppy seed oil, or, as would be the case if rope made from Indian hemp were still commercially important) such a law might not have to be passed. But where there is no special value seen in cultivating the plant, such a law, which maximizes the difficulties of enforcement, can be explained only on grounds unrelated to rational drug control.

Finally, as we will discuss at greater length later, the assignment of drugs to the various legal categories, while to a certain extent influenced by the dangers of the drug in question, also reflects many other factors as well. Some forty years ago, alcohol, in the United States, was treated according to a combination of various other models. It was available on prescription from a physician or for religious or sacramental purposes, but the manufacture, and sale, outside of these and a few other narrow exceptions, was criminal. It is interesting to note that at this same time a marijuana extract was treated according to the medical model. The assignment of models of control to drugs varies from nation to nation and as well as over time. Thus, heroin is treated under the medical model in England and some Western European countries today, while in Sweden amphetamines are prohibited almost entirely.

The question, of course, raised by the large variation in the models by which drug use is controlled is how a rational society should allocate drugs among the different methods of legal treatment.

In determining which variables should affect the legal classification—or model of control—suitable for a given drug, we must ask what social goals a society should have in mind in attempting such a classification. This is not an easy question, inasmuch as differing views of the nature of society might prompt different answers. For instance, one answer might be that a legal classification should be devised for the purpose of stating a moral position on the use of drugs. Such a view might be premised on the theory that the law is, in essence, a moral system. Alternatively, a drug classification might be adopted for the purpose of asserting the superiority of one life style or group in society over another.

These nonutilitarian goals are of considerable importance and merit consideration at some length. Space, however, forbids such an undertaking here. For the present, however, we need only point out that law is as much a means of social control as a moral or declarative scheme; that definitions of morality or the superiority of one group over another are often subject to great dispute; and that it is quite difficult, in any event, to show why one drug should be intrinsically more moral than another.

UTILITARIAN FUNCTION

Accordingly, the standard we will use here, at least as a first approximation, is a utilitarian one. More specifically we will ask what legal method of drug control maximizes a particular function over the society in question. This function can be represented by $(B_c - H_c - S_c)$, that is, the benefits attributable to the drug under the control system (B_c), minus the harm attributable to the drug under that system (H_c), minus the social costs of the control system itself (S_c). It is obvious that one or more of the variables will vary depending on the control system used—and our function merely indicates that the control system that maximizes the overall function is the most rational for the society to undertake.

Actually, this is not quite the case, since the maximization of the function is not a complete determinant even of a society's utilitarian position on drug control. As we will see, it is only an approximation and other factors not reflected in the function may rationally determine a nation's drug policies. These factors would include side payments or threats from other nations—and even political pressure and social conflict caused by those within a nation who would seek to use the drug-control law to vindicate their moral values or their position in society rather than for any utilitarian purpose. Nonetheless, the function is a first approximation, and we will begin by focusing upon it.

Benefits

It will be helpful if we begin our consideration of the function with its first term—B_c, the beneficial use of the drug—and its relation to the system of legal controls. The first point to make here is that whether the given effect of a drug is a benefit or not is often a political matter itself. Different groups within the society may agree on the benefits of a therapeutic use of a drug but may differ with great heat on whether the pleasure and relaxation attendant to normal alcohol or marijuana use should be regarded as a benefit. Similarly, the benefits of using cyclamates as weight-reducing aids may appear minimal to one who believes fat people should simply eat less. This is another matter that requires much more discussion. For the present, we will assume that a core of agreement can be reached on what effects of a drug should be considered beneficial.

We should note here that the indirect benefits of drug use must be considered along with the direct benefits. (The same point is more obvious with respect to the harm done by a drug, but should not be forgotten in that context, as well). Thus, a drug-related antianxiety effect, for example, does not just change the mood of an individual; it also has as a consequence the fact that this individual is again able to communicate better with his family and his friends, thereby improving the adjustment of these people and the societal functioning in general. An antidepressant drug, again, does not just relieve the medical conditions of a depressed patient; it integrates him anew into society with all the advantages that accrue from this fact for third persons and the community at large.

Another major point to make about the benefits of a drug is that although one can think of a legal control system actually designed to increase the good that a given drug would do over what it would do in the absence of any control at all, in practice this is rarely the case.

The simplest exception to this rule is fluoridation. In some parts of the United States, the use of sodium fluoride—a drug under most definitions of the term—is greatly increased by certain laws that require that the substance be added to municipal water systems for the purpose of preventing tooth decay. Note how different this is from the chlorination of the water supply, since the fluoride is actually intended to be taken into the body to produce changes rather than to prevent the ingestion of other harmful substances. If we take as given, then, that the intake of fluorides over the population as a whole does significant good, this type of legal arrangement increases that good more than would any other arrangement one might think of. Of course, before one could reach a decision on whether fluoridation of the water supply was a sensible means of drug control, one would have to know much more than this. One would have to know whether fluoridation does any harm as well, whether another control method (such as adding to milk in school lunches or the like) could accomplish most of the good without so much harm and at comparable social cost.

Another situation in which a control system is designed to increase the good done by a drug probably is that of the antibiotics in certain nations where purchase of these drugs is controlled by a prescription system. Here, it is not the purpose of the control system to increase the use of, and hence the benefits of, a substance. Rather, the control system is intended to place the user under medical supervision so that the potency of the drug will not suffer an attrition through promiscuous use, thus increasing the total good the drug can do in the society. Although very different from the fluoride example, this is another of the rare instances in which a control system can increase the beneficial use of a drug as compared with a system of no control at all.

Finally, it may be argued that the establishment of a medical profession is a method of increasing the good all medical drugs do over the society as a whole.

Here, it is not only promiscuous use of the particular drug that might lessen the good that the drug does. Rather, the enormous number of drugs that might be helpful in one situation or another demands some system in which a high degree of skill can be used to match up, as it were, the drug and the appropriate condition.

One final type of control, in part designed to increase the good the drugs do—though probably even more designed to decrease the harm—is a control system so loose that we often do not consider it a control at all. Nonetheless, the laws prohibiting misbranding, false advertising, and adulterants in drugs, insofar as they are enforced, certainly do help guarantee that beneficial uses of a drug otherwise intended do actually occur.

For the most part, however, a legal control apparatus—at least of the type usually thought of as such—does not attempt to increase the good a drug does over what it would do in the case of no regulation at all. Rather, a control system generally concerns itself with not decreasing significantly the benefit of a drug while at the same time trying to reduce its harm.

Sometimes this will be felt to be impossible, and a prohibition will be used that is designed to prevent any use of the drug, the beneficial along with the harmful. This will tend to occur, however, only where the good done by the drug is seen as small—at least in comparison to the harm. Thus, Sweden's banning of amphetamines for almost all purposes is an overt recognition that the law must prevent some of the good a drug does in order to prevent a greater harm. Where a drug is seen to be doing a significant amount of good, a regulation will usually be designed to save the greater part of that good while differentially preventing the harm. This is the case in most developed countries with respect to antibiotics and—though some nations are beginning to reevaluate this decision—barbiturates. By means of a prescription system, we turn over to the medical profession a decision as to which uses of the drug are beneficial and which are not. Those uses that are beneficial are to be supplied under medical prescription and all other uses are forbidden—typically criminalization of sale to anyone without a medical prescription but also, in the case of some drugs, by direct punishment of possession without a prescription. In the case of medical drugs, the fact that a drug is seen to do considerable good as well as harm invites us to use the medical profession—like Maxwell's demon—to allow the former use while inhibiting the latter. In some nations, a related kind of control is used, that is, supply through qualified pharmacists only with imposition on pharmacists of responsibility of supplying without prescription only to suitable individuals. This type of control, at least in the United Kingdom, where it is quite common, is reserved for drugs of some, but not great, danger.

A drug-control measure, however, unlike Maxwell's demon, is not completely selective, and as a result, any effort to reduce the harm done by a drug may well cause a reduction in the drug's beneficial use. This principle has been most often discussed with respect to medical drugs—even though the medical model seems best adapted to distinguishing between beneficial and harmful use, since it allows physicians to make the determination on a case-by-case basis. It is by no means restricted to the "medical" drugs, however.

It is possible also that this principle may have application to the cyclamates. There might be many people, for example, who should rationally take their chances on the relatively unlikely possibility of bladder cancer caused by cyclamates, rather than face the more certain health dangers of obesity. If the long-term health consequences of putting on too much weight are considered, it may be that the benefits of cyclamates to the large numbers of those who need these drugs to avoid being overweight outweigh the harm of cyclmate-caused cancer to the small percentage of such users.

The cyclamates point up another aspect of this problem. With the possible exception of some medical "wonder" drugs, the good that a drug does will tend to be more widespread, but far less dramatic, than the harm. Even in the case of alcohol, where the medical harm clearly outweighs the good, and in the case of marijuana, where the issue is subject to acrimonious debate, it is likely that many people cope successfully with serious mental problems by relaxing and reducing anxiety with one or other of these drugs. In the case of both alcohol and marijuana, then, one might still decide that a complete prohibition would be the best social response in terms of both the benefits (B_c) and harms (H_c) of the drug, if it could be made to work at a social cost proportional to the reduction in harm it caused. The point to be made here, however, is that in evaluating the function $B_c - H_c - S_c$ we must be careful to consider the first, as well as the last, two terms.

Attention will later be focused on the often neglected point that the greater the number of users who consider their drug use beneficial, the harder it will be to make a prohibition work and the higher will be the third variable of our function—the social cost of the legal control. At this point, it is necessary only to note that a prohibition may well discourage the beneficial use much more effectively than the harmful use. The person who is dependent on and desperately needs a drug is likely to be not only the one who will work hardest to get it but also the one most likely to injure himself with it. In some situations, the law works well to keep people from using a drug who might benefit from it but is relatively ineffectual to prevent use by those who harm themselves. The marijuana laws today and, so far as can be told, the alcohol prohibition of earlier years in a number of nations, most notably the United States, discouraged moderate use by older more stable and cautious members of society far more than they deterred the younger, more unstable, and less forward-looking, who in fact are much more likely to become abusers.

Although we will not go into the issue further here, we should note one additional complexity. The beneficial use of a drug may be a function of the legal treatment of other drugs. For instance, were heroin the only available opiate, nations that presently forbid it altogether might make it available under a rigid prescription scheme, as is generally the case with morphine. The existence of morphine, which is felt to be less abusable than heroin while having the same beneficial effects, allows us to treat the beneficial effects of heroin as negligible and to attempt to suppress that drug entirely.

That is not to say, of course, that the existence of morphine is a necessary and sufficient condition for the prohibition of heroin. First of all, some nations such as Britain and Belgium allow heroin to be prescribed for virtually the same purposes as morphine. Second, there are those who think that, regardless of the existence of morphine, heroin should be prohibited and follow this view to its logical conclusion by arguing for the ban on prescription—and hence manufacture, sale, distribution—of all opiates. Whether in fact such a drastic solution would have the effect of preventing significant amounts of harmful use along with the beneficial use is another question indeed. It might well be that such a solution —like others mentioned earlier—would destroy completely the beneficial use of opiates without affecting the harmful use significantly.

Harmfulness

The second variable in our function—H_c, the harmfulness of the drug— generally receives the most attention in debates about the appropriateness of differing legal controls. Just as with beneficial use, whether a given drug effect is or is not harmful can be a matter of intense political dispute. To see this, we need only to ask whether one should consider an addiction as harmful if it is unaccompanied by any other behavioral or psychological changes; or one might ask whether the allegedly increased emphasis on the internal rather than the external world that some have associated with marijuana use should be regarded as harmful. On the other hand, though this subject requires extended discussion, we will assume here that there exists a core of agreement as to what drug effects should be regarded as harmful.

In any event, it is clear that were a drug seen to cause absolutely no individual or social harm, there would be no utilitarian reason to attempt to control it through law at all (though, of course, one might still control it for the purpose of stating a moral principle or to stigmatize certain users). Probably tea and coffee come closest to this ideal today. For more than a century, neither of those drugs has been regarded in most places as an appropriate subject for any type of drug control at all.

On the other hand, a drug the ingestion of which causes serious harm to a sizable number of people is prima facie a candidate for a drug-control policy. In other words, if the second variable of our function, H_c, is high under a less stringent control, it is at least possible that a more stringent control could lower H_c and hence result in a higher value for the entire function. This is, of course, not to say that the mere fact that the drug does harm is enough of a reason to attempt any particular kind of control—or indeed any control at all.

This issue, however, is especially complex. We will return later to the problem of deciding what method of control minimizes our function, on the assumption that some control is advisable. At this point, we need only note that barbiturates, for instance, are an extremely harmful drug but are often regulated relatively loosely because it is felt—whether rightly or wrongly—that under medical supervision they also achieve a significant good that would be lost by more stringent regulation. Similarly, alcohol and tobacco are probably the two drugs most harmful to individuals in Western society; yet both are regulated far more leniently than, say, mescaline, simply because the ancillary costs of a much more stringent legal control system for those two popular social drugs might even exceed the harm they do in the society.

To return now to the harm the drug causes in the society—it is important to note that we typically lack many of the necessary data. First of all, with respect to the illegal drugs, we usually do not even have a simple head count of users, which might be a starting point for any estimates of the harm done by those drugs. Moreover, even as to the drugs distributed through legitimate channels, where we may know the total amount consumed and even the number of users, we need much more information before we can make a judgment as to the total harm. This would include the physical and psychological harm to individuals; harms to society caused by lessened productivity of the citizenry; damage from further drug abuse to the extent that the drug use may be regarded as a type of public health contagion, and many other harms. To estimate these harms at least where they are not measurable directly—as is the death rate from cirrhosis of the liver—we would have to know not only the distribution of drug use, but something about set, setting, and use-pattern in the society. It is possible to imagine that just about any drug might be quite harmful and a serious subject for legal control if its pattern of use in the society were harmful enough. We should also note that the pattern of use and effects of the same drug may vary widely from society to society.

Variations in use-patterns of a drug are important not only in determining the harm its use causes. They are also important in considering the more complicated concept of contingent harm. It has been pointed out that once a drug is introduced into a society, there is a tendency for more concentrated and abusable forms of the drug to gain use. Thus, tobacco (from pipe-smoking to cigarettes), alcohol (from beer or wine to distilled liquors), opiates (from opium to morphine and then to heroin), and cocaine (from coca leaves to cocaine) all fit this view. To be sure, there are counterexamples such as coffee, which at one time was consumed in far stronger and probably more damaging ways, and perhaps even alcohol, which in some societies today is merely extremely harmful, rather than devastating as it was a century or two ago. Nonetheless, the possibility that the use-pattern of a drug may become more harmful with time is obviously one with which a rational lawmaker must contend.

At the very least, a lawmaker should consider the possibility that, over time, the widespread benign use of a drug might weaken the cultural restraints against its over-use. Moreover, the widespread benign use of the drug over a substantial period might make the application of otherwise desirable controls either politically impossible or simply impracticable because of citizen noncooperation.

The alcohol prohibition experience of the United States may be an example of this latter phenomenon; some observers have asserted that alcohol had simply been too widely used for too long for such a prohibition to work. Obviously, a similar fear may be behind reluctance to change the control mechanism for marijuana. It has been argued that should a licensing system be adopted for cannabis that would increase considerably the moderate use of that drug, this might render impossible a later tightening up, and especially a reprohibition, should either more virulent patterns of use develop or new scientific data reveal as yet undocumented, or even unsuspected, harms done by that drug.

Social Costs

We will next consider the last term of our function—S_c, the social costs of the control system. As with both benefit and harm, whether an effect of a drug-control measure should be considered a social cost is subject to considerable dispute. Despite this, it can be argued that the social costs of drug-control measures deserve the greatest scrutiny, because they are most often ignored in considering drug control arrangements. Indeed, this is the case even as to drug regulations that the public tends to regard as extremely successful. For instance, the prescription system, even if it works properly and prevents significant amounts of harmful use while allowing the beneficial use, is nonetheless an extremely expensive one if nothing else, in terms of the millions and millions of dollars it costs to get prescriptions for drugs from physicians. Antibiotics are available over the counter in some nations and are controlled by a prescription system in others; yet we have no evidence that the prescription system is superior from the public health view, let alone when one considers its social cost.

Similarly, inventory provisions, quotas, and new-drug testing procedures may well successfully reduce harmful use while not affecting beneficial use and hence may maximize the value of $(B_c - H_c)$, our function, without its last term. Nonetheless these controls may be so expensixe to implement in practice that lesser controls might maximize the entire function $(B_c - H_c - S_c)$. Indeed, the social costs of stringent new-drug testing measures may be extremely high. The harms can include those of reduced competition among new drugs because of their diminished number, reduced competition for drugs already on the market caused by the diminished number of new drugs, the increased developmental cost of new drugs, and most important the costs of keeping valuable drugs off the market during the time necessary to satisfy a bureaucracy of their effectiveness. Several observers have commented that, although the protection afforded by new-drug testing against another thalidomide disaster is very important, the harm done to society by unnecessarily keeping beneficial drugs off the market may outweigh the more demonstrable harm caused by allowing the prescription of potentially harmful drugs. Whether or not these charges are correct, it must be remembered that the evaluation of medical drugs has been turned over to a bureaucracy and that there is a constant and strong tendency for a bureaucrat to prefer invisible to visible errors. Since he will suffer far less attack if he keeps a valuable drug off the market than if a drug he has passed does harm, the bureaucrat will always tend toward a caution that may be damaging to society as a whole.

Moreover, any changing control system that can tighten or loosen control creates uncertainties among both the users and the producers of drugs. In the former instance, these uncertainties may lead to hoarding. In the far more important latter situation, a proposed regulation, whether adopted or not, can have the effect of discouraging investment in and production of one drug while its competitors remain unaffected or even benefit from the threat. It should go without saying that this type of uncertainty is costly not only for the drug producer but for the public as well.

Despite these costs of a system in which almost everyone obeys the law, it is primarily when there is a sizable amount of law violation that the social cost of a drug control system becomes most significant.

At this point, we must consider as costs the harm done in arresting large numbers of citizens. In California, which operates under a marijuana prohibition system, 70,000 persons were arrested in 1971 for violation of the marijuana laws. The great majority of these were arrested for simple possession of the drug and hence their arrests must be acknowledged as a cost of making simple possession by the user illegal. Indeed, largely to avoid this several jurisdictions—such as Denmark and the Netherlands (and, as a practical matter, a number of American municipalities)—have determined that they will not arrest simple cannabis users.

Of course, it is arguable that the social costs of the arrests are not entirely a product of the marijuana law. This is probably true with respect to some drugs and must be kept in mind in evaluating the social costs of any drug law. Thus, many of those arrested for heroin offenses in the United States would probably be arrested for some other type of crime if they were not arrested for heroin offenses. Under this view, the cost of arrest is really in great part the general cost of dealing with inconvenient people rather than appropriate cost of drug law.

As to heroin, the matter is somewhat more complex than this since it is also likely that this system of legal control, which prohibits sale of heroin, also raises the price of the drug to such an extent that the user, who must somehow raise the increased price of his drug habit, becomes a much more "inconvenient" (and criminal) person than he would under a control system that permitted medical prescription of low-priced heroin to addicts.

As far as we can tell, however, this is not the case with the marijuana user, and the great majority of those arrested for marijuana use, in the United States at least, would not have been predicted to come into any other contact with the criminal system.

In any event, the pure numbers of arrested marijuana offenders are a significant factor in overburdening the criminal system of the United States. Although we have no data for the nation as a whole, approximately one-third of the felony cases in Los Angeles County are marijuana cases; and it has been estimated that in California alone approximately $50 million in law enforcement resources are required simply to process marijuana users each year. Probably the major cost of the marijuana possession offense is the adverse effect of a marijuana arrest and the large numbers of young people affected.

Of course, it is likely that if the enforcement system could apprehend a much higher percentage of violators, it might succeed in deterring widespread violation and hence considerably lower this social cost. The same result, too, would follow if the laws that are intended to prevent production, importation, and sale were effectively enforced. In that case, there would not be many who could use the drug, regardless of whether they themselves were deterred.

We have, heretofore, discussed laws against use of a drug and laws against its possession as if they were functionally equivalent. Although this is not quite correct, in the main, use and possession offenses cover the same conduct. First of all, possession typically includes use, as it is impossible to use a drug, at least voluntarily, without possessing it. One can, to be sure, possess a drug without using it, but, in almost all cases one might think of, the possession if not for use would be either for sale or to aid and abet use by another—each of which would almost certainly be a criminal offense along with use. The major exception to this rule is possession for a purpose other than use, and the most important such purpose is that of research. As a result, a social cost of a prohibition of possession of a drug—unless some exculpatory mechanism is provided—is that it hinders research. Indeed, the history both of cannabis and opiate regulation in the United States demonstrates that this problem can be quite serious. In any event, for many drugs, possession must be made illegal if a law against use is to be at all effective. Use is often difficult to test for and often is episodic in nature, while possession is generally much more subject to law enforcement efforts.

We should point out here that it may very well be that prohibition of either use or possession might be a relatively costly means of lowering use, and that the vice model may be almost as effective at a much lower social cost. It should be noted, however, that even if possession for personal use is permitted, a law prohibiting the manufacture, importation, and sale of a drug may be quite costly if it is unable to prevent a sizable degree of violation. The problems of inhibiting a consensual traffic with no victim complaints may force the police to adopt a whole range of practices that cause considerable resentment among the citizenry. Nor is it only the police who must impinge upon what many consider the civil liberties of the citizen. In many states, the legislatures have enacted laws in response to the illegal drug traffic. It is no coincidence that, in the United States, "no knock" laws, stop-and-search laws, and questions involving rights to remain silent and, in Sweden, wiretapping have all been argued against a background of concern over drugs. These problems are, perhaps, even more acute where possession is prohibited, but they are nonetheless quite serious even where the vice model laws are widely violated.

Moreover, the existence of large profits in the illegal drug trade, together with the absence of a complaining witness, may make police corruption a serious problem in the enforcement of such laws. The American prohibition experience is a good example of this. Indeed, most authorities date the major growth of American organized crime, with its many ties into law enforcement and political life, from the prohibition era.

Another significant cost of a prohibition on manufacture, sale, or importing is that it can call into existence a drug-dealing network that not only supplies the prohibited commodity but that can supply others as well. Marijuana selling in the United States has been shown to be a significant factor in the use and distribution of more dangerous drugs. The marijuana seller, to engage in business, must have both customers who are prepared to deal with him clandestinely and a source of supply "higher up" in drug dealing. As a result, he is an ideal conduit for drugs passing from the more sophisticated, drug-involved, and often criminalistic operators higher up the chain of manufacture, importing, or sale and his less sophisticated customers. Moreover, since he is already committing a crime by selling marijuana he risks relatively little if he deals in more profitable, and more harmful, drugs as well. Put another way, a prohibition on sale, importing, and manufacture gives a monopoly of what traffic there remains to those who are willing to violate the law; and, typically, they use their monopoly—as most monopolists do—to expand their product line.

Another social cost of the vice model (and, of course, a prohibition as well) has already been alluded to. Such laws create, in Herbert Packer's term, a "crime tariff," which raises the price of the drug to many times what it would be in a competitive market. Crime is necessary for so many American heroin addicts not so much because heroin prevents the addict from holding down a legitimate job, but because only crime can permit the relatively uneducated addict to earn enough to feed his habit at monopoly prices. Moreover, since heroin addicts develop a tolerance to that drug, they tend gradually to be *socialized* into criminality, while their need increases as they become more experienced criminals. Although many addicts support their habit through the sale of heroin, users cannot make a living by simply selling to each other. Sooner or later the community outside must be victimized through property crimes or the manufacture of new addicts—who in turn repeat the same process. On the other hand, lest this issue be thought simple, we must consider as a social cost an alternative method of heroin control, maintenance with methadone. Where the institutions are not present to control the use of this drug on large numbers of addicts the escape of that drug "onto the street" may cause a public health problem as serious as the criminal problem the maintenance system was meant to alleviate.

VARIABLES IN DETERMINING CONTROL MODELS

We have now discussed, albeit briefly, some of the social costs of various types of drug control. At this point then it is possible to consider in a slightly more systematic way the variables related to the drug and its use that are most crucial in determining the costs of differing control methods.

To begin with, we should note that an important factor in the success or failure of any method of drug control is the degree to which the users want the drug. This is one major reason why, when the United States government ordered cyclamates off the market, that drug simply disappeared, whereas alcohol during prohibition and marijuana, more recently, did not. The cyclamates could be successfully barred in great part because most users really did not want them very much. They were only used to save calories, and calories could be reduced almost as effectively in other ways. Although cyclamates did not have the bitter after-taste of saccharine, a combination of saccharine and a small amount of sugar was a sufficient substitute for most people. Nor did cyclamates, unlike heroin for instance, produce either addiction or psychological dependence to make its users seek the drug at substantial personal cost. Consequently, the illegal seller of cyclamates did not have a very good market.

Compare marijuana or alcohol with the cyclamates. Both cause dependence, though to only a relatively small number of users; and they give considerable pleasure to a high proportion of the rest. The users of each of these "social" drugs do not, in addition, seem to recognize substitutes for their drugs, as was the case with cyclamates. They are not, then, presented with easily available alternatives so as to make unnecessary their efforts to procure alcohol or marijuana.

A second point is that the technology of drug production and consumption is an important factor in the success or failure of a drug-control measure. Where the technology of drug production and distribution is not difficult to overcome, drug control will be very difficult, but where that is not the case, the control will be far more effective. Take, for example, the cyclamates. Their manufacture requires some, though not a great deal of, technology and invested capital; and, unlike amphetamines, they are not easily divertible from normal chains of commerce; unlike marijuana, they neither grow wild in nature nor are produced in less developed countries beyond the effective reach of law enforcement; and, unlike alcohol, they cannot easily be distilled in anyone's basement from relatively untraceable ingredients. Moreover, as long as cyclamates are consumed in cans of diet drinks selling for ten or fifteen cents each, it would hardly be economical to transport large quantities of such beverages illegally; a truckload of such diet drinks would be considerably less valuable than a pocketful of heroin, a small suitcase full of marijuana or a car full of alcohol. Of course, if there were a sufficient demand for cyclamates, and if the technology of production and marketing were simpler, it might be that legitimate business would produce nonsweet soft drinks to which the illegal drug user could add his cyclamates—much as large amounts of cigarette papers and water pipes are now sold and which, for the most part, end up being used with illegal marijuana. Until this level of use is reached, however, the technology of production and distribution can work in favor of effective drug control.

In addition to those variables that relate to the drug's popularity and its techniques of production, distribution, and use, there are other variables that are crucial in determining the social cost of a drug-control measure. These concern the nature of the society that is attempting to control the drug we use. We can divide societies in various ways but one axis is whether its legal system is capable of coping with and enforcing a sizable percentage of its criminal laws or whether it must concern itself merely with the bare essentials of attempting to govern a society. For instance, in many underdeveloped societies with primarily a subsistence economy the law must cope with the problems of poverty, weak governmental control, corruption of officials, and even rebellion. In this type of situation governmental resources are simply not sufficiently available for the control of drugs. In such societies, moreover, the attempted enforcement of drug-control measures might create so much resentment against the government that it not only would have insufficient power to enforce its rule but would also weaken its own chances of survival. This type of situation is especially likely to occur where the drug use and production are imbedded into the culture of a discrete geographical section of the population. Where the writ of a central government barely runs at all, attempting to interfere with established local customs may be a very dangerous move.

Even among developed countries, where poverty and the threat of revolution are not regarded as serious possibilities, there are great differences in the "hardness" of the social control systems. Different countries have widely differing ratios of police to population, citizen cooperation with police forces, and legal requirements on search and other kinds of surveillance over the individual by the institutions of the society. The greater the control over the individual the society maintains, the more likely it will be able to pursue a prohibitory drug-control policy at low cost. Indeed, since drug-control measures tend to produce the greatest social cost when they are inadequately enforced, the inability to enforce a law may be a good reason for not attempting a drug-control measure beyond the nation's grasp.

It is obvious that this is least likely to be the case as to nations where rigid controls are maintained over communications among citizens. Such controls and their attendant legal apparatus are ideally suited for preventing a drug subculture from developing, and as long as there are sufficient police to enforce ideological conformity, it is no great additional trouble to prevent drug use as well. Moreover, in such a situation one would expect the greater likelihood of apprehension to lead to less flouting of the drug-control law and hence lowered social costs of the control system. Finally, the greater adherence to the control system would probably produce a lessened harm attributable to the drug as well.

Another variable concerning the legal system of a nation that is relevant to the cost of its drug-control law is whether the legal system is highly formal with relatively little discretion accorded to its actors or whether the legal system operates to a sizable degree informally with considerable amounts of flexibility. This is a significant variable in determining the costs of a drug control apparatus. For instance, under a theoretically complete prohibition form of control, if the police have the discretion, and in fact will use it, to arrest only those who are abusing a drug, rather than merely all those who possess it, the benefits of the drug control will increase, while its costs go down. Moreover, the possession prohibition can also then be a powerful weapon against traffickers, either because they are also users or because they may possess the drug incident to trafficking. This, however, is the case only as long as the police can be trusted to devote their attention solely to apprehend traffickers and to ignore mere users. On the other hand, where the actors in the legal system either are not permitted, or do not choose, to act with such flexibility, one tends to get the very high level of arrestees such as previously discussed in the case of California—and even where the number of arrestees is not so high, the society may pay a price for such police discretion in discriminatory enforcement of the law.

It is likely, however, that both the Japanese success in controlling amphetamines and the Chinese success in controlling opium were due in great part to the combination of a "hard" legal system with one that is quite informal.

In addition, a further advantage of a relatively informal legal system is that **it is conductive** to experiments aimed at improving drug control through bringing about changes in any of the variables of our function. The more informal the legal system, the less the necessity of mobilizing political forces to secure formal changes in the law, and the more quickly any errors that become apparent in drug-control systems can be repaired. Moreover, an informal law enforcement apparatus can adapt more easily to changes in the variables that affect drug control, such as changes in drug use-patterns, technology, or knowledge as to long-term harm aimed at maximizing the function $(B_c - H_c - S_c)$.

On the other hand, we must note that the more informal the legal system, the more likely is its society to pay a price in diminished human rights for a more effective drug control.

INTERNATIONAL CONTROL

Up to this point we have been discussing the variables to be considered in determining the optimal drug policy in a nation in isolation. It is a fact of international life, however, that varying drug-control policies involve extranational benefits or detriments that are not encompassed in our original function. Thus, it might be rational for Turkey, in isolation, to allow cultivation of the opium poppy because the drug does little harm and would be very costly to suppress. However, if the United States not only pays for the costs of a prohibition on opium cultivation and throws in side payments of other types of aid, contingent upon the more restrictive drug-control policy, a utilitarian Turk might very well conclude that the most rational course would be to accept the American payment and modify his own law.

There are several problems with such an arrangement, however. It is not at all clear to what extent such a new drug-control policy would in fact be implemented. Once a sizable number of people in a nation feel that their drug-control policy is being dictated, or at least purchased, from the outside it may be that their attitude toward that policy may be even more hostile than toward a merely ill-advised policy of their own government. In such a case, it is quite likely that unless the legal system is both "hard" and formal the nation will merely accept the outside money but in fact will not put into effect the drug-control policy upon which it is contingent.

Nor need the external influence on a nation's drug policy be limited to side payments. A fear of international consequences may determine the policy. Not only is this merely a fear of the bilateral action implied in recent American threats to cut off any aid to any country that does not adopt certain drug-control measures, but it also can be as a consequence of an international compact already entered. Indeed, the legal system may be sufficiently formal that the international compact will have the same force as domestic law and hence be an important determinant of the drug-control policy itself. More likely, however, it will be seen that there are reasons to live up to the treaty obligations, which may require certain drug-control measures even apart from the threats of international sanction, which are at least becoming theoretically available in more recently drafted treaties in the drug area. However, it is by no means certain that a nation that feels its assent to a treaty was not completely free will attempt—or even be able—to implement a required drug-control policy at an acceptable social cost.

At this point, it might be appropriate to, as it were, step back and ask whether there is any way of determining whether an international drug-control program is appropriate, analogous to the consideration of our utilitarian function for a given nation. The chances are, however, that we cannot yet do this. All the issues involving the appropriate classification of drugs for the purpose of national control apply with far greater complexity when the issue is international control. Indeed, the variation of cultures among nations is such that it becomes extremely hard to even visualize an appropriate quantification for the good a drug does, the harm a drug does, or the social cost of a drug control measured across national boundaries.

Within a nation we might use as a standard the total number of people in the nation who would be injured by the drug, but it is obvious that no such "one man one vote" would be held to prevail in the international area. The demands of national sovereignty clearly would forbid this.

Another way of putting this is that the very concept of a utilitarian function becomes difficult when one considers only two countries. Even if there were some way to measure the total good that the drug did, the total harm it did, and the total social cost of the drug-control policy in the two countries, a simple maximization of the function over both countries would not be seen as just if the drug-control measure helped one nation while hurting the other. And if side payments were to be used to compensate a nation for the harm a drug-control policy caused, we would run into all the problems we have just discussed.

To be sure, it is possible to conceive of an international drug-control arrangement between two nations, each having identical ratios of the three variables in the function. However, insofar as the international drug-control arrangement required a domestic law in two such nations, it would properly duplicate only what the nations should do anyway. If the two nations were in very different situations, however, an international drug arrangement that required a particular law of both of them might very well operate to the advantage of one and the disadvantage of the other. If only two nations were involved, the matter could perhaps be settled by bilateral side payments. When a drug arrangement is entered into by many countries, it will tend to be further from optimal in the case of some nations than in the case of others. It might be that a mechanism could be set up by those nations benefiting most from the international control system to compensate those hurt most by it. It is possible that this would not prove sufficient to render the agreement acceptable (or more likely to guarantee good-faith enforcement), but any other method would seem even less likely to prove effective.

It should be noted that our present international agreements in the drug area tend for the most part to slide over these difficult issues. There are a number of concessions, to be sure, to the different nations, most clearly in those provisions that allow nations to opt out of certain of the control features. For the most part, however, international drug regulation proceeds on the model of the criminal law—which merely forbids or permits certain conduct—and does not take account of the much more complex considerations that we have attempted to sketch out in this chapter.

Administrative Considerations

Jasper Woodcock

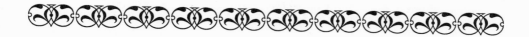

XVI

In the sixty years since the first international agreement on opium, the spread of the nonmedical use of drugs has been accompanied by a ramification in the administration measures aimed at its limitation. Today, a confusing array of international and intergovernmental organs concern themselves with drugs to a greater or lesser extent. They fall into four main categories:

1. Bodies forming an integral part of the United Nations Organization and funded, though not necessarily exclusively, from the UN budget.
2. Intergovernmental agencies related to the UN through specific agreements covering, as a rule, reciprocal representation at meetings, exchange of information, uniform personnel arrangements, and coordination of statistical, budgetary, and financial arrangements. These agencies have separate memberships and separate budgets and are separately

Besides the references cited in the text, the material on which this section is based was drawn chiefly from published and unpublished UN and WHO documents available for reference in UN libraries, including: Reports of the Commission on Narcotic Drugs (published as Supplements to the Official Records of the UN Economic and Social Council); Annual Reports of the International Narcotics Control Board, New York, United Nations; Reports of the WHO Expert Committee on Drug Dependence. Published in the WHO Technical Report Series, Geneva; "Twenty Years of Narcotics Control under the United Nations." *UN Bulletin on Narcotics,* 1966, *18*(i), 1–60; "How New Drugs Are Brought under International Narcotics Control by the Procedure of the Single Convention on Narcotic Drugs, 1961." *UN Bulletin on Narcotics,* 1968, *20*(ii), 51–52; Rules of Procedure of the Functional Commissions of the Economic and Social Council, New York, United Nations, 1971.

funded by contributions from their members. In UN parlance, they are often called the "specialized agencies." Some of them, such as the International Labour Office and the Universal Postal Union, were established decades before the UN.

3. Organs specifically established by the international agreements on psychoactive drugs.

4. Intergovernmental organs independent of the UN. Some of these, such as the International Criminal Police Organization (Interpol) and the Customs Cooperation Council, have a worldwide membership.

In this chapter, the organization and interrelationship of these organs, in so far as they concern themselves with the control of drugs will be described. Their functions in the classification of drugs and in the consequent process of control are outlined in other chapters. Organs wholly devoted to drug problems have their titles in bold characters.

ECONOMIC AND SOCIAL COUNCIL (ECOSOC)

The Economic and Social Council is one of the six principal organs of the United Nations established by the UN Charter.* It is empowered by the Charter (Article 62) to make or initiate studies and reports, and to prepare draft international conventions concerning international, economic, social, cultural, educational, health, and related matters. The authority for the establishment of most of the administrative machinery of international control is derived from ECOSOC.

ECOSOC has a rotating membership of twenty-seven states† drawn from the members of the UN, and elected by the General Assembly. It meets twice a year in New York and Geneva.

ECOSOC works through commissions, committees, and other subsidiary organs to which it delegates responsibility for specific areas of its manifold concerns. In 1946, it established the Commission on Narcotic Drugs to deal with problems arising from the abuse of drugs. In practice, ECOSOC devotes an average of less than 2 percent of its sessional time to drugs, roughly in proportion to the budget allocation for narcotics of the Department of Economic and Social Affairs of the UN Secretariat (See Table 1).

The resolutions ECOSOC adopts have usually been debated and drafted by the Commission on Narcotic Drugs and usually receive only a brief discussion in ECOSOC's sessions.

COMMISSION ON NARCOTIC DRUGS

The Commission on Narcotic Drugs is one of six "functional commissions"** established by ECOSOC. It was set up in 1946 "in order to provide

---

* The others are: the General Assembly, the Security Council, the Trusteeship Council, the International Court of Justice, and the Secretariat.

† The membership is shortly to be increased to fifty-four.

** The others are the Statistical Commission, the Population Commission, the Com-

Table 1. BREAKDOWN OF PROGRAM ACTIVITIES OF UNITED NATIONS
DEPARTMENT OF ECONOMIC AND SOCIAL AFFAIRS FOR 1968

Chief Parts of the Program	Expenditures in Millions of Dollars
Development planning, projection, and policies	10
Development of natural resources	18.5
Transport and communications	3
Fiscal and financial	1.5
Social development	3.4
Population	1.6
Housing, building, and planning	3.5
Statistics	5
Public administration	0.6
Narcotics	0.9

SOURCE: Adapted from Bertrand (1969).

machinery whereby full effect may be given to the international conventions relating to narcotic drugs, and to provide for continuous review of and progress in international control of such drugs" (Resolution of first session).

Since 1968, the Commission has been composed of twenty-four states,[†] elected by ECOSOC for a term of four years. Membership of the Commission is not confined to members of the UN, but may include members of the specialized agencies and parties to the Single Convention who do not belong to the UN. In the choice of members, account must be taken of the following factors: (1) the adequate representation of countries that (a) are important producers of opium and coca, (b) are important manufacturers of narcotic drugs, (c) have an important problem of drug addiction or illicit traffic; and (2) equitable geographical distribution.

The practical consequence of these requirements is that, first, certain countries are assured of what is effectively permanent membership of the Commission and, second, countries with very little firsthand experience of dealing with the problems of drugs may be members. (See Table 2.) The former tend to be represented at the Commission's meetings by senior administrators from government departments with a long experience with drug-related problems, and the latter by individuals with general diplomatic experience.

Besides the elected members of the Commission, countries are also invited

mission for Social Development, the Commission on Human Rights, and the Commission on the Status of Women.

[†] Increased to thirty in 1973.

Table 2. MEMBERSHIP OF THE COMMISSION OF NARCOTICS, 1950–1972

Country	50	51	52	53	54	55	56	57	58	59	60	61	62	63	64	65	66	67	68	69	70	71	72
Argentina																/	/	/					
Austria								/	/	/													
Brazil													/	/	/	/	/	/	/	/	/	/	/
Canada			/	/	/	/	/	/	/	/	/	/	/	/	/	/	/	/	/	/	/	/	/
China			/	/	/	/	/	/	/	/	/	/	/	/	/	/	/	/	/	/	/	/	/
Dominican Republic																			/	/	/	/	/
Egypt	/	/	/	/	/	/	/	/	/	/	/	/	/	/	/	/	/	/	/	/	/	/	/
Federal Republic of Germany													/	/	/	/	/	/	/	/	/	/	/
France	/	/	/	/	/	/	/	/	/	/	/	/	/	/	/	/	/	/	/	/	/	/	/
Ghana													/	/	/	/	/	/	/	/	/	/	/
Greece					/	/	/																
Hungary								/	/	/	/	/	/	/	/	/	/	/	/	/	/	/	/
India	/	/	/	/	/	/	/	/	/	/	/	/	/	/	/	/	/	/	/	/	/	/	/
Iran	/	/	/	/	/	/	/	/	/	/	/	/	/	/	/	/	/	/	/	/	/	/	/
Jamaica																	/	/	/	/	/	/	/
Japan													/	/	/	/	/	/	/	/	/	/	/

Korea, Republic of

Lebanon

Madagascar

Mexico

Morrocco

Nigeria

Netherlands

Pakistan

Peru

Poland

Sweden

Switzerland

Togo

Turkey

United Kingdom

United States

Soviet Union

Yugoslavia

Number of Observer Nations: 1967 (21st session)—14; 1968 (22nd session)—22; 1969 (23rd session)—23; 1971 (24th session)—27.

to send observers to its sessions. The invitations are sent out by the Division of Narcotic Drugs, which acts as the Commission's secretariat (see below), in consultation with the chairman. The number of countries invited as observers has grown steadily over the years, and at the Commission's 1971 meeting they outnumbered the members. Observers have the right to intervene in the Commission's debates, but not to vote.

Governments nominate themselves for election to the commission, one quarter of whose seats fall vacant each year; the election of members to fill them is the prerogative of ECOSOC. Whereas with the other functional commissions of ECOSOC governments are required to name, and the UN Secretary-General to approve, the individuals who will attend the Commission's meetings, they are not required to do so in the case of the Commission on Narcotic Drugs, since individuals attend the Commission's meetings as representatives of their governments and not as independent experts.

The Commission meets in the Palais des Nations at Geneva. The frequency and length of its meetings are decided by ECOSOC. Until 1969 it met annually for about three weeks. In that year, however, as part of an economy drive within the UN, ECOSOC decided, very much against the Commission's wishes, that the Commission should meet every other year (see Table 3 for budget). The next regular session of the Commission was accordingly not held until 1971. However, two special sessions, together lasting twenty-one days, were held in 1970; the first to finalize the draft of the Convention on Psychotropic Substances, and the second to make short- and long-term recommendations for integrated international action against drug abuse and to consider a United States proposal for the establishment of a special UN fund for drug abuse.

The meetings are public. However, certain items of the agenda may be discussed in closed session, with the public, and sometimes the observers, excluded. Discussions of trends in illicit traffic are usually closed, as are those concerning delicate matters relating to individual countries. For example, in 1971 the discussions of Iran's decision to resume opium production was confined to members of the Commission and representatives of some of the specialized agencies.

The 1971 session of the Commission was attended by representatives of twenty-four member states, invited observers from twenty-seven states, and representatives from seventeen UN and other international bodies (see Table 4). There appears to be no limit to the number of alternates and advisers by whom a country's representative may be accompanied, and the size of some of the delegations suggests that the Commission's meetings are an occasion for a great deal of extrasessional activity on the part of governments.

At the commencement of each session, the Commission elects a chairman, two vice-chairmen, and a rapporteur, who remain in office until the next session. There is usually only one candidate for each office, and the votes are usually unanimous. The nomination of candidates for office is in the hands of the Commission's "Bureau," an informal body consisting of the four officeholders. However, past chairmen attending the session as representatives of member governments are always invited to attend the Bureau's meetings, an effective way of ensuring the representation of influential "permanent" members of the Commission at the Bureau's deliberations. At recent sessions, the informal Bureau appears to have been replaced by a formal Steering Committee. This innovation occurred at the first session for many years at which the United States was represented by an individual who was not a past chairman of the Commission; the Steering Committee at this session had the same composition as the Bureau, but in addition the representatives of four countries (including the United States) were elected to it. At the 1971 sessions, when the United States representative was elected first vice-chairman, the composition of the Steering Committee was identical with the Bureau—that is, present officers and past chairmen only. Apart from this recently established Steering Committee, the Commission has no regular committees, though ad hoc committees and working parties may be appointed at a particular session to consider specific items of the agenda and to draft resolutions.

The provisional agenda for the Commission's session is drawn up by the Division of Narcotic Drugs in consultation with the chairman of the previous session. Sometimes, the Commission will propose certain items for inclusion in the agenda of its next session, but usually it does not. Additional items may be proposed (subject to adequate notice) by members of the UN and the specialized agencies, by the UN General Assembly, ECOSOC, the Security Council, and the Trusteeship Council, and by Interpol.

The proceedings of the Commission are recorded in the form of minutes, except for particularly important items of the agenda for which summary records are produced. At the 1971 session, for example, only two agenda items, one dealing with Iran's decision to resume opium production and the other with the amendment of the 1961 Single Convention, were considered important enough to warrant summary records. This reliance upon minutes is a consequence of the measures of economy imposed on all UN bodies since 1968.

The reports of the Commission's sessions are presented to ECOSOC and are published as supplements to the latter's official records.

The actions of the Commission take the form of resolutions directed to other UN organs, the specialized agencies, or to governments. Most of these resolutions are in the form of drafts for consideration and adoption by ECOSOC, suggesting that the Commission's authority is not considered weighty enough on its own.

Apart from those relating to the Commission's own internal functioning (setting up committees, laying down voting procedures), the Commission's (and ECOSOC'S) resolutions can only "recommend," "invite," "request," or "urge" governments and other bodies to act. The Commission, like all the international bodies in this field, has no executive apparatus. Whatever actual effects flow from its deliberations are the product of actions by individual national administrations. One consequence of this executive impotence of the Commission is the tendency to draw on extraneous authority to add force to its resolutions, as noted above. Another is the difficulty of securing public acknowledgment or attention to its

Table 3. INTERNATIONAL NARCOTICS CONTROL EXPENDITURE UNDER THE REGULAR BUDGET FOR 1969, 1970, AND 1971
(in thousands of United States dollars)

Established posts		Division $	n	Commission $	INCB $	n
Salaries and wages	1969	374.2	17;14ᵃ	—	163.2	9;6
	1970	390.6	17;14	—	166.1	9;6
	1971	403.1	17;14	—	180.0	10;7
Temporary assistance	1969	4.8		7.9	4.9	
	1970	13.5		23.9	3.0	
	1971	14.0		20.0	5.5	
Common staff costs	1969	91.4		—	39.9	
	1970	98.1		—	41.7	
	1971	103.1		—	46.0	
Travel:						
Representatives	1969	—		9.3	38.4	
	1970	—		12.0	59.5	
	1971	—		14.0	59.5	
Staff	1969	6.1		3.4	2.9	
	1970	8.0		—	3.5	
	1971	8.0		—	4.0	

	Year			
Printing	1969	19.1	8.2	1.5
	1970	24.4	—	7.3
	1971	23.9	—	8.0
Other costs	1969	0.3	—	0.4
	1970	0.3	—	0.5
	1971	0.3	—	0.5
Total direct cost	1969	268.7	28.8	478.4
	1970	298.5	35.9	518.0
	1971	319.2	34.0	536.7
Distribution of conference service costs	1969	44.8	221.6	—
	1970	50.0	230.0	—
	1971	50.0	240.0	—
Total costs under regular budget	1969	313.5	250.4	478.4
	1970	348.5	265.9	518.0
	1971	369.2	274.0	536.7

[a] First figure refers to number of posts in professional category and above; second figure refers to number in general service.

Table 4. Number of Representatives at the 24th Session of the Commission on Narcotic Drugs, Geneva, September 27–October 21, 1971

Members of Commission		Observers	
Brazil	3	Algeria	2
Canada	6	Argentina	1
Dominican Republic	3	Australia	2
Egypt	6	Austria	2
Federal Republic of Germany	4	Belgium	2
France	5	Bolivia	1
Ghana	2	Burma	1
Hungary	3	Chile	1
India	2	Colombia	1
Iran	2	Denmark	3
Jamaica	2	Greece	1
Japan	3	Holy See	1
Lebanon	2	Iraq	2
Mexico	3	Israel	1
Pakistan	3	Italy	5
Peru	2	Netherlands	2
Sweden	6	New Zealand	1
Switzerland	4	Nigeria	1
Togo	1	Panama	2
Turkey	8	Philippines	1
Soviet Union	2	Poland	1
United Kingdom	4	Singapore	1
United States	16	South Africa	2
Yugoslavia	2	Spain	1
		Thailand	4
	94	Venezuela	2
		Republic of Vietnam	2
			46

UN Organs		
UN Special Fund for Drug Abuse		4
Interagency Affairs Office		1
UNCTAD		1
UNDP		1
Treaty Bodies		
INCB		5
Specialized Agencies		
WHO		5
ILO		1
FAO		1
UNESCO		1
Other Intergovernmental Bodies		
Interpol		3
Custom Cooperation Council		1
Arab Antinarcotic Bureau		1
Nongovernmental Bodies		
League of Red Cross Societies		2
Friends World Committee for Consultation		1
World Young Women's Christian Association		1
International Federation of Women Lawyers		1
International Council on Alcohol and Addictions		1
		31

work, which has led the Commission (as some other international bodies) at times to couch its resolutions in exaggerated and overdramatic language (Edwards, 1971).

The cost of the Commission in 1971 was $274,000 (see Table 3).

DIVISION OF NARCOTIC DRUGS

The Division of Narcotic Drugs is an integral part of the Secretariat of the UN. Its activities are official actions of the Secretary-General of the UN, and are accordingly usually ascribed to him in the international treaties and other documents.

The Division is housed in the Palais des Nations at Geneva. It has a staff of thirty-one under the control of a director, and an annual budget of more than $500,000 (see Table 3).

Internally, the Division is organized into the Office of the Director, the General Section, the Scientific and Technical Section (otherwise known as the UN Narcotics Laboratory), and the Commission.

UN DEVELOPMENT PROGRAM

The United Nations Development Program (UNDP) is set up to provide funds for technical assistance to the less developed countries. It is financed by voluntary contributions from members of the UN and disburses its funds through UN organs and the specialized agencies. In 1970, out of a total budget of about $200 million, UNDP allocated $27,231 to technical assistance in the field of narcotics control. The smallness of this allocation reflects the low priority given to this field by many of the less developed nations, reinforced by the fact that there is a limit to each country's allocation of funds from UNDP, and the use of these funds for drug programs would cut into the amount available for agricultural and economic development.

Drug problems are of minor importance in comparison with the other social and economic needs of the less developed countries, even those that produce the raw materials (opium, cannabis, and coca) that sustain the serious drug problems of highly industralized societies. It is scarcely to be expected, therefore, that scarce UNDP funds should be devoted to programs such as crop substitution that would mainly benefit the developed nations, while involving the recipient country in, on balance, substantial social and financial costs.

UN SPECIAL FUND FOR DRUG ABUSE CONTROL (UNFDAC)

The UN Special Fund was established in April 1970, largely through the initiative of the United States. It is financed by voluntary contributions, and it disburses its resources through existing UN and other agencies. Its function is thus very similar to UNDP; it was established partly to remedy the inapplicability of UNDP funds to drug problems.

The Fund is administered directly by the Secretary-General of the UN (not by the Division of Narcotic Drugs). Until 1973, he exercised control through a Personal Representative with a staff of three, assisted by three consultants. In February 1973, however, a reorganization of UNFDAC was announced, which will give it a bureaucracy of its own under an exective director still directly responsible to the Secretary-General. UNFDAC will thus become a new section of the UN secretariat wholly concerned with drug problems, but administratively independent of the Commission and the Division.

In February 1973, the total either actually paid or pledged to the Fund amounted to just under $4,750,000; the initial contribution of the United States represents more than two-fifths of this sum.

Programs totaling $98 million over the next five years have been prepared in the expectation that the Fund would have reached its target of $20 million annually.

WORLD HEALTH ORGANIZATION

Membership of the World Health Organization (WHO) is open to any member of the UN by the simple act of accepting WHO's constitution; nonmembers of UN can be elected by a simple majority vote of the World Health Assembly. Territories that do not have responsibility for their international relations can become associate members. WHO is financed by contributions from its members: in 1971 its budget amounted to $72,230,000.[*]

WHO is administered by an Executive Board made up of twenty-four individual experts in public health designated by member states and elected by the World Health Assembly. The Board meets regularly twice a year to prepare the work of the Assembly, and to give effect to its decisions. The secretariat is housed in Geneva.

Only a small part of WHO's activities is concerned with drug abuse. The Drug Dependence Unit of the secretariat's Division of Pharmacology and Toxicology has a staff of four and a budget in 1971 of $52,551 (see Table 5).

The WHO draws on the medical and scientific expertise of the world by the device of expert advisory panels, consisting of individual experts appointed, with the agreement of their governments, by the director-general. Appointment to a panel is usually for a period of five years, with the possibility of reappointment subject to an age limit (except in special cases) of sixty-five. The function of a panel is to provide a pool of experts who can be called upon to serve as members of an expert committee. Membership of an expert advisory panel carries no remuneration.

[*] WHO Official Records No. 179, 1971, p. 20.

Table 5. WHO Drug Dependence Section, Budget Estimates

	1970	1971	1972
Salaries and Wages (2;2)[a]	$44,110	$45,151	$46,467
Consultants' Fees	2,700	2,700	3,600
Travel:			
Duty	2,000	2,000	2,000
Consultants	2,700	2,700	3,600
	$51,510	$52,551	$55,667
Expert Committee	14,600	16,000	17,000

[a] First figure refers to number of posts in professional category; second to number in general service category.
Source: WHO Official Records # 187, pp. 72–73.

EXPERT COMMITTEE ON DRUG DEPENDENCE

The Expert Committee on Drug Dependence has a membership of nine, chosen from the twenty-four members of the Expert Advisory Panel on Drug Dependence by the WHO Secretariat. The choice of members of the Committee is dictated by the content of the Committee's agenda (which is drawn up by the Drug Dependence Unit), and within these limitations by the principle of equitable geographical distribution. The composition of the Committee thus varies from meeting to meeting according to the main subject matter of the agenda. Like all WHO expert committees it has no real continuity of existence of its own, and functions much more like an ad hoc committee than a permanent one. Besides the appointed members of the Committee, its meetings are usually attended by up to three approved consultants, who are not necessarily members of the Expert Advisory Panel. Members of the Committee are specifically debarred from receiving instructions from their governments; their appointments are wholly in their capacity as experts in their field and limited to the session of the Committee. The range of scientific disciplines represented on the Committee tends to be limited, with medicine and pharmacology predominating (Edwards, 1971).

Though the WHO budget makes provision for an annual meeting of the Expert Committee, the interval between meetings may be more than a year. It has met on average in only two years out of every three (eighteen times in the past twenty-five years).

The Committee meets in the WHO headquarters in Geneva and its meetings usually last a week. Besides the members of the Committee, the meetings are attended by representatives of the Division of Narcotic Drugs and of the International Narcotics Control Board. A chairman and a rapporteur are elected on the first day. No minutes or shorthand notes are kept of the discussions. The draft of the Committee's official report is prepared by the rapporteur and considered and approved by the Committee at the end of the session. The consultants attending the Committee's meeting have usually been asked to prepare papers for the Committee dealing with one or another item on the agenda. These papers, and any other documentation, may be circulated to members of the Committee before they arrive in Geneva. The Committee's reports are published in the WHO Technical Report Series, after scrutiny by the WHO Directorate for any "statements of opinion that might be considered prejudicial to the best interests of the Organisation or any Member State" (Regulations for Advisory Panels, 1970, pp. 88–96), which may be deleted, though not amended, by the chairman without reference to the members of the Committee. Publication of the Committee's report is authorized by the WHO directorate. None of the documentation submitted to the Committee is published.

OTHER AGENCIES RELATED TO UN

In UN documents, frequent reference is made to liaison with other specialized agencies besides WHO. The chief of these are Food and Argiculture Organization (FAO), International Labour Office (ILO), United Nations Children's Fund (UNICEF), United Nations Conference on Trade and Development (UNCTAD), United Nations Educational Scientific and Cultural Organization (UNESCO), United Nations Social Defense Research Institute (UNSDRI), and Universal Postal Union (UPU).

Though no doubt valuable exchanges of information and advice result from liaison among these organizations and the organs directly concerned with drug programs, up to the time of writing no substantial budgetary commitments on the part of these organizations have been traced. The FAO has been involved for some years in discussions on the problems of substituting other cash crops for opium, particularly in Thailand, and the ILO in problems of rehabilitation and employment of former addicts in the same area. However, so far the active involvement of both these organizations, which are the two most frequently mentioned in the documents, seems to have been limited to the supply by ILO of one expert to help in the establishment of a welding shop in a prison for addicts, at the request of the Hong Kong government.

UNICEF and UNESCO have expressed interest and concern in developing educational and other programs for the prevention of drug abuse.

The UPU is concerned only with problems arising from the sending of controlled drugs, licitly and illicitly, through the international postal system.

Though the practical involvement of these agencies is at present minimal, the establishment of the UN Special Fund for Drug Abuse, with its promise of substantial funds to be channeled through UN agencies, has encouraged all of them (except the UPU and UNCTAD) to draw up programs in the field of drugs. However, the huge discrepancy between the estimated cost of all the programs hopeful of funding from the Special Fund, and the actual cash available, makes it impossible at this stage to forecast the likely practical involvement of any particular agency in the immediate future.

INTERNATIONAL NARCOTICS CONTROL BOARD (INCB)

The International Narcotics Control Board is a quasi-judicial body established by the 1961 Single Convention. Though in its present form it has been in existence only since 1968, it is directly descended from bodies with similar powers but different names (Permanent Central Opium Board, Permanent Central Narcotics Board, Drug Supervisory Body), going back to 1928. Of all the international bodies concerned with drug control, the INCB has the longest continuous experience with the problem (see Table 6).

Table 6. YEARS OF MEMBERSHIP IN INCB AND ITS PREDECESSORS OF BOARD MEMBERS IN 1972

Number of years	Number of Members	Total member/years
9 and over	4	69
3 to 8	3	12
Fewer than 3	4	4

The Board's authority derives directly from the international conventions; though it meets, and its secretariat is housed, in the Geneva headquarters of the UN, its terms of reference cannot be modified by any UN organ. This independence extends even to questions of interpretation of the treaty clauses governing the Board's activities. In the event of a dispute between the Board and another party, it is probable that the only possible outside arbiter would be the International Court of Justice.

The Board monitors world production, manufacture, trade, and distribution of substances controlled under the 1961 Single Convention on Narcotics and the 1971 Convention on Psychotropic Drugs. To this end, the Board regularly examines and collates statistical returns from governments throughout the world and is empowered to demand explanations of discrepancies. It is charged also with the duty of dealing with any country whose shortcomings appear likely to endanger the aims of the Conventions, and is armed with the power of reporting an offending country to ECOSOC and to other parties to the treaties, and in extreme circumstances of recommending the imposition of an embargo on the export of controlled drugs to the offender. In practice, the Board and its predecessors have very rarely resorted to the first of these sanctions and have never had occasion to recommend an embargo. The 1972 Protocol amending the 1961 Convention (which has yet to come into force) will to some degree extend the Board's powers of scrutiny and its capacity to impose sanctions.

The eleven members of the INCB are elected for a term of three years by ECOSOC under a complex set of restraints. By the terms of the Single Convention (Article 9) the Board must consist of:

> 1. (a) Three members with medical, pharmacological or pharmaceutical experience from a list of at least five persons nominated by the World Health Organisation; and (b) eight members from a list of persons nominated by Members of the United Nations and by Parties [to the Single Convention] which are not members of the United Nations.
>
> 2. Members of the Board shall be persons who, by their competence, impartiality and disinterestedness, will command general confidence. During their term of office they shall not hold any position or engage in any activity which would be liable to impair their impartiality in the exercise of their functions. . . .
>
> 3. The Council [ECOSOC], with due regard to the principle of equitable geographic representation, shall give consideration to the importance of including on the Board, in equitable proportions, persons possessing a knowledge of the drug situation in the producing, manufacturing, and consuming countries, and connected with such countries.

Impairment of impartiality (paragraph 2 above) is interpreted in practice as disqualifying anyone who holds an office that places him in a position of direct dependence on his government, unless upon election he resigns or is granted leave of absence for the term of his membership of the Board and does not act under the instructions of his government. Judges, university professors, doctors, lawyers, and other professional people have not had to give up their positions under this requirement; nor, surprisingly, has an ambassador.

Nominations for election to the Board are sifted first by ECOSOC's Committee on Candidatures. At the last election, in 1970, WHO nominated the minimum five persons required by the Single Convention; the twenty-two nominations received from governments were whittled down to a panel of sixteen by the Committee. While governments usually nominate only one of their own nationals, the same person may be, and occasionally is, nominated by more than one government or by both WHO and a government. The election is conducted in two stages; first, three members are elected from among the WHO nominees, then eight members are elected from the panel of government nominees. If an unsuccessful WHO nominee has also been nominated by a government, then he is added to the panel of government nominees, and thus has a second chance of election. In the 1970 election, both the candidates with such a dual nomination were in fact elected in the first ballot and both received more votes than anyone else in either ballot.

How, under this system of election, due weight is given to the requirements of paragraph 3 above is unclear; nevertheless, the Board's present membership appears to satisfy them well enough.

Membership of the Board is not a sinecure and all members are expected to attend all its meetings, for which the quorum is seven. These are held two (and sometimes three) times a year and each occupies between two and four weeks. In addition, members are expected to possess knowledge and experience of narcotics control at both national and international levels. These requirements, coupled with the bar on direct dependence on governments, weight the choice of nominees heavily toward individuals nearing or past retirement from their main careers, and the average age of the Board is consequently high. A further consequence is that the scientific expertise represented on the Board is confined to disciplines, such as pharmacology and medicine, with a long-standing concern with narcotic drugs, while the social and behavioral sciences that have only begun to take an interest in more recent years are not represented.

The Board elects a president and two vice-presidents annually, and re-election of officeholders is usual. The present president, for example, has occupied that office since 1953.

Besides travel and per diem expenses in connection with the Board's meetings, members of the Board receive a small honorarium ($1,000 annually). In 1971, payments to members under all heads totaled $59,500. (See Table 2.)

INCB SECRETARIAT

Administratively, the INCB secretariat is part of the secretariat of the UN and its costs are met out of UN funds. However, its functional independence is required by the 1961 Single Convention and assured in practice by a detailed resolution of ECOSOC (1196 XLII) which lays down, among other things that (1) The INCB secretariat is bound to carry out the decisions of the INCB; (2) it must have a separate budget prepared by itself, approved by the INCB, and submitted directly to the General Assembly of the UN by the UN Secretary-General as part of the total UN budget; (3) its budget must include provisions for the travel of INCB members, salaries of the secretariat, printing of reports, and other items necessary for it to function effectively; (4) all payments out of the budget require the INCB's authority; (5) the INCB's correspondence is subject to no outside control, its incoming mail must reach its secretariat unopened, and outgoing mail must be sealed by the secretariat before dispatch; and (6) the appointment of the head of its secretariat is subject to the approval of the INCB.

Though the INCB secretariat is housed in the same building, the Palais des Nations at Geneva, as the Division of Narcotic Drugs, its offices are separate from those of the Division.

The secretariat has a staff of seventeen and an annual budget in 1971 of $370,000 (see Table 3).

INTERNATIONAL CRIMINAL POLICE ORGANIZATION (INTERPOL)

Interpol was established in 1923 with the aim of enabling police forces in different countries to coordinate their work and cooperate in law enforcement and crime prevention. Until 1956, it was primarily a Western European organization, but since then it has developed a worldwide membership with the exception of Eastern European nations. It has been based in Paris since 1946.

Interpol is governed by a general assembly of delegates from its 111 member countries working through an executive committee of thirteen. It is financed by contributions from its member governments. It has a staff of 108, of whom 12 are assigned to drug problems. Its 1971 budget was a little less than $1 million.

Interpol always sends observers to the sessions of the Commission on Narcotic Drugs and has for many years cooperated with the Division on Narcotic Drugs in supplying information on illicit traffic to the Commission. In 1971, it came to an agreement with ECOSOC that provides for even closer cooperation. The amount of time spent at Interpol's annual conferences in discussing resolutions concerning drugs is very much greater than the proportion of staff assigned to this field would suggest.

Interpol's functions are limited to the collection, collation, and dissemination of information about international criminal activities. It has no enforcement or investigational powers. Its effectiveness thus depends upon the efficiency of reporting by its members.

CUSTOMS COOPERATION COUNCIL

The Customs Cooperation Council was established in 1953 with a principal function of coordinating and resolving technical problems relating to customs and to facilitate the expansion of international trade. It also provides a channel for exchange of information between national customs administrations about violations of customs laws. In 1971, it adopted a recommendation for the spontaneous exchange of information among its members about illicit traffic in psychoactive substances.

Sixty-seven nations, from all parts of the globe, are members of the CCC. Its budget for 1972 was $1 million, and its headquarters are in Brussels.

CLASSIFICATION FOR INTERNATIONAL CONTROL

This section seeks to answer two questions. First, how do psychoactive drugs come to be included in the schedules (classifications) of the Conventions as adopted by Plenipotentiary Conference? Second, how are the schedules, once adopted, amended by the addition, deletion, or transfer between schedules of substances?

Drafting of Schedules

The draft schedules presented to the conferences called to agree upon final texts of both the 1961 and 1971 Conventions were prepared by WHO with the assistance of its Expert Committee on Drug Dependence. At both conferences, a technical committee was appointed to examine the drafts.

For the 1961 Convention, WHO introduced what was virtually a consolidated list of the substances controlled under previous international treaties. The Conference recast the order and the definitions of certain drugs but made no major alterations to the substances proposed for control.

For the 1971 Convention, WHO put forward a draft based on a compilation of Isbell and Chrusciel (1970), the main contribution of the Expert Committee being the selection and allocation of psychoactive drugs from that list to one of four schedules, according to their presumed medical usefulness and dependence-producing potential. The technical committee of the 1971 conference retained the four-schedule structure, but made a number of amendments to the list of drugs included in the "less dangerous" categories and did not include the drugs that the Expert Committee had considered on grounds, not of demonstrated potential for abuse, but of analogy with drugs known or suspected to be abused.

Schedules of 1961 Single Convention

The procedure for amending its schedules is set out in Article 3 of the 1961 Convention.

The first step is the reception by the Division of Narcotic Drugs of a proposal to add, delete, or alter the scheduling of, a psychoactive drug. In practice, the great majority of proposals have been for the addition of new drugs. Proposals may originate either from parties to the Single Convention or from WHO; however, in practice, WHO has not originated any proposals relating to single drugs (as opposed to classes of drugs); they have all come from individual governments.[*]

[*] WHO has originated only one proposal under Article 3—for the inclusion in Schedule I of a generic description of a class of drugs that had featured in the schedules of the 1931 Convention. This proposal had already once been rejected by the Conference on the 1961 Convention, which had preferred to specify drugs individually; it was rejected again by the Commission on Narcotic Drugs on legal grounds.

However, there are occasions when WHO appears to originate a proposal relating to an individual drug. This comes about when a government that is a party to earlier conventions but not to the 1961 Convention proposes a drug for control under the earlier convention. Under the pre-1961 treaties, the WHO Expert Committee on Drug Dependence is sole arbiter of whether a drug should be internationally controlled or not. When it places a drug under control under one of the earlier treaties, it simultaneously makes a recommendation for its inclusion in the 1961 Single Convention. For example, in 1968, Belgium, which at that time had not ratified the 1961 Convention, proposed bezitramide for inclusion under the 1948 Protocol to which she was a party. The Expert Committee decided that bezitramide should be controlled under the 1948 Protocol, and also proposed that it should

Proposals for the addition of individual new drugs usually have their origin with the pharmaceutical manufacturer responsible for its development, who will wish to clarify the drug's status under both national and international law before developing it further for therapeutic use. In the early days of the control of synthetic narcotic analgesics (by the 1948 Protocol), the practice was to report all newly developed drugs with dependence liability, irrespective of the likelihood of their proving of value in actual clinical use. As a result, between 1951 and 1960, fifty-one new drugs were brought under international control, though the majority were never marketed, or even manufactured on anything larger than an experimental laboratory scale. More recently, it has become the practice to put forward new drugs for international control only if there is a real expectation that they will possess sufficient advantages over existing drugs to warrant manufacturing them on a commercial scale. Consequently, only eighteen new drugs have been controlled under the Single Convention between 1961 and 1970.

The notification received from a government by the Division of Narcotic Drugs will thus usually be based on information supplied by a manufacturer and supported by evidence from the same source. The Division translates the notification and the directly relevant parts of the supporting evidence into the four UN official languages and circulates them to all the parties to the Single Convention and to WHO.

WHO places the proposal on the agenda of the next meeting of the Expert Committee on Drug Dependence. Originally, the Expert Committee was formed for the sole purpose of classifying drugs under the international treaties, but in recent years its agenda has been broadened considerably so that classification proposals form only a minor part of its work. The Committee's recommendations are based on a consideration of the notification transmitted by the Division of Narcotic Drugs, and data prepared by the WHO secretariat from the evidence submitted with the notification and from other sources, sometimes accompanied by the views of an acknowledged expert. The Committee's role is confined to a consideration of the evidence submitted to it; neither it nor WHO have facilities for any kind of experimental investigation of the dependence liability of drugs. Usually, the Committee is able to reach a decision, but occasionally it will conclude that the evidence is insufficient and will defer the matter to its next meeting.

Proposals to free drugs from international control are uncommon. Only one, dextropropoxyphene, has been deleted from the schedules of the 1961 Convention. The evidence needed to support such a proposal must clearly be of a different kind from that required to support a proposal for control. In the case of dextropropoxyphene, it consisted of evidence of widespread clinical use over a period of five years with a low incidence of reported dependence, coupled with the

---

be controlled under the 1961 Convention. At the time of writing, some thirty countries, including the Federal Republic of Germany, Greece, and Switzerland, are parties to the older international treaties, but have not yet ratified the 1961 Convention. So this anomalous procedure is likely to recur.

results of repeated observations on human volunteers at the Addiction Research Center at Lexington, Kentucky, in the United States (World Health Organization Technical Report #273, 1964).

The final stage in the process of classification is the consideration of the WHO recommendations by the Commission on Narcotic Drugs, which has the final authority for deciding whether a drug should be controlled under the 1961 Convention (but see previous footnote). This decision is made either at the Commission's session or, to avoid delay, by a postal ballot of member governments of the Commission if the next session is not due to start within three months from the receipt of WHO's recommendation by the Division of Narcotic Drugs.

The Commission's power of decision is limited to accepting or rejecting the WHO recommendation; it may not amend it. The Commission cannot, for example, decide to place a drug in a different schedule, and thus subject it to a different degree of control, from that recommended by WHO. This is a consequence of the criteria for inclusion of a new substance under the 1961 Convention, that is, whether it has a potential for abuse similar to that of drugs already included in one or another of the schedules. This is supposed to be a matter of scientific fact, and WHO is the only body recognized by the Convention as having competence in matters of scientific fact.

In practice, the Commission has always accepted WHO's recommendations when they have been confined to the allocation of individual drugs to particular schedules. When, however, WHO's recommendation strays beyond this and is in a form that could be interpreted as an amendment to the Convention rather than to its schedules or could set a precedent affecting future classification decisions, the Commission has always either rejected the WHO recommendation in toto or reduced it to a simple recommendation for the control of an individual substance. It is on these matters that the Commission will seek the advice of the UN Office of Legal Affairs to establish whether the WHO recommendation would constitute an amendment to the Convention rather than to its schedules.

The example of etorphine and acetorphine illustrate this point. These two drugs appear to possess a high potential for abuse and are not used in human medicine, facts that render them candidates for the most severe controls, that is, inclusion in both Schedules I and IV along with heroin, cannabis, and two lesser known drugs. However, etorphine and acetorphine have an important role in veterinary medicine: they are used to immobilize large wild animals, like elephants and elks, so that a veterinary surgeon can examine or treat them without risk of attack. The Expert Committee, therefore, besides recommending the inclusion of these drugs in Schedules I and IV, added a rider making their inclusion in the stricter Schedule IV dependent upon this not unduly restricting their use in animals. The Office of Legal Affairs ruled that the wording of the 1961 Convention did not permit a distinction to be drawn between human and veterinary medicine, and that to give effect to the Expert Committee's rider would require the Convention to be amended. WHO then reiterated its former recommendation that these drugs should be controlled under Schedules I and IV, this time adding a further recommendation that the Convention should be amended so that a drug could be subjected to the strictest control as far as its use in humans, while remaining subject to less severe control with respect to its use in animals. The Commission on Narcotic Drugs confirmed the inclusion of etorphine and acetorphine in Schedules I and IV, and took no action on the question of amending the Convention.

It is pertinent to observe that during the two years (1967 and 1968) that the Commission was considering the classification of etorphine and acetorphine, the WHO Expert Committee did not meet. The revised recommendation (that the Single Convention should be amended) therefore emanated from WHO without having been considered by the Expert Committee. There is, indeed, no requirement in the Single Convention that WHO's recommendations on the classification of drugs should be made with the assistance of the Expert Committee. Moreover, the published reports of the Expert Committee carry a statement on the cover in which WHO disclaims responsibility for the views expressed within; it would therefore seem that there is no requirement that WHO's recommendations to the Commission should accord with the Expert Committee's advice, though in practice they always have.

When the Commission on Narcotic Drugs has decided whether or not to adopt the WHO's recommendation, the process of classification is in practice completed, and governments are bound to apply the appropriate controls as soon as they are notified of the Commission's decision by the Division of Narcotic Drugs. For though the Single Convention does provide for an appeal to ECOSOC against a classification decision taken by the Commission, such an appeal has never been made. Nor, since no one can imagine any circumstances in which ECOSOC would overturn a decision of the Commission on so technical a matter as classification, is an appeal ever likely to be made.

Schedules of 1971 Convention

The 1971 Convention has not yet come into force so any discussion of its machinery for classification must be theoretical.

In general, the procedures laid down are similar to those of the 1961 Convention. The important differences are that the respective areas of competence of WHO and the Commission are spelled out in the 1971 Convention (WHO to take account of medical and scientific considerations; the Commission to concern itself with economic, social and other factors) and that the wording gives the Commission much increased authority in matters of classification. The first would seem a natural extension and codification of a division of responsibility that has emerged in practice under the 1961 Convention, rather than an innovation. The second represents a new development whereby the Commission could become the effective classifying body, with WHO reduced to a merely advisory role. It remains to be seen in what circumstances the Commission will overrule WHO's advice and what kind of evidence will form the basis of the Commission's classification decisions.

CLASSIFICATION CRITERIA OF INTERNATIONAL CONVENTIONS

Single Convention on Narcotic Drugs, 1961, Article 3, paragraph 3

3. . . . . Where a notification relates to a substance not already in Schedule I or in Schedule II, (i) . . . (ii) . . , (iii) If the World Health Organisation finds that the substance is liable to similar abuse and productive of similar ill effects as the drugs in Schedule I or Schedule II or is convertible into a drug, it shall communicate that finding to the Commission which may, in accordance with the recommendation of the World Health Organisation, decide that the substance shall be added to Schedule I or Schedule II.

4. If the World Health Organisation finds that a preparation because of the substances which it contains is not liable to abuse and cannot produce ill effects (paragraph 3) and that the drug therein is not readily recoverable, the Commission may, in accordance with the recommendation of the World Health Organisation, add that preparation to Schedule III.

5. If the World Health Organisation finds that a drug in Schedule I is particularly liable to abuse and to produce ill effects (paragraph 3) and that such liability is not offset by substantial therapeutic advantages not possessed by substances other than drugs in Schedule IV, the Commission may, in accordance with the recommendation of the World Health Organisation, place that drug in Schedule IV.

Convention on Psychotropic Substances, 1971, Article 2, paragraph 4

4. . . . . If the World Health Organisation finds: (a) that the substance has the capacity to produce (i) (1) a state of dependence, and (2) central nervous system stimulation or depression, resulting in hallucinations or disturbances in motor function or thinking or behavior or perception or mood, or (ii) similar abuse and similar ill effects as a substance in Schedule I, II, III or IV, and (b) that there is sufficient evidence that the substance is being or is likely to be abused so as to constitute a public health and social problem warranting the placing of the substance under international control the World Health Organisation shall communicate to the Commission an assessment of the substance, including the extent or likelihood of abuse, the degree of seriousness of the public health and social problem and the degree of usefulness of the substance in medical therapy, together with recommendations on control measures, if any, that would be appropriate in light of its assessment.

5. The Commission, taking into account the communication from the World Health Organisation, whose assessments shall be determinative as to medical and scientific matters, and bearing in mind the economic,

social, legal, administrative and other factors it may consider relevant, may add the substance to Schedule I, II, III or IV. The Commission may seek further information from the World Health Organisation or from other appropriate sources.

ANALYSIS OF CLASSIFICATION PROCESSES

The process of classifying drugs for the purposes of international control is worthy of study for many reasons, not least the worldwide impact of its decisions. The classifications recommended by WHO and confirmed by the Commission on Narcotic Drugs play a decisive role not only in international legislation, but also in the legislation of individual countries. Though only the parties to the international treaties are bound to act on the Commission's classification decisions, in practice most nations treat any drug controlled under the international treaties as ipso facto in need of national control within their own jurisdictions. Indeed, countries with little nonmedical use of drugs tend to rely entirely on the international classification system and to have no separate classification process of their own. Thus until 1964 the schedules of drugs controlled under United Kingdom dangerous drugs laws were strictly linked to the schedules of the Single Convention and could not be altered independently of international classification decisions; special legislation had to be introduced in 1964 to bring the misuse of drugs not covered by the Single Convention, such as amphetamines and LSD, under legal control. More recently, Argentina and Ghana adopted the schedules of the 1971 Convention, before ratification, as a basis of national legislation. There are also indications that some countries intend to lump together all substances covered by both the 1961 and 1971 Conventions, designating them all as "narcotics" to be controlled with the same severity. Such developments illustrate the classificatory force that UN decisions may exert on national legislation to an extent not intended by the international treaties.

The tendency toward automatic adoption of international classification decisions as an appropriate basis for national legislation thus makes the impact of these decisions wider and more immediate than that of the treaties under which they are made. As a consequence they lead to the imposition of a considerable burden of regulation, licensing, quota-fixing, and other control measures. This burden falls alike on government administrations and producers, manufacturers, and distributors of classified drugs as well as on the medical and pharmaceutical professions. For a first objective of drug legislation has always been to control licit manufacture and trade in order to prevent diversion of classified drugs into the illicit market, licit operations being naturally more amenable to regulation than illicit.

So far as illicit trade is concerned, international classification decisions do not seem to have great impact, perhaps because the controls they impose on new substances do in fact prevent their entry into the illicit market or perhaps because, as long as the old and tried drugs are available, the illicit market feels no need to experiment with alternatives. Certainly, if illicit supplies of the traditional opium derivatives were successfully curtailed, the schedules of the Single Convention would provide illicit users with a handy shopping list of alternatives.

The criteria laid down in the Single Convention (Article 3), on the basis of which WHO is to make its classificatory recommendations, are threefold: liability to abuse, production of ill effects, and therapeutic usefulness. As is well documented elsewhere in this volume, the arrival at a scientifically based, objective assessment of these three criteria is fraught with difficulties and perhaps not achievable at the present time; however, it is not a priori impossible. The shortcomings imputed to the WHO Expert Committee on Drug Dependence, are usually in terms of inadequate representation of relevant expertise other than traditional medical and pharmacological or of the inadequacy of the scientific resources available to it. It is assumed that scientific assessment is not impossible, and that it is therefore not impossible that the Expert Committee or some body of scientists could bring genuine objectivity to bear on classification decisions made for the purpose of international legislation and control.

However, a closer reading of Article 3 of the Single Convention reveals that the substances WHO is asked to classify are a *selected* sample of psychoactive substances, and that WHO need not have any say in the criteria by which they are selected. In other words, there is a process of classification that is superordinate to the classification work of WHO. In actual fact, there are, not one, but two such superordinate classification processes.

The existence of the first is indicated by the words "in its opinion" in paragraph 1 of Article 3, which reads: "Where a Party or the World Health Organisation has information which in its opinion may require an amendment to any of the schedules (of controlled drugs), it shall notify the Secretary General . . ."

The decision whether a drug should be reported to the UN as a possible candidate for international control is made by national governments, as has been described earlier, often at the instance of the manufacturer responsible for its development. Though a consideration of the criteria specifically mentioned in the Single Convention will clearly play an important part in forming this decision, other criteria, such as potential marketability, may enter.

The second classification superordinate to WHO has much more profound implications and goes back to the genesis of the entire system of international control. Its existence is signalled in the Single Convention by a significant qualification of the criteria of liability to abuse and production of ill effects: the abuse and the ill effects must be "similar" to those that attend substances *already* in the schedules of the Convention. This proviso has prevented any proposal that, for example, alcohol or tobacco should be controlled under the Single Convention and has also prevented consideration of amphetamines and other psychotropic drugs for inclusion in its schedules. What this proviso means is that WHO may make classification decisions only about the kind of psychoactive substances that the Single Convention is meant to cover.

What kind of psychoactive substances, then, is the Single Convention meant to cover? As has already been pointed out, all the substances in its original schedules had already been subject to control under various earlier treaties. Moreover, a closer examination reveals that, with the exception of cannabis, all these drugs are derived from or related to the two drugs—opiates (specifically opium, morphine, and heroin) and cocaine—that were listed in the first international treaty to deal with psychoactive substance, the Hague International Convention for the Suppression of Abuse of Opium and Other Drugs of 1912. The reasons these drugs were singled out at that time as in need of international control are complex and confused: undoubtedly moral indignation and political, social, and mercantile considerations all played a part. What is certain is that this original classification decision was not based on an objective examination of statistical or scientific evidence, but on the kind of value judgments that have always gone to the making of political decisions about social problems, and on the then-existing balance of international power (King, 1972). (One might speculate, for instance, that had the Moslem nations wielded greater influence, a combination of pressure from them and from the powerful Christian temperance movements of the period might have led to alcohol becoming the first psychoactive substance subject to an international agreement.)

Whether political decisions can, or even should, be determined by objective examination of scientific or statistical evidence is a topic well beyond the scope of this discussion. The point to be made is that, as a matter of historical fact, the Single Convention on Narcotic Drugs is the end product of a value judgment about what kinds of drugs should be the subject of an international system of control. The determinants of this judgment are to be found in the 1912 climate of moral opinion and the complexities of international diplomacy and trade at that time. Scientific knowledge and objective assessment are called in only for the purpose of elaborating the detailed consequences, and providing insofar as possible a justification, of the original judgmentally based classification.

The Convention on Psychotropic Substances appears to give a freer hand to WHO. Besides the criteria of "similarity" to substances already covered by the Convention, an alternative set of criteria is laid down that on the face of it would appear to allow the inclusion of, for example, tobacco and alcohol in the schedules of the Convention. At the same time, however, the power of the Commission on Narcotic Drugs to enter into the classification process is substantially increased, and with it the opportunity for politically determined value judgments to override conclusions reached by the logical application of objective tests. Until—and assuming that—the 1971 Convention comes into force, it must remain a matter of speculation how far the pursuit of objective criteria in classification will be limited by preselection of the substances put forward for consideration, and how far by rejection by the Commission using its broad authority untrammeled by canons of evidence. Of the two constraints, the latter is to be preferred if only because it may enable the conflict between conclusions arrived at by scientific endeavor and those reached by the exercise of political judgment to be exposed and even fruitfully discussed. This would, of course, require something more than brief minutes to report the dynamics of the Commission's deliberations.

Conflict of this kind is likely to be present in any attempt to use scientific and objective methods in classifying psychoactive substances for the purposes of imposing legislative controls. Such difficulties are by no means a peculiarity of the international system; undoubtedly they are present in equal or greater degree in national systems of classification. The international system has been singled out for description because it has the virtue that its manner of working is at least capable of scrutiny and can thus serve to exemplify the difficulties and dilemmas of classifying drugs for purposes of public policy.

Issues and
Recommendations

James Moore

XVII

The complexity of the issues involved in devising drug-classification schemes makes it abundantly clear that no simple and single approach can be anticipated. Some guidelines can be offered, however, which can go far to alleviate many of the difficulties that have plagued both nations and international bodies for decades.

In all drug classification, the first decision must be whether a substance is to be considered a drug. At the present time the drugs that command most legislative attention are those substances that affect the mind (psychoactive drugs). However, it must not be forgotten that no classification scheme linked to a control system can effectively contain the distribution of all psychoactive substances. Many commonly available household and industrial solvents, for example, do not lend themselves to such controls, even though it is recognized that their use can and sometimes does give rise to problems.

The majority of psychoactive drugs constitute valuable and sometimes indispensable therapeutic agents. But the benefits of their legitimate medical administration must be weighed against possible risks arising from their non-medical use. A realistic assessment of that balance in relation to the objectives of control policies presupposes, however, the existence of appropriate criteria and adequate methods in order to estimate the nature and importance of these risks and benefits.

It follows, then, that as new information emerges, new assessments will have to be made and, perhaps, new judgments based on the new data. Therefore, control efforts, classification schemes, and, indeed, all forms of intervention do well to be permanently provisional. They must have built-in mechanisms for evaluation and revision. Likewise, programs that are not intended to be evaluated should contain self-terminating mechanisms as part of their formal procedure.

Unfortunately, it must be said that little attention has been paid to the impact of existing treaties and regulations. This situation need not continue. There is general agreement that legislative and other social responses to drug use can be evaluated, and evaluated in ways by which we can learn something of the conditions that contribute to either effective or ineffective intervention. This process can also provide information about what corrective courses should be pursued. Laws without action are of little value. Likewise, laws and action without evaluation cannot provide a sound basis for drug control. Continuous evaluation is essential.

Classification schemes themselves are useful only insofar as they are designed for a specific purpose and attempt to rank substances according to defined criteria or concepts (for example, chemical, biological, therapeutic, or toxicological). But it must be kept in mind that such classifications cannot automatically be applied to social controls. There are many ways to control the production, marketing, and use of drugs—by prohibition or regulation; by taxing or issuing licenses or franchises; by punishing, educating, or providing alternatives. Do not assume that one form of social response—criminal sanctions—is the only one deserving of national or international recommendation or requirement. Nor can one assume that the same response or intervention works equally well for each drug, user, or setting, nor that a form of intervention will always succeed as long as one of these elements remains constant. The passage of time often introduces important changes that will alter the impact of that intervention.

Unfortunately, national laws and international agreements apparently have placed the emphasis on administrative and penal controls, and administrators have rarely, if at all, conducted systematic analyses to determine which models are appropriate to various national and local conditions. In national laws and international agreements, the scope of all alternative courses must be considered if policies are to be comprehensive and flexible.

Where are these alternatives to be found? While scientific methods and understanding of drug effects and drug use are still imprecise, nevertheless science can play an important role in the building of classification schemes and of the controls and other social responses linked to those schemes. True, scientists do not always agree on what are the best methods for studying drug uses and drug effects or on what data are the most appropriate and adequate for such studies. Nevertheless, there is unanimous agreement that many different factors influence the use of drugs. These include chemical, physiological, psychological, social, and cultural factors.

One difficulty arises, of course, from the lack of standards to govern the kind and quantity of information that should be available to policy-makers before they classify drugs or devise control measures. They must, therefore, set explicit standards regarding this evidence. When it is insufficient they must establish procedures for obtaining it. They must devise methods for financing the required research; they must identify the pool or pools of scientists and scholars available for the studies; they must specify the settings in which they wish to have observations conducted; and they must anticipate that their findings will have varying levels of probability.

The information upon which most existing classification schemes are based varies not only among schemes prepared by different agencies (for example, national or international), but even among the classifications into subcategories within a single scheme. Although, for example, they may purport to be based on pharmacological principles, all too often they are incomplete, inconsistent, or illogical, even within this limited framework. They seldom take account of well-known evidence that drug effects depend upon such factors as formulation, dose, frequency, or route of administration and that they are subject to statistical (sampling) error. The principles upon which any drug classification system is based should be explicitly stated and logically applied. If they are based on pharmacological principles they should explicitly take account of formulation, dose, frequency, and route of administration. They should also state the permissible limits of tolerance (in a statistical sense), as do other internationally accepted measures for the estimation of drug concentration and purity (for example, pharmacopoeial standards for antibiotics, hormones, and vitamins).

It is also evident that the scope, vocabulary, sanctions, and logic of existing classification schemes and of the controls that are linked to the schemes are often inadequate. One need only consider the imprecision and ambiguity that arise from the use of such terms as *misuse, risk, benefits, efficacy.*

Considering this multitude of complexities and taking account of the serious shortcomings in present approaches, the classification schemes currently employed for legislative purposes should be abandoned. New schemes must be developed that are suited to the goals of policy-makers. These should deal explicitly with the array of criteria and assumptions that present themselves when policy-makers wish to achieve classificatory objectives for purposes of social control. However, before they adopt new schemes of classification, they should consider and systematically evaluate the many alternative methods and perspectives that are available to them. They must recognize the many factors that are implicit in all of this—pharmaceutical chemistry, pharmacodynamics, purposes of drug use, settings of drug use, the characteristics of the users, and the different kinds of controls that might be employed, as well as sanctions and other social response measures that are available. They must consider risks, benefits, costs of all kinds, feasibility of implementation, and the likely impact of all the various policy approaches. Again, they should not look for absolute and final solutions, but should keep in mind that probability rather than certainty is the proper language of estimation.

Nor should it be forgotten that present drug classification and control schemes exclude some important, problem-creating drugs. Because they have a history of social use that antedates international controls, we cannot ignore the problems posed by the use of such powerful drugs as alcohol and tobacco.

In a similar context, existing classification schemes are also prone to assume, without demonstration, the prevalence and severity of the problems that arise from the nonmedical use of certain drugs. Inadequate though it may be, any and all information about the size of the problems created by the use of such drugs and the comparative success of the different measures that have been adopted to deal with the problem should be employed. This information can be used to create a quantitative basis on which model systems can be constructed, which, in turn, can replace conjecture and unjustified assumptions about the prevalence, severity, or outcomes of drug use.

Present schemes are also defective when they attribute observed drug effects solely to the pharmacological properties of the drug, ignoring profound modifications of behavior that arise from variations in the responses of individuals to a drug. These modifications may arise from differences in the will, knowledge, expectations, and the environment of both the person who receives the drug and the person who gives it. Therefore, classification schemes should not be based solely upon pharmacological principles. Because social and individual factors often modify responses to drugs as much as their chemical structure, these must also be taken into account. As a result of these factors, some groups may merit either exemption from controls or stricter control. In any event, the measures adopted should be sufficiently flexible to allow variation in either of these directions as well as modifications when changing circumstances require them.

Those responsible for classification must keep in mind that minor differences in the chemical structure of drugs may bring about different desirable or undesirable effects, giving rise to new and different social problems or degrees of problem. This requires special attention. Whatever control criteria are explicitly adopted to cope with this factor, whether they be chemical, pharmacological, clinical, or social, they should be in sufficient detail to permit an appropriately differentiated control of substances that may resemble each other in respect to one criterion, but not in respect to others. The criteria should not, however, be so minutely descriptive as to result in a topheavy, uneconomic, and unworkable administrative apparatus.

Although explicitly based upon one set of criteria (for example, pharmacological), some classification schemes may implicitly incorporate other concealed criteria. Some of these may concern, for example, whether the uses to which the substances are put are licit or illicit, or whether the control measures are workable in practice. Some measures may also, in fact, discriminate between the kinds of people who use drugs, or the kinds of places in which drugs are used. Control measures should not seek to control or free from control groups of individuals for reasons that are not explicitly related to their actual use of drugs.

Factors such as age, health, and degree of maturation may modify individual responses to psychoactive drugs and the resulting risks. These and other factors may need to be considered in preparing classification and drug control measures. Before they are used as a permanent basis for discriminatory measures, adequate information about their relevance should be obtained.

We must also be aware of the danger that political leaders at times may act, in drug matters, under pressures that are unrelated, in fact, to drug-associated problems. They may, for example, associate drug use with crime, family disruption, youthful unrest, or other social difficulties. If such complications are expressed in international policy, they may very well inhibit effective intervention in genuine drug problems.

The type of control to be applied must depend not only on the effects of the drugs, but also on the effects of the control policies themselves. The outcome of these policies will vary according to national and even local conditions. Treaties and laws, therefore, should be flexible enough to permit the flexible application of policies.

The difficulties faced by policy-makers in devising classification schemes and control systems are further compounded by the rapid development of new psychoactive drugs, new means of administering them, and new standards for both their medical and nonmedical use. The expectation of such rapid change should be reflected not only in classification schemes, but also in information systems, methods of research, control measures, or other social responses. Flexibility is absolutely essential. Personnel engaged in drug classification must have uptodate information available to them so that fundamental revisions in the schemes, when needed, can be anticipated. Such revisions will effect, of course, the control systems linked to the classification schemes as well as other social responses. Essentially, it is a question of learning to anticipate the advent of new kinds of drugs, new standards of behavior, new expectations regarding both desired and undesired outcomes, new forms of nonmedical drug use (both licit and illicit), and medical use and new mechanisms of action. In summary, they must expect new problems.

The virtually universal nature of drug use makes the formulation of international classification schemes having common objectives and policies that can be implemented extremely difficult. There are no cross-cultural or within-society agreements regarding preferences for forms of drug use, the propriety of drug use, or for the lifestyles that may be associated with drug use. For this reason it is highly unlikely that experiences (successes or failures) in one setting or country can be applied automatically in another setting or country, let alone find uniform application on an international scale.

At the international level, those who plan classification schemes must consider what range of responses will be relevant to all those persons, communities, regions, and nations that constitute the world community. They must determine which responses are capable of being facilitated by national or international action. They must know what practical steps must be taken. They must gather and interpret information about the operation and impact of each of the various forms of response in order to estimate costs and benefits of various responses in specific populations in specific settings.

It must be kept in mind, too, that genetic and cultural factors modify responses to drugs to an extent that drug-related problems may differ substantially from one people to another.

History demonstrates that policy-makers have often been prone to recommend harsh sanctions to combat practices that are foreign to their own customs. Restraint should therefore be exercised in proposing interventions that are adverse to either nonrepresented groups or to disinterested parties. A golden rule in planning international drug policy might be: discuss the classification and control of others' drugs as you would have them discuss the classification and control of yours. Such an ethic might help to sensitize policy-makers to the inequities in control practices that are based on the drug customs of another culture.

Nor should it be forgotten that a variety of interest groups seek to influence the course of national and international drug programs. These groups include users as well as commercial, religious, and political institutions and experts in the various fields of intervention, to mention only a few. Therefore, independent evaluations of international policies and operations are essential. The alternative is to permit narrow interests to create policies that not only may fail to benefit but also may bring harm to nonrepresented parties. Independent evaluations, on the other hand, can expedite the termination of ineffectual programs and enhance workable ones. Evaluators should also be encouraged to study the interests that generate and oppose programs, so that we may better understand the political, economic, and social dynamics of drug-policy development.

By failing to examine their own drug use and responses to it, for example, nations have tended not to formulate objectives in the national interest. The effects of this omission are compounded when they fail to assess how international collaboration may best serve national interests. Likewise, apathy or failure by governments to perceive the utility of involving themselves from the beginning in treaty planning can give rise, at a later date, to international ineffectiveness or national discontent. This arises when parties that were formerly disinterested find themselves confronted with drug-related problems of their own, or when they discover that their own interests are affected by the control measures employed by parties outside their jurisdiction.

It cannot be denied that, given the diversity of national interests, any international scheme for control is likely to be in conflict with some national interests. It is also true that practices will exist within nations that, while not identified as a national interest, represent local commerce or customs that do not align themselves with uniform international policy. In consequence, international policies should be sufficiently broad to entertain a diversity of national programs. In such situations, when local practices are antithetical to national and international objectives, methods can be devised to cooperate with the nation in question to influence or change local practices. One could consider, for example, steps by which those nations that are beneficiaries of international policies might compensate nations whose interests are compromised by those policies.

In addition policy-makers should not forget that although precedent may provide a useful basis for achieving agreement among those trained in law and diplomacy, it may very well prove quite inadequate in anticipating drug-related problems or responses to those problems.

The administration of international drug programs requires a competent administrative apparatus. It must be geared to gather, communicate, and utilize new information in the drafting of classification schemes and the designing of control and intervention programs. But one should not, in advance, assume the most desirable approach—centralized or decentralized administrative units, the finances that will be required, or the skills of the personnel that will be needed. These judgments should come only after a systems study that will take account of both present and anticipated program objectives.

Obviously, however, a need exists for a resource pool or technical facility to serve international bodies by identifying drugs, outcomes, settings, and users of special interest. This entity must have clear channels of communication to policymakers and must have the capability to conduct or support needed research. It should routinely develop alternate classification schemes, identify all forms of social response to and intervention in drug problems, and ensure the evaluation of the various responses within the framework of drug, setting, and population.

Once a systems study has indicated the appropriate structure and needs of this international entity, it can be formalized and its coordinating function can begin. But its endeavors should not be limited to those resources that are within the conventional framework of the United Nations and its affiliated institutions. Other resources, international and national, should be utilized to meet national, regional, or local needs. The potential utility of all those human and technical resources that can be involved in drug response programs should be considered. Essentially, a service-oriented network should be constructed through a process of search, registration, recruitment, coordination, and dispatch. These resources (scientists, physicians, educators, administrators, police, and the like) need not be incorporated into the bureaucratic structure of either the United Nations or national governments. Maximum flexibility should be provided for their time and work, and logistical-tactical support should be forthcoming from the coordinating agency.

At the present time, international bodies are straitjacketed by the requirement that, with the exception of medical and laboratory data, their information must come from national governments. National governments, in turn, often tend to recognize only information emerging from within their own bureaucratic framework. As a consequence, when making decisions respecting classification and other responses, they have access only to data that are often incomplete and unreliable. At the same time, they are denied the use of more relevant data established by sound research. One solution would be for governments to encourage, with technical and financial assistance from the UN, if necessary, epidemiological and other studies to establish the nature and extent of drug use within their territories. The annual reports of governments, as required by the international treaties, should incorporate findings from any reputably conducted studies, whether carried out under governmental auspices or not. The international bodies should also be authorized to collect and collate data on drug use from non-governmental sources.

As has been already noted, new data about drug effects, drug use, and the efficacy of control systems are accumulating continuously. However, little provision is made in the present international system for a continuing review of these new data or for adequate responses to change. Therefore, international bodies should institute means whereby independent and expert advice—sociological, criminological, legal, economic, and so forth—could be made available to them. This might well be patterned on the system of expert panels and expert committees by which the World Health Organization has access to medical and pharmacological advice, independent of governments. The WHO expert committees and these proposed new sources of expert advice should be given the resources to enable them to gather relevant information and, when necessary, to sponsor special studies and research.

Though the United Nations does collect, translate, and summarize drug laws enacted by individual countries, little information is available about the administration and practical application of these laws or about their effectiveness in achieving their objectives. As much, if not more, attention should be paid to the administrative effectiveness as to the context of the laws themselves. Given the great disparity among countries in the resources available to them for administration of the laws, the UN should take steps to acquire from governments information about the cost effectiveness of their control and intervention systems. This activity should be undertaken not with the aim of embarassing or castigating governments whose programs are ineffectual, but rather of discovering examples of effective, low-cost programs suitable for various economic and sociocultural conditions. Assistance could then more easily be given to countries to enable them to introduce the most effective control methods appropriate to their individual situations.

But the improved flow of sound, objective information to international bodies will not obviate disagreements about the classification of individual drugs. At present, there is only a rudimentary system of appeal against classification decisions. This is available only to governments and has no practical apparatus for either reviewing the data on which a decision is based or for considering fresh evidence. The Economic and Social Council should elaborate the apparatus by which it will deal with appeals from classification decisions made by the Commission on Narcotic Drugs. This apparatus should include provision for review by a suitably qualified independent tribunal of the data on which the Commission based its decision and other relevant data not considered by or not available to the Commission.

One further broad consideration is in order. A principal objective of drug control in the past has been the protection of society as a whole from the consequences of certain individual or minority acts. But an equally important consideration has been neglected, bearing on the protection of individuals, minorities, or, perhaps, the majority from governmental violation through the use of drugs. Therefore, the development of international collaboration to protect individuals and society from the abuse of power through the use of pharmaceuticals is needed now and will be, in the future, an even more serious requirement.

Given the opportunities for mistakes and failure when attempting to cope with broad social problems, there is a tendency for the public to lay the blame on individuals within national and international organizations, rather than on the difficulties under which they work in massive, complex, and often uncoordinated bureaucracies. It is imperative, then, that actions taken to create an international drug administration apparatus that can implement new approaches and programs must be accompanied by a program of public education about the complexities of international action. In this way the United States and other personnel can be relieved of the burden of false blame that arises from public misunderstanding.

To date, funds for the support of international efforts in the field of drugs have been extremely limited. Even with the advent of the United Nations Fund for Drug Abuse Control, there is no assurance that money for broad programs will be forthcoming. In consequence, restrictive priorities are set and administrative machinery is necessarily limited. Under these conditions, expectations for performance cannot be grandiose. At the outset, participating nations and the world community must be made aware of this. These considerations, however, do not preclude much more sophisticated international endeavor or work attuned to realities rather than myths or self-serving interests. On the contrary, they emphasize the themes of the acceptance of uncertainty, the appreciation of alternatives and diversity, the need for evaluation of what is done and why it is done, and the need for knowledge as the basis for action.

Bibliography

ABERLE, D. F. *The Peyote Religion Among the Navajo.* Chicago: Aldine, 1966.

ABRAHAM, M. J., ARMSTRONG, I., AND WHITLOCK, F. A. "Drug Dependence in Brisbane." *Medical Journal of Australia,* 1970, *2,* 397.

ACKERLY, W. C., AND GIBSON, G. "Lighter Fluid Sniffing." *American Journal of Psychiatry,* 1964, *120,* 1056–1061.

ADAMS, B. G., HORDER, E. J., HORDER, J. P., STEIN, C. A., AND WIGG, J. W. "Patients Receiving Barbiturates in an Urban General Practice." *Journal Royal College of Practitioners,* 1966, *12,* 4.

ADVISORY COMMITTEE ON DRUG DEPENDENCE. *Cannabis: A Report.* (Commonly known as the *Wooton Report.*) London: Her Majesty's Stationery Office, 1968.

AHRENS, U., KIHLBOM, M. AND NAS, N. "Studenter och narkotika," *SOU,* 1969, 53.

ALCOHOLISM AND DRUG ADDICTION RESEARCH FOUNDATION. *Eighteenth Annual Report.* Addiction Research Foundation of Ontario, Canada, 1969.

ALLENTUCK, S., AND BOWMAN, K. M. "The Psychiatric Aspects of Marijuana Intoxication." *The American Journal of Psychiatry,* September 1942, *99* (2), 248–251.

A.M.A. Drug Evaluations. Chicago: American Medical Association, 1971.

AMSEL, Z., FISHMAN, J. J., RIVKIND, L., KAVALER, F., KRUG, D., CLINE, M., BROPHY, F., AND CONWELL, D. "The Use of the Narcotics Register for Follow-up of a Cohort of Adolescent Addicts." *International Journal of the Addictions,* 1971, *6,* 225–239.

ANGRIST, B. M., AND GERSHON, S. "The Phenomenology of Experimentally Induced Amphetamine Psychosis—Preliminary Observations." *Biological Psychiatry,* 1970, *2,* 95–107.

APPLETON, W. S. "Snow Phenomenon." *Psychiatry,* 1965, *28,* 88–93.

ARMITAGE, P. *Statistical Methods in Medical Research.* Oxford: Blackwell, 1971.

341

ASH, P. "The Reliability of Psychiatric Diagnosis." *Journal of Abnormal and Social Psychology,* 1949, *44,* 272–276.

BADEN, M. "Medical Aspects of Drug Use." *New York State Journal of Medicine,* March 24, 1968, 464–468.

BALINT, M., HUNT, J., JOYCE, C. R. B., MARINKER, M., AND WOODCOCK, J. *Treatment or Diagnosis: A Study of Repeat Prescriptions in General Practice.* Philadelphia: Lippincott, 1970.

BALL, J. C. AND CHAMBERS, C. D. *The Epidemiology of Opiate Addiction in the United States.* Springfield, Ill.: Thomas, 1970.

BECKER, GARY S. "Crime and Punishment: An Economic Approach." *Journal of Political Economy,* March/April 1968, 169–217.

BECKER, H. S. "Becoming a Marijuana User." *American Journal of Sociology,* 1953, *59,* 235–242.

BECKER, H. S. *The Outsiders: Studies in the Sociology of Deviance.* New York: Free Press, 1963.

BEECHER, H. K. *Measurement of Subjective Responses: Quantitative Effects of Drugs.* New York: Oxford University Press, 1959.

BEESE, D. H. (Ed.). *Tobacco Consumption in Various Countries.* Research paper 6. London: Tobacco Research Council, 1968.

BEJEROT, N. "Aktuell Toxikomaniproblematik." Unpublished paper, 1965.

BEJEROT, N. *An Epidemic of Phenmetrazine Dependence—Epidemiological and Clinical Aspects.* Paper given at the Symposium on the Pharmacological and Epidemiological Aspects of Adolescent Drug Dependence, London Hospital Medical College, September 1–3, 1966.

BEJEROT, N. *An Epidemic of Drug Abuse in Arrestees in Stockholm between 1965–70.* Paper read at the Fifth World Congress of Psychiatry at Mexico City, 1971.

BENTEL, D. J., AND SMITH, D. E. "The Year of the Middle Class Junkie." *California's Health,* 1971, *28* (10), 1–5.

BENZI, M. *Les Derniers adorateurs du Peyotl.* Paris: Gallimard, 1972.

BERG, D. F. "The Non-Medical Use of Dangerous Drugs in the U.S.A.—A Comprehensive View." *International Journal of the Addictions,* 1970, 777–834.

BERGER, F. M. "Classification of Psychoactive Drugs According to Their Chemical Structures and Sites of Action." In L. Uhr, and J. G. Miller (Eds.), *Drugs and Behavior,* New York: Wiley, 1960, 86–105.

BERTRAND, M. *Report on Programmes and Budgets in the U.N. Family of Organisations.* New York, Joint Inspection Unit, United Nations, 1969.

BEWLEY, T. H. "Heroin Addiction in the United Kingdom 1954–64." *British Medical Journal,* 1965, *2,* 1284.

BEWLEY, T., FAMES, I. P., AND MAHON, T. "Evaluation of Effectiveness of Prescribing Clinics for Narcotic Addicts in United Kingdom 1968–70." C. Zarafonetis (Ed.), *Proceedings of the International Conference.* Philadelphia: Lea and Febiger, 1972.

BINNIE, H. L. "Attitude to Drugs and Drug Takers of Students at University and Colleges of Further Education in an English Midland City." *Vaughan Papers,* 1964.

BIRDWOOD, G. "It All Depends What You Mean." *Drugs & Society,* June 1972, *1* (9), 7–11.

BLACKER, K. H., JONES, R. T., STONE, G. C., AND PFEFFERBAUM, D. "Chronic Users of LSD: The Acidheads." *American Journal of Psychiatry,* 1968, *125* (3), 341–351.

BLACKWELL, B. "MAO Inhibitors and Cheese." In F. J. Ayd and B. Blackwell (Eds.), *Discoveries in Biological Psychiatry,* Philadelphia: Lippincott, 1970.

BLUM, E. M. "The Uncooperative Patient: The Development of a Test to Predict Uncooperativeness in Medical Treatment." In *Supplementary Studies on Malpractice.* San Francisco, California Medical Association, 1958.

BLUM, E. M., AND BLUM, R. H. *Alcoholism: Modern Psychological Approaches to Treatment.* San Francisco: Jossey-Bass, 1967.

BLUM, E. M., AND BLUM, R. H. *The Dangerous Hour.* New York: Scribner, 1970.

BLUM, E. M., AND DE TOBAL, C. "Hippie Families." In R. H. Blum and Associates, *Horatio Alger's Children: The Role of the Family in the Origin and Prevention of Drug Risk.* San Francisco: Jossey-Bass, 1972.

BLUM, R. H. *The Management of the Doctor-Patient Relationship.* New York: McGraw-Hill, 1960.

BLUM, R. H. "Case Identification in Psychiatric Epidemiology." *Milbank Quarterly,* 1962, *15,* 253–288.

BLUM, R. H. *Task Force Report: Narcotics and Drug Abuse.* Report to the President's Commission on Law Enforcement and the Administration of Justice. Washington, D.C.: Government Printing Office, 1967.

BLUM, R. H. *Social and Epidemiological Aspects of Psychopharmacology: Dimensions and Perspectives."* Philadelphia: Lippincott, 1968, 243–282.

BLUM, R. H. "To Wear a Nostradamus Hat: Drugs and America." *Journal of Social Issues,* 1971, *27* (3), 89–106.

BLUM, R. H. (Ed.). *Origins of Drug Use and Drug Problems.* Report to the National Strategy Council of the Special Action Office for Drug Abuse Prevention, Executive Office of the (U.S.) President, 1972a.

BLUM, R. H. (Ed.). *Societal Response to Drug Problems: Issues and Recommendations for Research.* Report to National Commission on Marijuana and Drug Abuse, 1972b.

BLUM, R. H. "Children's Drug Use: Educational and Other Correlates." Personal communication on current project, 1973.

BLUM, R. H., AND ASSOCIATES. *Utopiates: A Study of the Use and Users of LSD—25.* New York: Atherton, 1964.

BLUM, R. H., AND ASSOCIATES. *Society and Drugs.* San Francisco: Jossey-Bass, 1969a.

BLUM, R. H., AND ASSOCIATES. *Students and Drugs.* San Francisco: Jossey-Bass, 1969b.

BLUM, R. H., AND ASSOCIATES. *Horatio Alger's Children: Role of the Family in the Origin and Prevention of Drug Risk.* San Francisco: Jossey-Bass, 1972a.

BLUM, R. H., AND ASSOCIATES. *The Dream Sellers: Perspectives on Drug Dealers.* San Francisco: Jossey-Bass, 1972b.

BLUM, R. H., AND BALBAKY, M. L. F. "Social and Cultural Observations." In R. H. Blum and Associates, *Society and Drugs.* San Francisco: Jossey-Bass, 1969.

BLUM, R. H., AND BLUM, E. M. *Health and Healing in Rural Greece.* Stanford, Calif.: Stanford University Press, 1965.

BLUM, R. H., GORDON, A., AND EGAN, T. "Enforcement Realities." In R. H. Blum and Associates, *Drug Dealers—Taking Action.* San Francisco: Jossey-Bass, 1973.

BLUM, R. H., AND MUNSON, N. In R. H. Blum and Associates, *The Dream Sellers: Perspectives on Drug Dealers.* San Francisco: Jossey-Bass, 1972.

BLUM, R. H., AND SMITH, J. P. "Pharmacists." In R. H. Blum and Associates, *The Dream Sellers.* San Francisco: Jossey-Bass, 1972.

BLUM, R. H., AND WAHL, J. "Police Views on Drug Use." In R. H. Blum and Associates, *Utopiates: The Use and Users of LSD—25.* New York: Atherton, 1964.

BLUM, R. H., AND WOLFE, J. In R. H. Blum and Associates, *The Dream Sellers: Perspectives on Drug Dealers.* San Francisco: Jossey-Bass, 1972.

BLUMBERG, A., COHEN, M., HEATON, A. M., AND KLEIN, D. "Covert Drug Abuse Among Voluntary Hospitalized Psychiatric Patients." *The Journal of the American Medical Association,* 1971, *217,* 1659–1661.

BOSTON COLLABORATIVE DRUG SURVEILLANCE PROGRAM. "Drug Induced Deafness." *Journal of the American Medical Association,* 1973, *224,* 515–516.

BOURNE, P. *Alcoholism: Progress in Research and Treatment.* New York: Academic Press, 1972.

BOVET, D., BOVET-NILTI, F., AND OLIVERIO, A. "Genetic Aspects of Learning and Memory in Mice." *Science,* January 1969, *163,* 139–149.

BOWMAN, K. M., AND JELLINEK, E. M. "Alcoholic Mental Disorders." In E. M. Jellinek (Ed.), *Alcohol Addiction and Chronic Alcoholism.* New Haven, Conn.: Yale University Press, 1942.

BRANSBY, E. R. "A Study of Patients Notified by Hospitals as Addicted to Drugs: First Report." *Health Trends,* 1971, *3,* 75–78.

BRECHER, E. M., AND THE EDITORS OF CONSUMER REPORTS. *Licit and Illicit Drugs: The Consumer Union Report on Narcotics, Stimulants, Depressants, Inhalants, Hallucinogens, and Marijuana.* Boston: Little, Brown, 1972.

BRENT, R. L. "Protecting the Public from Teratogenic and Mutagenic Hazards." *Journal of Clinical Pharmacology,* 1972, *12,* 61–70.

BRESSLER, R. R. "Combined Drug Therapy." *The American Journal of Medical Sciences,* 1968, *225,* 89–93.

BROSS, I. D. J., SHAPIRO, P. A., AND ANDERSON, B. B. "How Information Is Carried in Scientific Sub-languages." *Science,* 1972, *176,* 1303–1307.

BROTMAN, R., AND FREEDMAN, A. "A Community Mental Health Approach to Drug Addiction." U.S. Department of Health, Education and Welfare. Washington, D.C.: U.S. Government Printing Office, 1970.

BROWN, C. C., AND SAVAGE, C. *The Drug Abuse Controversy.* Baltimore: National Educational Consultants, 1971.

BROWN, S. "Addiction to Amphetamines." *British Medical Journal,* 1964, *2,* 1204.

BRUUN, K. *Alkoholi, Kaytto, Vaikutus Kontrolli.* Finland: Tammi, 1972a.

BRUUN, K. "Dilemmas in Drug Control Policy." Fifth Leonard Ball Oration, Alcoholism Foundation of Victoria, 1972b.

BUICKHUISEN, W., AND TIMMERMAN, H. "The Development of Drug Taking Among School Children in the Netherlands." *UN Bulletin on Narcotics,* July 1972, *24,* 317.

BUNZEL, R. "The Role of Alcoholism in Two Central American Cultures." *Psychiatry,* 1940, *2,* 361–387.

BURTON, R. F. *First Footsteps in East Africa.* London: Dent, 1910.

CADELL, T. E., AND CRESSMAN, R. J. "Group Social Tension as a Determinant of

Alcohol Consumption in Macaca Mulatta." *Journal of Medical Primatology.* In press.

CAFFREY, E. M., HOLLISTER, L. E., KLETT, C. J., AND KAIM, S. C. "Veterans Administration Cooperative Studies in Psychiatry." In W. G. Clark and J. del Guidice (Eds.), *Principles of Psychopharmacology,* New York: Academic Press, 1970.

CAHALAN, D. *Problem Drinkers: A National Survey.* San Francisco: Jossey-Bass, 1970.

CAHN, C. H. "The Effects of Drugs on Group Therapy: An Experiment." *Journal of Nervous and Mental Diseases,* 1953, *118,* 516.

CAMERON, D. C. "Drug Dependence—Some Research Issues." *Bulletin W.H.O.,* 1970, *43,* 589.

CAMERON, M. *The Reform Movement in China.* Stanford, Calif.: Stanford University Press, 1931.

CAMPBELL, A. M. G., EVANS, M., THOMSON, J. L. G., AND WILLIAMS, M. J. "Cerebral Atrophy in Young Cannabis Smokers." *Lancet,* 1971, *2,* 1219–1224.

CAMPBELL, A. M. G., EVANS, M., THOMSON, J. L. G., AND WILLIAMS, M. J. "Cerebral Atrophy in Young Cannabis Smokers." *Lancet,* 1972, *1,* 202–203.

CAMPS, F. E. "Investigation of the Cause of Death in Cases of Drug Dependency." Lecture presented at the International Conference on Drug Dependence, OPTAT, Quebec, 1968.

CAMPS, F. E. "Drug Dependence—A Social and Pharmacological Problem." *International Journal of the Addictions,* March 1970, *5,* 1.

CAPLAN, G. *An Approach to Community Mental Health.* New York: Grune & Stratton, 1961.

CAPPELL, H., LE BLANC, A. E., AND ENDRENYI, L. "Aversive Conditioning by Psychoactive Drugs: Effects of Morphine, Alcohol and Chlordiazepoxide." *Psychopharmacologia* (Berlin), 1973, *29,* 239–246.

CARSTAIRS, G. M. "Daru and Bhang: Cultural Factors in the Choice of Intoxicants." *Quarterly Journal of Studies on Alcohol,* 1954, *15,* 220–237.

CATTELL, H. W. *"606": Ehrlich's New Preparation, Arsenobenzol ("606"), in the Treatment of Syphilis.* Vol. 4, 20th series, in *International Clinics,* Philadelphia: Lippincott, 1910.

CHAMBERS, C. D., AND HECKMAN, R. D. *Employee Drug Abuse—A Manager's Guide for Action.* Boston: Cahners Publishing, 1971.

CHANCE, M. R. A. "Ethology and Psychopharmacology." In C. R. B. Joyce (Ed.), *Psychopharmacology: Dimensions and Perspectives.* London: Tavistock, 1968.

CHAPLE, P. A. L., SOMEKH, D. E., AND TAYLOR, M. E. "Follow-up Cases of Opiate Addiction from Time of Notification to Home Office." *British Medical Journal,* June 17, 1972, 680–683.

CHEIN, I., GERARD, D. L., LEE, R. S., AND ROSENFELD, E. *The Road to H: Narcotics, Delinquency and Social Policy.* New York: Basic Books; London: Tavistock (under the title *Narcotics, Delinquency and Social Policy*), 1964.

CHERUBIN, C., MC CUSKER, J., BADEN, M., KAULER, F., AND AMSEL, Z. "Epidemiology of Deaths in Narcotic Addicts." *American Journal of Epidemiology,* 1972, *1,* 96.

CHILD, I. L., BACON, M. K., AND BARRY, H. "A Cross-cultural Study of Drinking." *Quarterly Journal of Studies on Alcohol,* 1965, Supplement 3.

CHRISTIE, N. AND BRUUN, K. "Alcohol Problems: The Conceptual Framework." In

Proceedings of the Twenty-eighth International Congress on Alcohol and Alcoholism, vol. 2. Rutgers, N.J.: Hillhouse Press, 1969.

CITRON, B. P., HALPERN, M., MC CARRON, M., LUNDBERG, G. D., MC CORMICK, R., PINCUS, I. J., TATTER, D., AND HAVERBACK, B. J. "Necrotizing Angiitis Associated with Drug Abuse." *New England Journal of Medicine,* 1970, *283,* 1003–1011.

CLARK, W. G., AND DEL GUIDICE, J. (Eds.) *Principles of Psychopharmacology.* New York: Academic Press, 1970.

"Clinical Toxicology." Editorial quoted by J. Wenger and S. Einstein, "Use and Misuse of Aspirin—A Contemporary Problem." *International Journal of the Addictions,* 1970, *5* (4), 757.

CLUFF, L. E., THORNTON, G., SEIDL, L., AND SMITH, J. "Epidemiological Study of Adverse Drug Reactions." *Transactions of the Association of American Physicians,* 1965, *78,* 255–268.

COCHRAN, W. G., AND COX, G. M. *Experimental Designs.* (2nd ed.) New York: Wiley, 1957.

COHEN, A. "Relieving Acid Indigestion: Educational Strategies Related to Psychological and Social Dynamics of Hallucinogenic Drug Use." In *Management of Adolescent Drug Use: Clinical, Psychological and Legal Perspectives.* Beloit, Wis.: Stash, 1973.

COHEN, H. "Multiple Drug Use Considered in the Light of Stepping Stone Hypothesis." *International Journal of the Addictions,* 1972, *7,* 11.

COHEN, S. *The Drug Dilemma.* New York: McGraw-Hill, 1969.

COLE, J. O. "Behavioral Toxicity." In L. Uhr and J. M. Miller (Eds.), *Drugs and Behavior,* New York: Wiley, 1960, 166–183.

COLE, P., AND MAC MAHON, B. "Attributable Risk Percent in Case-Control Studies." *British Journal of Preventive and Social Medicine,* 1971, *25,* 242–244.

COMMISSION OF ENQUIRY INTO THE NON-MEDICAL USE OF DRUGS. *Interim Report.* Ottawa: Ministry of National Health and Welfare, 1970.

COMMISSION OF INQUIRY INTO THE NON-MEDICAL USE OF DRUGS. *Final Report.* Ottawa: Ministry of National Health and Welfare, 1972.

COMMISSION ON NARCOTIC DRUGS. *Report of the Twenty-Fourth Session.* New York: U.N. Economic and Social Council, 1971.

COMMITTEE ON CRIME PREVENTION AND CONTROL OF THE UNITED NATIONS ECONOMIC AND SOCIAL COUNCIL. "Drug Abuse and Criminality—Part I." *UN Bulletin on Narcotics,* 1972, *24,* 35–46; "Part II," *ibid.,* 1973, *25,* 49–60.

CONNELL, P. H. *Amphetamine Psychosis.* Maudsley Monograph 5. London: Oxford University Press, 1958.

CONNELL, P. H. "Amphetamine Misuse." *British Journal of Addiction,* 1965a, *60,* 9.

CONNELL, P. H. "Ether Drinking in Ulster." *Quarterly Journal Studies of Alcohol,* 1965b, *26,* 629–653.

CONNELL, P. H. "The Use and Abuse of Amphetamines." *The Practitioner,* 1968, *200,* 234–243.

CONNELL, P. H. "Clinical Aspects of Drug Addiction." *Journal of the Royal College of Physicians* (London), 1970, *4,* 254–263.

CONNELL, P. H. "Clinical, Ethical and Legal Implications of Clinical Trials of Dependence or Potentially Dependence Producing Drugs." Paper presented at Bayer Symposium IV, London, n.d.

CONNELL, P. H., AND BOWMAN, M. J. "The Value of Screening Urines for the Presence of Drugs in an In-Patient Unit for Drug Dependent Persons." Unpublished manuscript, 1973.

CONWELL, D. P., FISHMAN, J. J., AND AMSEL, Z. "New York City Narcotics Register: A Brief History." *International Journal of the Addictions,* 1971, *6,* 561–569.

COOK, S. *Variations in Response to Illegal Drug Use: A Comparative Study of Official Narcotic Drug Policies in Canada, Great Britian, and the· United States from 1920 to 1970.* Addiction Research Foundation Substudy 1—Co & 11—70. Ottawa.

COPPERSTOCK, R. "Sex Differences in the Use of Mood Modifying Drug: An Explanatory Model." *Journal of Health and Social Behavior,* 1971, *12,* 238.

CORNFIELD, J., AND HAENSZEL, W. "Some Aspects of Retrospective Studies." *Journal of Chronic Diseases,* 1960, *11,* 523.

CORTI, C. *A History of Smoking.* New York: Harcourt, Brace, 1932.

COSTELL, J. T., LEWIS, J. M., AND PHILLIPS, V. A. "Extent and Prevalence of Illicit Drug Use, as Reported by 56,745 Students." *Journal of the American Medical Association,* 1971, *216* (9), 1464–1470.

CUTTING, W. (Ed.). *Annual Review of Pharmacology.* Palo Alto, Calif.: Annual Reviews, 1964.

DALE, A. (Ed.). *The Role of the Drinking Driver in Traffic Accidents.* Bloomington, Ind., Indiana University, Department of Police Administration, 1964.

DANGEROUS DRUGS ACT. London: Her Majesty's Stationery Office, 1967.

DANTO, B. L. "A Bag Full of Laughs." *American Journal of Psychiatry,* 1964, *121,* 612–613.

DE ALARCON, R. "The Spread of Heroin Abuse in a Community." *UN Bulletin on Narcotics,* July/September 1969, *21* (3), 17–22.

DE ALARCON, R. "Epidemiological Evaluation of a Public Health Measure Aimed at Reducing the Availability of Methylamphetamine." *Psychological Medicine,* 1972, *2,* 293–300.

DE ALARCON, R., AND RATHOD, N. H. "Prevalence and Early Detection of Heroin Abuse." *British Medical Journal,* 1968, *2,* 549–553.

DE ANGELIS, G. G. "Testing for Drugs—Advantages and Disadvantages." *International Journal of the Addictions,* 1972, *7,* 365–385.

DE ANGELIS, G. G. "Drug Testing—Techniques and Issues." Unpublished manuscript, 1973.

"Declaration of Helsinki: Recommendations Guiding Doctors in Clinical Research." *British Medical Journal,* 1964, *2,* 177–178 (also in *World Medicine Journal,* September 1964).

DELAY, J. (Ed.). "Colloque international sui le chlorpromazine." *Encephale,* special number, 1956.

DELGADO, J. "Pharmacological Modifications of Social Behavior." *Proceedings of the First International Pharmacological Meeting,* vol. 8. New York: Pergamon Press, 1962, 265–292.

DE LINT, E., AND SCHMIDT, W. "Distribution of Alcohol Consumption in Ontario." *Quarterly Journal of Studies on Alcohol,* 1968, *29,* 968.

DELISLE BURNS, B. *The Mammalian Cerebral Cortex.* London: Arnold, 1958.

DE MONFRIED, H. *Hashish.* London: 1935.

DENEAU, G., YANAGITA, T., AND SEEVERS, M. H. "Self-administration of Psychoactive Substances by the Monkey: A Measure of Psychological Dependence." *Psychopharmacologia*, 1969, *16*, 30–48.

DEPARTMENT OF HEALTH AND SOCIAL SECURITY. *Annual Report for the Year 1971*. London: Her Majesty's Stationery Office, 1972.

DEPARTMENT OF NATIONAL HEALTH AND WELFARE. *Consumption of Barbiturates and Amphetamines, Sept. 1969*. Quoted in interim report of the Commission of Enquiry into Non-Medical Use of Drugs. Ottawa: Ministry of National Health and Welfare, 1970.

DIEM, K. (Ed.). *Documenta Geigy Scientific Tables*. Ardsley, N.Y.: Geigy Pharmaceuticals, 1962.

DI PALMA, J. R. *Drill's Pharmacology in Medicine*. New York: McGraw-Hill, 1965.

DOWNING, R., AND RICKELS, K. "Personality and Attitudinal Correlates of Response to Drug Treatment in Psychiatric Out-patients." *Journal Psychology*, 1962, *54*, 345–361.

Drug Usage and Arrest Charges: A Study of Usage and Arrest Charges Among Arrestees in Six Metropolitan Areas of the United States. Washington, D.C.: Bureau of Narcotics and Dangerous Drugs, U.S. Department of Justice, December 1971.

DUNLOP, D. "Use and Abuse of Psychotropic Drugs." *Proceedings Royal Society of Medicine*, 1970, *63* (12), 1279–1282.

DUNNELL, K., AND CARTWRIGHT, A. *Medicine Takers, Prescribers and Hoarders*. London: Routledge and Kegan Paul, 1972.

DUPONT, R. L. "Profile of Heroin Epidemic." *New England Journal of Medicine*, 1971, *285*, 320.

DURANDINA, A. I., AND ROMASENKO, V. A. "Functional and Morphological Changes in Experimental Acute Poisoning by Resinous Substances Prepared from Yujnochuisk Cannabis." *Bulletin on Narcotics* (United Nations), October/December 1971, *23* (4), 1–9.

DUREMAN, I. Discussion of E. Jacobsen, "An Analysis of the Gross Action of Drugs on the Central Nervous System." In O. Walaas, (Ed.), *Molecular Basis of Some Aspects of Mental Activity*. New York: Academic Press, 1967.

EDDY, N. B., FRIEBEL, H., HAHN, K. J., AND HALBACH, H. *Codeine and Its Alternates for Pain and Cough Relief*. Geneva: World Health Organization, 1970.

EDDY, N. B., HALBACH, H., ISBELL, H., AND SEEVERS, M. H. "Drug Dependence: Its Significance and Characteristics." *Bulletin of the World Health Organization*, 1965, *32*, 721–733.

EDDY, N. B., AND MAY, E. L. *Synthetic Analgesics pt. 2 (B) 6, 7 morphens*. London: Pergamon, 1966.

EDWARDS, G. *Unreason in an Age of Reason*. Edwin Stevens Lectures for the Laity. London: Royal Society of Medicine, 1971.

EDWARDS, G., AND HAWKS, D. *Terminology and Criteria of Drug Dependence*. Geneva: World Health Organization Expert Committee on Drug Dependence, 1972.

EDWARDS, G., HENSMAN, C., AND PETO, J. *Drinking Problem Amongst Recidient Prisoners*. London: William Heineman Medical Books, 1971.

EDWARDS, G., KELLOG-FISHER, M., HAWKER, A., AND HENSMAN, C. "Clients of Alcoholic Information Centre." *British Medical Journal*, 1967, *4*, 346.

EISENLOHR, L. *International Narcotics Control.* London: Allen and Unwin, Ltd., 1934.

EMMERSON, D. K. (Ed.). *Students and Politics in Developing Nations.* New York: Praeger, 1968.

ENGLISH, J. M. *Cost-Effectiveness.* New York: Wiley, 1968.

ERICKSON, EDWARD. "The Social Costs of the Discovery and Suppression of the Clandestine Distribution of Heroin." *Journal of Political Economy,* July/August 1969, 484–486.

ETIENNE, ROBERT. *A Study of the Cost of Narcotics and Drug Law Enforcement in California.* Palo Alto, Calif.: Stanford Law School, 1970.

EVANS, W., AND KLINE, N. *Psychotropic Drugs in the Year 2000.* Springfield, Ill.: Thomas, 1971.

FABING, H. D. "Toads, Mushrooms and Schizophrenics." *Harpers,* May 1957, 50–55.

FEINGLASS, S. "A Street Pharmacopeia." Unpublished manuscript, 1972.

FEINSTEIN, A. R. "Clinical Biostatistics XIV: The Purposes of Prognostic Stratification." *Clinical Pharmacology and Therapeutics,* 1972a, *13,* 285–297.

FEINSTEIN, A. R. "Clinical Biostatistics XV: The Process of Prognostic Stratification." *Clinical Pharmacology and Therapeutics,* 1972b, *13,* 442–457.

FELDMAN, H. "Ideological Supports to Becoming and Remaining a Heroin Addict. *Journal Health and Social Behavior,* 1968, 9, 131–139.

FELDMAN, H. "Street Status and Drug Preference." In V. L. Patch (Ed.), *Heroin Addiction,* Boston: Little, Brown, 1972.

FENNESSY, M. R., HEIMANS, R. L. H., AND RAND, M. J. "Comparison of Effect of Morphine-like Analgesics on Transmurally Stimulated Guinea-Pig Ileum:" *British Journal of Pharmacology,* 1969, *37,* 436–449.

FERNANDEZ, R. A. "The Clandestine Distribution of Heroin, Its Discovery and Suppression." *Journal of Political Economy,* July/August 1969, 487–488.

FIELD, P. B. "A New Cross-cultural Study of Drunkenness." In D. J. Pittman and C. R. Snyder (Eds.), *Society, Culture and Drink Patterns.* New York: Wiley, 1962.

FINNEY, D. J. "Statistical Aspects of Monitoring for Dangers in Drug Therapy." *Methods of Information in Medicine,* 1971, *10,* 1–8.

FREEDMAN, A. In C. C. Brown and C. Savage (Eds.), *The Drug Abuse Controversy.* Baltimore: National Educational Consultants, 1971.

FREEDMAN, D. X. *Societal Features of Repetitive Drug Use.* Statement at Salk Conference, La Jolla, California, July 14, 1972.

FRIEBEL, H. "Drug Safety in Theory and Practice." *WHO Chronicle,* 1973, *27,* 89–93.

FRIEBEL, H., AND KUHN, H. F. "Über den Nachweis von "Physical Dependence' bei Codein-behandelten Meerschweinen." *Medical Pharmacology,* 1965, exp. 12., 92.

FRIEDMAN, G. D. "Screening Criteria for Drug Monitoring: The Kaiser-Permanente Drug Reaction Monitoring System." *Journal of Chronic Diseases,* 1972, *25,* 11–20.

FRIEDMAN, G. D., COLLEN, M. F., HARRIS, L. E., VAN BRUNT, E. E., AND DAVIS, L. S. "Experience in Monitoring Drug Reactions in Out-patients: The Kaiser-Permanente Drug Monitoring System." *Journal of the American Medical Association,* 1971, *217,* 567.

FUJII, E. T. *Public Investment in the Rehabilitation of Heroin Addicts.* Unpublished doctoral dissertation. Stanford, Calif.: Stanford University, 1972.

GABER, I. "The Don'ts of Drug Surveys." *Drugs and Society,* 1972, *1,* 10–13.

GARDNER, R. "Deaths in the United Kingdom of Opioid Users (1965–69)." *Lancet,* September 1970, *2,* 650.

GARDNER, R., AND CONNELL, P. H. "One Year's Experience in a Drug Dependence Clinic." *Lancet,* 1970, *2,* 455–459.

GARDNER, R., AND CONNELL, P. H. "Opioid Users Attending a Special Drug Dependence Clinic 1968–69." *UN Bulletin on Narcotics,* 1971, *23* (4), 9–15.

GARDNER, R., AND CONNELL, P. H. "Amphetamine and Other Non-opioid Drug Users Attending a Special Drug Dependence Clinic." *British Medical Journal,* 1972, *2,* 322–326.

GIBBINS, R. J. "Role of Tolerance and Physical Dependence in Drug Taking." Audio-tape-cassette produced by Addiction Research Foundation. Toronto, 1971.

GLICK, S. D., JARVIK, M. E., AND NAKAMURA, R. K. "Inhibition by Drugs of Smoking Behavior in Monkeys." *Nature,* 1970, *227,* 969.

GLUECK, S., AND GLUECK, E. *Predicting Delinquency and Crime.* Cambridge, Mass.: Harvard University Press, 1960.

GODBER, G. E. *On the State of Public Health.* Annual report of the Chief Medical Officer of the Ministry of Health for the year 1969. London: Her Majesty's Stationery Office, 1969.

GOLDBERG, L. "Drug Abuse in Sweden." *UN Bulletin on Narcotics,* January–March 1968, *20* (1), 1–31; April–June 1968, *20* (2), 9–36.

GOLDBERG, S. C., COLE, J. O., AND KLERMAN, G. L. "Differential Prediction of Improvement Under Three Phenothiazines." In J. R. Wittenborn and P. R. A. May, (Eds.), *Prediction of Response to Pharmacotherapy,* Springfield, Ill.: Thomas, 1966.

GOLDBERG, S. C., SCHOOLER, N. R., DAVIDSON, E. M., AND KAYCE, M. M. "Sex and Race Differences in Response to Drug Treatment among Schizophrenics." *Psychopharmacologia* (Berlin), 1966, *9,* 31–47.

GOLDBERG, S. R. "Cocaine Self-administration in the Squirrel Monkey." *Report of the Thirty-Fourth Annual Scientific Meeting, Committee on Problems of Drug Dependence,* 1972, *34,* 234.

GOODE, E. *The Marijuana Smokers.* New York: Basic Books, 1970.

GOODE, E. *Drugs in American Society.* New York: Knopf, 1972.

GOODMAN, L. S., AND GILMAN, A. *The Pharmacological Basis of Therapeutics.* New York: Macmillan, 1965–1968.

GOODWIN, D. W., POWELL, B., BREMER, D., HOINT, H., AND STERN, J. "Alcohol in Recall: State-Dependent Effects on Man." *Science,* March 21, 1969, *163,* 1358–1360.

GORDON, R. A., BRITT, B. A., AND KALOW, W. (Eds.). *Malignant Hyperthermia.* Springfield, Ill.: Thomas, 1973.

GÖTESTAM, K. G., AND GUNNE, LARS M. "A Follow-up of Amphetamine Addicts Participating in Clinical Drug Trials." *Lakartidningen,* 1972, *69,* 1103–1105.

GREENBLAT, M., SOLOMON, M. H., EVANS, A. S., BROOKS, G. W. *Drug and Social Therapy in Chronic Schizophrenia.* Springfield, Ill.: Thomas, 1965.

GRIFFITH, J. D., CAVANAUGH, J. H., HELD, J., AND OATES, J. A. "Experimental Psychosis Induced by d-Amphetamine." In E. Costa and S. Garatlini (Eds.), *Amphetamines and Related Compounds.* New York: Raven Press, 1970.

GRIFFITH, J. D., CAVANAUGH, J., HELD, J., AND OATES, J. A. "Dextroamphetamine: Evaluation of the Psychotomimetic Properties in Man." *Archives of General Psychiatry,* 1972, *26,* 97–100.

GRIMLUND, K. "Phenacetin and Renal Damage at a Swedish Factory." *Acta Medica Scandinavia,* 1963, supplement 405, 1–26.

GRINSPOON, L. *Marijuana Reconsidered.* Cambridge: Harvard University Press, 1971.

GRUPP, S. E. "Addict Mobility and the Nalline Test." *British Journal of Addiction,* 1968, *63,* 227.

GRUPP, S. E. "Narcotic Control and the Nalline Test: The Addict's Perspective." *Journal of Forensic Sciences,* 1970a, *15,* 34.

GRUPP, S. E. "Drug Users' Attitudes Toward the Nalline Test." *International Journal of the Addictions,* 1970b, *5,* 661.

GRUPP, S. E. "The Nalline Test I—Development and Implementation." *Journal of Criminal Law, Criminology and Police Science,* 1970c, *61,* 296.

GRUPP, S. E. "The Nalline Test II—Rationale." *Journal of Criminal Law, Criminology and Police Science,* 1970d, *61,* 463.

GRUPP, S. E. "The Nalline Test III—Objections, Limitations and Assessment." *Journal of Criminal Law, Criminology and Police Science,* 1971, *62,* 286.

GUERTIN, W. H. "Do the Different Methods of Factor Analysis Still Give Almost Identical Results?" *Perceptual and Motor Skills,* 1971, *33,* 600–602.

HAERTZEN, C. A., HILL, M., AND BELLEVILLE, R. "Development of the Addiction Research Center Inventory: Selection of Items That Are Sensitive to the Effects of Various Drugs." *Psychopharmacologia,* 1963, *4,* 155–156.

HAKANSSON, K. Memorandum to the Swedish National Board of Health regarding definition of drug addiction. October 24, 1966.

HALBACH, H. "Drug Abuse and Drug Dependence—A Matter of Terminology?" *Pharmakopsychiatrie and Neuro-Psychopharmakologie,* 1968, *1,* 233–238.

HALBACH, H. *The Non-medical Use of Drugs.* Paper presented to the International Congress on Alcohol and the Addictions. Hong Kong, 1971.

HALBACH, H., AND EDDY, N. B. "Tests for Addiction (Chronic Intoxication) of Morphine Type." *Bulletin World Health Organization,* 1963, *28,* 139–173.

HALD, J., JACOBSEN, E., AND LARSEN, V. "The Sensitizing Effects of Tetraethylthiuram Disulfide (Antabuse) to Ethyl Alcohol." *Acta Pharmacologica Toxicologica,* 1948, *8,* 285–296.

HAWKS, D. V. "The Dimensions of Drug Dependence in the United Kingdom." *International Journal of the Addictions,* 1971, *6* (1), 135–160.

HAZARD, R., CHEYMOL, J., LEVY, J., BOISSIER, J. R. AND LECHAT, P. *Manuel de Pharmacologie.* Paris: Masson, 1969.

HINDMARCH, I. "The Patterns of Drug Abuse Among School Children." *Bulletin on Narcotics* (United Nations), July–September 1972, *24* (3), 23–26.

HINKLE, L. E., AND WOLFF, H. G. "The Nature of Man's Adaptation to His Total Environment and the Relation of This to Illness." *A.M.A. Archives of Internal Medicine,* 1957, *99,* 442–460.

HOLAHAN, J. F., AND HENNINGSEN, P. A. "The Economics of Heroin." In *Dealing with Drug Abuse: A Report to the Ford Foundation.* New York: Praeger, 1972.

HOLLIDAY, A. R., AND DILLIE, J. "The Effects of Meprobamate, Chlorpromazine,

Pentobarbital and a Placebo on a Behavioral Task Performed Under Stress Conditions." *Journal of Comparative Physiological Psychology,* 1958, *51,* 811–815.

HOLLINGSHEAD, A. B., AND REDLICH, F. C. *Social Class and Mental Illness.* New York: Wiley, 1958.

HOLLISTER, L. E. *Chemical Psychoses: LSD and Related Drugs.* Springfield, Ill., Thomas, 1968.

HOLMSTED, B., AND LILJESTRAND, G. (Eds.). *Readings in Pharmacology.* Elmsford, N.Y.: Pergamon, 1963.

HOME OFFICE, Drugs Branch. *Statistics on Drug Addiction.* London, 1972.

HORDERN, A. "Psychopharmacology: Some Historical Considerations." In C. R. B. Joyce (Ed.), *Psychopharmacology: Dimensions and Perspectives.* Philadelphia: Lippincott, 1968.

HORDERN, A., AND CALDWELL, ANNE E. "History of Psychopharmacology." In W. G. Clark and J. del Guidice (Eds.), *Principles of Psychopharmacology.* New York: Academic Press, 1970.

HORTON, D. "The Function of Alcohol in Primitive Societies: A Cross-cultural Study." *Quarterly Journal Studies of Alcohol,* 1943, *4,* 199–320.

"How New Drugs Are Brought Under International Narcotics Control by the Procedure of Single Convention on Narcotic Drugs, 1961." *United Nations Bulletin on Narcotics,* 1968, *20* (ii), 51–52.

HOWARD, R. A. *Decision Analysis: Applied Decision Theory.* Speech given at the Fourth International Conference on Operational Research. Boston, Mass., 1966.

HOWARD, R. A. "The Foundations of Decision Analysis." *IEEE Transactions on Systems Science and Cybernetics,* September 1968, SSC–4, No. 3, 211–219.

HUGHES, P. H. "The Social Structure of a Heroin Copping Community." In R. H. Blum and Associates, *The Dream Sellers.* San Francisco: Jossey-Bass, 1972.

HUGHES, P. H., BARKER, N. W., CRAWFORD, G. A., AND JAFFE, J. "The Natural History of a Heroin Epidemic." *American Journal of Public Health,* 1972, *62,* 995–1001.

HUGHES, P. H., AND CRAWFORD, G. A. "A Contagious Disease Model for Researching and Intervening in Heroin Epidemics." *Archives of General Psychiatry,* 1972, *27,* 149–155.

HUGHES, P. H., SENAY, E. C., AND PARKER, R. "The Medical Management of a Heroin Epidemic." *Archives of General Psychiatry,* 1972, *27,* 585–591.

HURST, P. M., AND WEIDNER, M. F. *Drug Effects upon Cognitive Performance Under Stress.* ONR Report H 66–3, Division of Psychobiology. University Park, Pa.: Pennsylvania State University, Institute of Research, 1966.

INGLEBY, D. "Ideology and Human Sciences." *The Human Context,* July 1970, *2,* 159.

INMAN, W. H. W., AND EVANS, D. A. "Evaluation of Spontaneous Report of Adverse Reactions to Drugs." *British Medical Journal,* 1972, *2,* 746–749.

IRWIN, S. *Drugs of Abuse: An Introduction to Their Actions and Potential Hazards.* Beloit, Wis.: Student Association for the Study of Hallucinogens, 1970.

ISBELL, H., AND CHRUSCIEL, T. L. *Dependence Liability of "Non-Narcotic" Drugs.* Geneva: World Health Organization, 1970.

ISBELL, H., WOLBACH, A. B., WIKLER, A., AND MINER, E. J. "Cross Tolerance between LSD and Psilocybin." *Psychopharmacologia* (Berlin), 1961, *2*, 147–159.

JACOBSEN, E. "Studies on the Subjective Effects of the Cephalotrophic Amines in Man: II. A Comparison between Beta-Phyenylisopropylamine Sulphate and a Series of Other Amine Salts." *Acta Medica Scandinavica,* 1939, *100*, 188–202.

JACOBSEN, E. "The Pharmacological Classification of Central Nervous System." *Journal of Pharmacy and Pharmacology,* 1958, *10*, 273–294.

JACOBSEN, E. "Tranquillizers and Sedatives" in D. E. G. Lawrence and A. C. Bacharach (Eds.), *Evaluation of Drug Activities: Pharmacometrics.* New York: Academic Press, 1964.

JACOBSEN, E. "An Analysis of the Gross Action of Drugs on the Central Nervous System." In *Molecular Basis of Some Aspects of Mental Activity.* Vol. 2. New York: Academic Press, 1967.

JAFFE, J. H. "Treatment of Drug Abusers." In W. G. Clark and J. del Guidice (Eds.), *Principles of Psychopharmacology,* New York: Academic Press, 1970.

JAFFE, J. H. *White House Special Action Office Report.* Washington, D.C., 1972.

JAMES, I. P. "Suicide and Mortality Amongst Heroin Addicts in Britain." *British Journal of Addictions,* 1967, *62*, 391.

JAWETZ, E. "The Use of Combinations of Antimicrobial Drugs." *Annual Review of Pharmacology,* 1968, *8*, 151–170.

JEFFREYS, M., BROTHERSTON, J. H. F., AND CARTWRIGHT, A. "Consumption of Medicine on a Working Class Housing Estate." *British Journal of Preventive and Social Medicine,* 1960, *14*, 64–67.

JELLINEK, E. M. *Disease Concept of Alcoholism.* New Haven, Conn.: College and University Press, 1966.

JOFFE, J. M. "Environmental Agents II. Drugs." In H. J. Eysenck (Ed.), *Prenatal Determination of Behavior.* Elmsford, N.Y.: Pergamon, 1969, 61–94.

JOHNSON, B. D. *Social Determinants of the Use of 'Dangerous Drugs' by College Students.* Doctoral dissertation. Columbia University, 1971.

JOHNSON, J., AND CLIFF, A. D. "Dependence on Hypnotic Drugs in General Practice." *British Medical Journal,* 1968, *4*, 613.

JONES, D. I. R. "Self-Poisoning from Drugs—A View from a General Medical Unit." *Practitioner,* 1969, *203*, 73.

JONES, M. K. "A Report of Three Growth Studies at the University of California." *The Gerontologist,* 1967, *7*, 49–54.

JONES, M. L. "Accuracy of Pulse Rates Counted for Fifteen, Thirty and Sixty Seconds." *Military Medicine,* 1970, 1127.

JONGSAMA, T. "Problems of Alcohol, Drugs, and Tobacco in the Netherlands." Response to WHO Enquiry, 1971.

Journal of the Addiction Research Foundation (Toronto). August 1, 1972, p. 1.

JOYCE, C. R. B. "Patient Co-operation and the Sensitivity of Clinical Trials." *Journal Chronic Disease,* 1960, *11*, 484–495.

JOYCE, C. R. B. "Cannabis." *British Journal of Hospital Medicine,* August 1970, 162–166.

JOYCE, C. R. B., AND SWALLOW, J. M. "The Controlled Trial in Dental Surgery: Premedication of Handicapped Children with Carisoprodol." *Dental Practitioner and Dental Records,* 1964, *15*, 44–47.

KALANT, H., AND KALANT, O. *Drugs, Society and Personal Choice*. Addiction Research Foundation. Toronto: University of Toronto Press, 1971.

KALANT, H., LE BLANC, A. E., AND GIBBONS, R. J. "Tolerance to and Dependence on, Some Non-opiate Psychotropic Drugs." *Pharmacological Reviews,* 1971, *23,* 135–191.

KALANT, O. J. *The Amphetamines*. (1st ed.) Springfield, Ill.: Thomas, 1966.

KALANT, O. J. *An Interim Guide to the Cannabis (Marijuana) Literature*. Toronto: Alcoholism and Drug Addiction Research Foundation, 1968, 162–165: "Cannabis."

KALANT, O. J. "Moreau, Hashish and Hallucinations." *International Journal of the Addictions,* 1971, *6,* 553–560.

KALANT, O. J. *The Amphetamines*. (2nd ed.) Toronto: University of Toronto Press, 1973.

KAPLAN, J. *Marijuana, The New Prohibition*. New York: World Publishing, 1970.

KAPLAN, J. *Criminal Justice: Introductory Cases and Materials*. Mineola, N.Y.: Foundation Press, 1973.

KENDALL, R. S., AND PITTEL, S. "Three Portraits of the Young Drug User: Comparison MMPI Group Profiles." Paper presented at meeting of Western Psychological Association, Los Angeles, April 1970.

KESSEL, N. "Self-Poisoning." *British Medical Journal,* 1965, *2* (5473), 1265; (5474), 1336.

KESSEL, N., AND GROSSMAN, G. "Suicide in Alcoholics." *British Medical Journal,* 1961, *2,* 1671.

KILOH, L. G., AND BRANDON, S. "Habituation and Addiction to Amphetamines." *British Medical Journal,* 1962, *2,* 40.

KING, R. *The Drug Hang-up: America's Fifty-Year Folly,* New York: W. W. Norton, 1972.

KLERMAN, G. "Staff Attitudes, Decision Making and Use of Drug Therapy in the Mental Hospital." In H. C. B. Denber, (Ed.), *Research Conference on the Therapeutic Community*. Springfield, Ill.: Thomas, 1960.

KNUPFER, G., AND ROOM, R. "Age, Sex and Social Class as Factors in Amount of Drinking in a Metropolitan Community." *Social Problems,* 1964, *12,* 225–240.

KOCH, J. V., AND GRUPP, S. E. "The Economics of Drug Control Policies." *International Journal of the Addictions,* December 1971, *6* (4), 571–584.

KOGAN, N., AND WALLACH, M. A. *Risk Taking: A Study in Cognition and Personality*. New York: Holt, Rinehart & Winston, 1964.

KOK, J. C. M., FROMBERG, E., GEERLINGS, P. J., VAN DER HELM, H. J., KAMP, P. E., VAN DER SLOOTEN, E. P. J., AND WILLEMS, M. A. M. "Analysis of Illicit Drugs." *Lancet,* 1971, *1,* 1065–1066.

KOLB, L. *Drug Addiction*. Springfield, Ill.: Thomas, 1962.

KOSVINER, A., MITCHESON, M. C., MYERS, K., OGBORNE, A., STIMSON, Z., ZACUNE, J., AND EDWARDS, G. "Heroin Use in a Provincial Town." *Lancet,* 1968, *1,* 1189–1192.

KRAEPELIN, E. *Ueber die Beeinflussung einfacher psychischer Vorgange durch einige Arzneimittel*. Jena: Fischer, 1892.

KRUTILLA, J. V. "Welfare Aspects of Benefit-Cost Analysis." *Journal of Political Economy,* June 1961, 226–235.

LA BARRE, W. *The Peyote Cult.* Yale University Publications in Anthropology 19. New Haven, Conn.: Yale University Press, 1938.

LA BARRE, W. "Le complexe narcotique de l'Amérique autochtone." *Diogéne,* 1964, 120–124.

LADD, E. C., AND LIPSET, S. M. "Politics of Academic National Scientists and Engineers." *Science,* 1972, *176,* 1091–1100.

LANQUETTE, W. "Legislative Control of Cannabis: A Comparison of the Use of Information about Cannabis by Members of the U.K. House of Commons and the U.S. House of Representatives in the Course of Legislating for Drug Control, 1969–1971." Unpublished doctoral dissertation, London School of Economics, 1972.

LASAGNA, L., AND VON FELSINGER, J. "The Volunteer Subject in Research." *Science,* 1954, *120,* 359–361.

LAUFER, B. *Tobacco and Its Use in Asia.* Pamphlet 18. Chicago: Field Museum of Natural History, 1924a.

LAUFER, B. *Introduction of Tobacco into Europe.* Anthropology Leaflet 19. Chicago: Field Museum of Natural History, 1924b.

LAUFER, B., HAMBLY, W. D., AND LINTON, R. *Tobacco and Its Use in Africa.* Leaflet 29. Chicago: Field Museum of Natural History, 1930.

LAWSON, A. A. M., AND MITCHELL, I. "Patients with Acute Poisoning seen in a General Medical Unit (1960–71)." *British Medical Journal,* 1972, *5,* 583.

LE DAIN, G. *Interim Report of the Commission of Inquiry into the Non-Medical Use of Drugs.* Ottawa: Information Canada, 1970.

LEAKE, C. "The Scientific Status of Pharmacology." *Science,* December 29, 1971, p. 10.

LEE, J. A. H. "Prevention of Cancer." *Postgraduate Medicine,* 1972, *51,* 84.

LEGGE, D., AND STEINBERG, H. "Actions of a Mixture of Amphetamine and Barbiturate in Man." *British Journal of Pharmacology,* 1962, *18,* 490–500.

LENNARD, H. L., EPSTEIN, L. J., BERNSTEIN, A., AND RANSOM, D. C. *Mystification and Drug Misuse: Hazards in Using Psychoactive Drugs.* San Francisco: Jossey-Bass, 1971.

LERNER, M., AND NUCRO, D. N. "Drug Abuse Deaths in Baltimore, 1951–66." *International Journal of the Addictions,* 1970, *5* (4), 693–715.

LEVINE, H. R. Unpublished paper, 1971.

LEVINE, J. "The Nature and Extent of Psychotropic Drug Usage in the U.S." Statement before the Subcommittee on Monopoly of the Select Committee on Small Business, U.S. Senate, 1969.

LEWIN, L. *Phantastica: Narcotic and Stimulating Drugs.* New York: Dutton, 1964. Originally published by Stilke, Berlin, 1924.

LEWIS, A. "Historical Perspective." *British Journal of Addiction,* 1968, *63,* 241.

LEWIS, V. S., PETERSON, D. M., GEIS, G., AND POLLACK, S. "Ethical and Social-Psychological Aspects of Urinalysis to Detect Heroin Use." *The British Journal of Addiction,* 1972, *67,* 303–308.

LIGHT, R. J., AND SMITH, P. V. "Accumulating Evidence: Procedures for Resolving Contradictions Among Different Research Studies." *Harvard Educational Review,* 1971, *41,* 429.

LIND, R., AND LIND, J. *The Identification and Measurement of Drug Control Objectives.* Unpublished paper. Stanford, Calif.: Stanford University, 1972.

LIND, R. C. "Benefit-Cost Analysis: A Criterion for Social Investment." In Thomas H. Cambell and Robert O. Sylvester (Eds.), *Water Resources Management and Public Policy.* Seattle: University of Washington Press, 1968.

LIPSET, M. S., AND DOBSON, R. B. "The Intellectual as Critic and Rebel: With Special Reference to the U.S. and Soviet Union." *Daedalus,* Summer 1972, 137–198.

LITT, J. F., COHEN, M. I., SCHONBERG, S. K., AND SPIGLAND, I. "Liver Disease in the Drug Using Adolescent." *Journal of Pediatrics,* August 1972, 238.

LITTLE, ARTHUR D., INC. *Drug Abuse and Law Enforcement.* Cambridge, Mass. President's Commission on Law Enforcement and the Administration of Justice, 1967.

LITTLE, ARTHUR D., INC. *A Study of International Control of Narcotics and Dangerous Drugs.* Submitted to Bureau of Narcotics and Dangerous Drugs, U.S. Department of Justice, 1971.

LOEB, E. M. "Primitive Intoxicants." *Quarterly Journal of Studies on Alcohol,* 1943, 387–398.

LOLLI, G., SERIANNI, E., GOLDER, G. M., AND LUZZATO-FEGIZ, P. *Alcohol in Italian Culture.* New York: Free Press, 1958.

LOUHIVUORI, K. "Drug Addicts and Nonaddicts Among Finnish Pubertal Adolescents: A Comparative Sample Study." Monograph from the Psychiatric Clinic of Helsinki University Central Hospital. #3. 1971.

LOVETRUP, S. "On the Correlation Between Psychic Action, Chemical Effects and Physical Properties of Chlorpromazine and Imipramine. In O. Walaas (Ed.), *Molecular Basis of Some Aspects of Mental Activity,* New York: Academic Press, 1967, 39–73.

LOWES, P. D. *The Genesis of International Narcotics Control.* Geneva: Librairie Droz., 1966.

LUBBOCK, B. *The Opium Clippers.* Boston: Lauriat, 1933.

LUDWIG, A. M., AND LEVINE, J. "Patterns of Hallucinogenic Drug Abuse." *Journal of the American Medical Association,* 1965, *191,* 92–96.

LUSTED, L. *Introduction to Medical Decision Making.* Springfield, Ill.: Thomas, 1968.

MACCOBY, M. "Alcoholism in a Mexican Village." In D. McClelland, W. Davis, R. Kalin, and E. Wanner (Eds.), *The Drinking Man.* New York: Free Press, 1972.

MAC MAHON, B., PUGH, T. F., AND IPSEN, J. *Epidemiological Methods.* Boston: Little, Brown, 1960.

MAKELA, K. "Consumption Level and Cultural Drinking Patterns as Determinants of Alcohol Problems." *Proceedings of 30th International Congress on Alcoholism and Drug Dependence.* Amsterdam, 1972.

MANHEIMER, D. I., MELLINGER, G. D., AND BALTER, M. B. "Marijuana Use Among Urban Adults." *Science,* 1969, *166,* 1544–1545.

MANNERING, G. J. "Drug Interactions—Principles and Problems in Relation to Drugs of Abuse." In S. S. Epstein (Ed.), *Drugs of Abuse: Their Genetic and Other Chronic Nonpsychiatric Hazards.* Cambridge, Mass.: M.I.T. Press, 1971.

MARIATEGUE, A. S. J. "Epidemiology and Alcoholism in Latin America." In R. E. Popham (Ed.), *Alcohol and Alcoholism.* Toronto: Addiction Research Foundation, Canadian University of Toronto Press, 1970.

Marijuana and Health. Second annual report to the Congress by the Secretary of

Health, Education and Welfare. Washington, D.C.: U.S. Government Printing Office, May 1972.

MARKS, J. "Predrug Behavior as a Predictor of Response to Phenothiazines Among Schizophrenics." *Journal of Nervous Mental Diseases,* 1963, *137,* 597–601.

MARKS, V., AND CHAPLE, P. A. L. "Hepatic Dysfunction in Heroin and Cocaine Users." *British Journal of the Addictions,* 1967, *62,* 189.

MARSHMAN, J. D., AND GIBBINS, R. J. "The Credibility Gap in the Drug Market." *Addictions,* 1969, *16,* 22–25.

MARTENS, S., NETZ, B., AND SUNDWALL, A. Analys av risker vid bruk av LSD–25, *Lakartidningen,* May 3, 1967, *64,* 1856–61.

MARTIN, W. R. "Assessment of the Dependence Producing Potentiality of Narcotic Analgesics." *Encyclopedia of Pharmacology and Therapy,* 1966, *1,* 155.

MARTINEZ, T., ROSS, L., SPAAN, R., AND BLUM, R. H. "College Faculty." In R. H. Blum and Associates, *The Dream Sellers: Perspectives on Drug Dealers,* San Francisco: Jossey-Bass, 1972.

MATHEW, H., PROUDFOOT, A. T., BROWN, S. S., AND AITKIN, R. C. B. "Acute Poisoning— Organization and Workload of a Treatment Centre." *British Medical Journal,* 1969, *3,* 489.

MAY, L., AND CHI-LI, T. K. "Total Analysis of an Illicit or 'Street' Narcotic Sample by Thin-layer Chromatography." *Bulletin on Narcotics* (United Nations), 1972, *24* (3), 35–36.

MC ARTHUR, C., WALDRON, E., AND DICKINSON, J. "The Psychology of Smoking." *Journal of Abnormal and Social Psychology,* 1958, *56,* 267–275,.

MC ARTHUR, J. N., DAWKINS, P. D., AND SMITH, M. J. H. "Of Mice and Means." *Nature,* 1971, *229,* 66.

MC CLELLAN, D., DAVIS, W., KALEN, R., AND WANNER, E. *The Drinking Man: Alcohol and Motivation.* New York: Free Press, 1972.

MC GEER, P. L. "The Chemistry of Mind." *American Scientist,* 1971, *59,* 221–229.

MC GLOTHLIN, W. "Marijuana: An Analysis of Use, Distribution and Control." In R. H. Blum and Associates, *Drug Dealers—Taking Action,* San Francisco: Jossey-Bass, 1973.

MC GLOTHLIN, W. H., COHEN, S., AND MC GLOTHLIN, M. *Personality and Attitude Changes in Volunteer Subjects Following Repeated Administration of LSD.* Paper presented before the Fifth International Congress, Collegium Neuropsychopharmacologicum, Washington, D.C., March 1966.

MC GLOTHLIN, W., JAMISON, K., AND ROSENBLATT, S. "Marijuana and the Use of Other Drugs." *Nature,* December 19, 1970, *228* (5277), 1227–1228.

MC GLOTHLIN, W. H., TABBUSH, V. C., CHAMBERS, C. D., AND JAMISON, K. *Alternative Approaches to Opiate Addiction Control: Costs, Benefits and Potential.* Paper prepared for the Bureau of Narcotics and Dangerous Drugs, Department of Justice, Contract No. J–70–33, February 1972.

MC NAMEE, H. B., MELLO, N. K., AND MENDELSON, J. H. "Experimental Analysis of Drinking Patterns of Alcoholics: Concurrent Psychiatric Observations." *American Journal of Psychiatry,* 1968, *124,* 1063–1075.

"Medical Ethics: The Editor's Responsibility." Editorial. *Lancet,* 1972, *2,* 237–238.

MEDICAL RESEARCH COUNCIL. *Responsibility in Investigations on Human Subjects.* Medical Research Council Annual Report, M.R.C. Comnd. 2382. London: Her Majesty's Stationery Office, 1962–1963.

MENDEL, W. "Tranquilizer Prescribing as a Function of the Experience and Ability of the Therapist." *American Journal of Psychiatry,* 1967, *124* (1), 16–22.

MERCER, G. W., AND SMART, R. G. "The Epidemiology of Psychoactive and Hallucinogenic Drug Use." In *Recent Advances in Drug Abuse Research.* New York: Wiley, 1972.

MISHAN, E. F. *Cost-Benefit Analysis: An Introduction.* New York: Praeger, 1971.

MITCHESON, M., DAVIDSON, J., HAWKS, D., HITCHIN, L., AND MALONE, S. "Sedative Abuse by Heroin Addicts." *Lancet,* 1970, *1,* 606.

MODELL, W. "Hazards of New Drugs." *Science,* 1963, *139,* 1180–1185.

MODELL, W. "Mass Drug Catastrophes and the Roles of Science and Technology." *Science,* April 21, 1967, *156* (3773), 346–351.

MOLOF, M. J. "Differences Between Assaultive and Non-assaultive Juvenile Offenders in the California Youth Authority." Research Report 51. Sacramento: State of California Department of the Youth Authority, February 1967.

MONTALVO, J. G., JR., SCRIGNAR, C. B., ALDERETTE, E., HARPER, B., AND EYER, D. "Flushing, Pale-Colored Urines, and False Negatives—Urinalysis of Narcotic Addicts." *International Journal of the Addictions,* 1972, *7,* 355–364.

MOORE, M. *Policy Concerning Drug Abuse in New York State.* Vol. 3, *The Economics of Heroin Distribution.* New York: Hudson Institute, 1970.

MOREAU, J. J. "Du hachisch et de l'alienation mentale." In *Etudes Psychologiques.* Paris: Librairie de Fortin, Masson et Cie, 1845.

MORRIS, J. *Uses of Epidemiology.* Edinburgh: Livingstone, 1957.

MORRIS, J. N. *Uses of Epidemiology.* (2nd ed.) Edinburgh: Livingstone, 1964.

MORTIMER, W., AND GOLDEN, M. D. *History of Coca.* New York: Vail, 1901.

MOSS, M. C., AND BERESFORD-DAVIES, E. *"A Survey of Alcoholism in an English County."* British Journal of Psychiatry, 1966, *112,* 1223–1230.

MUDGE, G. H. "Diuretics and Other Agents Employed in the Mobilization of Edema Fluid." In L. S. Goodman and A. Gilman (Eds.), *Pharmacological Basis of Therapeutics* (4th ed.) New York: Macmillan, 1970.

MUNCH, J. C., AND CALESNICK, B. "Laxative Studies: I. Human Threshold Doses of White and Yellow Phenolphthalein." *Clinical Pharmacology and Therapy,* 1960, *1,* 311–315.

MUSTO, D. *The American Disease.* New Haven, Conn.: Yale University Press, 1973.

Narkotikaforskning, Nordiska Radet, Stockholm, November 1970.

NATIONAL ACADEMY OF SCIENCES. "United States Procedures for Screening Drugs." *UN Bulletin on Narcotics,* 1970, *22,* 11.

NATIONAL COMMISSION ON MARIJUANA AND DRUG ABUSE. *Marijuana: A Signal of Misunderstanding.* Washington, D.C.: Superintendent of Documents, U.S. Government Printing Office, 1972.

NEUFELD, R. J. "Generalization of Results Beyond the Experimental Setting: Statistical Versus Logical Considerations." *Perceptual and Motor Skills,* 1970, *31,* 443–446.

NILSSON, L., AND LINDROTH, C. H. *Myror.* Stockholm: Forum, 1959.

NISBETT, R. E. "Hunger, Obesity and the Ventromedial Hypothalamus." *Psychological Review,* November 1972, *79,* 433–453.

NOBLE, P., AND BASNES, G. G. "Drug Taking in Adolescent Girls: Factors Associated with Progression to Narcotic Use." *British Medical Journal,* June 1970, 620.

NOBLE, P., HART, T., AND NATHAN, R. "Correlates and Outcome of Illicit Drug Use by Adolescent Girls." *British Journal of Psychiatry,* 1972, *120* (558), 497.

NURCO, DAVID N. "An Ecological Analysis of Narcotic Addicts in Baltimore." *International Journal of the Addictions,* 1972, *7,* 341–353.

NURCO, DAVID N., AND LERNER, MONROE. "The Feasibility of Locating Addicts in the Community." *International Journal of the Addictions,* 1971, *6,* 51–62.

OKUN, R. "General Principles of Clinical Pharmacology and Psychopharmacology and Early Clinical Drug Evaluations." In W. G. Clark and J. del Guidice (Eds.), *Principles of Psychopharmacology,* New York: Academic Press, 1970.

OTIS, S. O., AND CRISMAN, C. A. *Animal Research in Psychopharmacology: Index for Psychopharmacology Handbooks, Volumes I–IV.* Washington, D.C.: Public Health Service, U.S. Department of Health, Education, and Welfare, 1966.

OWEN, P. E. *British Opium Policy in China and India.* New Haven, Conn.: Yale University Press, 1934.

PARISH, P. "Prescribing of Psychotropic Drugs in General Practice." *Journal of the Royal College of General Practicioners,* 1971, Supplement No. 4, *92.*

PATON, W. D. "Guide to Drugs." *Drugs and Society,* 1972, *1* (9), 17–19.

PATON, W. D. M., AND PAYNE, J. P. *Pharmacological Principles and Practice.* London: Churchill, 1968.

PEARLIN, L. I. "Treatment Values and Enthusiasm for Drugs in a Mental Hospital." *Psychiatry,* 1962, *25,* 170–179.

PEEL, J., AND SKIPWORTH, G. "Sample Size: An Innovatory Procedure in Survey Analysis." *Sociology,* 1970, *4,* 385.

PETRIE, H. G. "Theories Are Tested by Observing the Facts: Or Are They?" In *Seventy-first Yearbook.* Washington, D.C.: National Society for the Study of Education, 1972, Part 1, 47–74.

PICHOT, P., AND BUCHSENSCHUTZ, P. J. *La Personnalité du Toxicomane.* Unpublished manuscript, delivered in Milan, 1972.

PLATT, J. "Strong Inference." *Science,* 1964, *146,* 347–353.

PREBLE, E., AND CASEY, J. J., JR. "Taking Care of Business—The Heroin User's Life on the Street. *International Journal of the Addictions,* 1969, *4* (1) 1–24.

PREST, A. R. AND TURVEY, R. "Cost-Benefit Analysis: A Survey." *Surveys of Economic Theory,* 1967, *3,* 155–207.

PRINZMETAL, M., AND BLOOMBERG, W. "The Use of Benzedrine for the Treatment of Narcolepsy." *Journal of the American Medical Association,* 1935, *105,* 2051–2054.

RAIFFA, H. *Decision Analysis: Introductory Lectures on Choices Under Uncertainty.* Reading, Mass.: Addison-Wesley, 1968.

RASKIN, A. A. "A Comparison of Accepters and Resisters of Drug Treatment as an Adjunct to Psychotherapy." *Journal of Consulting Psychology,* 1961, *25,* 366.

RATHOD, N. H. *Early Experiences in the Life of a Narcotic User.* Paper read at the International Institute on the Prevention and Treatment of Drug Dependence, Lausanne, June 1970.

RATHOD, N. H. "Use of Heroin and Methadone by Injection in a New Town: Progress Report." *British Journal of the Addictions,* 1972, *67,* 113.

RATHOD, N. H., DE ALARCON, R., AND THOMSON, I. G. "Signs of Heroin Usage Detected by Drug Users and Their Parents." *Lancet,* December 30, 1967, 1411–1414.

RAY, O. S. *Drugs, Society and Human Behavior.* St. Louis, Mo.: Mosby, 1972.

REGULATIONS FOR EXPERT ADVISORY PANELS AND COMMITTEES. In *WHO Basic Documents,* 21st Ed. Geneva, 1970.

RENBORG, B. "International Control of Narcotics." In *Law and Contemporary Problems.* Durham, N.C.: Duke University School of Law, 1957.

Report of the Departmental Committee on Liquor Licensing. Her Majesty's Stationery Office, 1972.

RICHARDS, L. *National Conference on Research in School Health.* Detroit: American Association for Health, Physical Education and Recreation, 1971.

RICHMAN, A. "Follow-up of Criminal Narcotics Addicts." *Canada Psychological Association Journal,* 1966, *11* (2), 107–115.

RICKELS, K., AND CATTELL, R. B. "Drug and Placebo Response as a Function of Doctor and Patient Type." In R. A. May and J. R. Wittenbord (Eds.), *Psychotropic Drug Response,* Springfield, Ill.: Thomas, 1969.

ROBERTSON, L. "The Drug Laws: Problems of Overcriminalization." In C. C. Brown and C. Savage (Eds.), *The Drug Abuse Controversy.* Baltimore: National Educational Consultants, 1971.

ROBINS, L. N., AND MURPHY, G. E. "Drug Use in a Normal Population of Young Negro Men." *American Journal of Public Health,* September 1967, *9,* 69.

ROGERS, F. B. (Ed.) *Studies in Epidemiology: Selected Papers of M. Greenberg.* New York: Putman, 1965.

ROSENTHAL, R. *Experimenter Effects in Behavioral Research.* New York: Appleton-Century-Crofts, 1966.

ROSNOW, L., ROSENTHAL, R., MC CONOCHIE, R., AND ARMS, R. "Volunteer Effects on Experimental Outcomes" in *Educational and Psychological Measurements,* 1969, *29* (4) 825–846.

ROTTENBERG, S. "The Clandestine Distribution of Heroin, Its Discovery and Suppression." *Journal of Political Economy,* January/February 1968, 78–90.

ROTTENBERG, S. "The Social Cost of Crime and Crime Prevention." In *Crime and Urban Society.* New York: Dunellen, 1970.

ROYAL COLLEGE OF PHYSICIANS OF LONDON. *Report of the Committee on the Supervision of the Ethics of Clinical Investigations in Institutions.* London: Royal College of Physicians of London, 1967.

ROYAL COLLEGE OF PHYSICIANS. *Smoking and Health Now.* London, 1971.

Rules of Procedure of the Functional Commissions of the Economic and Social Council. New York: United Nations, 1971.

RUMBAUGH, C. L., BERGERON, R. T., FANG, H. C. H., AND MC CORMICK, R. "Cerebral Angiographic Changes in the Drug Abuse Patient." *Radiology,* November 1971, *101* (2), 335–344.

RUSSELL, H. M. A. "The Smoking Problem 1 and 2." *Nursing Times,* May 18 and 25, 1972.

SACKMAN, B. S. "Drug Abuse in Washington, D.C." unpublished study, 1971.

SADOUN, R., LOLLI, G., AND SILVERMAN, M. *Drinking in French Culture,* New Brunswick, N.J.: Rutgers Center of Alcohol Studies, 1965.

SAELENS, J. K., GRANAT, F. R., AND SAWYER, W. K. "The Mouse Jumping Test—A Simple Screening Method to Estimate the Physical Dependence Capacity of

Analgesics." *Archives Internale de Pharmacodynamie et de Thérapie,* 1971, *190,* 213.

SAMUELS, J. W. "International Control of Narcotic Drugs and International Economic Law." *Canadian Yearbook of International Law,* 1969, *7,* 192–217.

SATLOFF, A. "Patterns of Drug Usage in a Psychiatric Patient Population." *American Journal of Psychiatry,* 1964, *121,* 382–384.

SCHACHTER, S. "Some Extraordinary Facts About Humans and Rats." *American Psychology, February* 1971, *26,* 129–144.

SCHELLING, T. C. "Economics and Criminal Enterprise." *The Public Interest,* Spring 1967, 61–78.

SCHMIDT, W., AND DE LINT, J. E. E. "Causes of Death of Alcoholics." *Quarterly Journal of the Studies on Alcohol,* 1972, *33,* 171–185.

SCHOU, M. "Lithium, Sodium and Manic Depressive Psychosis." In O. Walaas (Ed.), *Molecular Basis of Some Aspects of Mental Activity.* New York: Academic Press, 1967.

SCHUMAN, H. "Attitudes vs. Actions versus Attitudes vs. Attitudes." *Public Opinion Poll,* 1972, *36,* 347–354.

SCHUSTER, C. R., AND JOHANSON, C. E. "The Use of Animal Models for the Study of Drug Abuse." Unpublished manuscript, 1973.

SCHUSTER, R. C., AND THOMPSON, T. "Self-administration of and Behavioral Dependence on Drugs." *Annual Review of Pharmacology,* 1969, *9,* 483–502.

SECRETARY GENERAL. *Drug Abuse.* New York: United Nations Economic and Social Council Commission on Narcotics, 1964–71.

SELTZER, C. C. "Critical Appraisal of the Royal College of Physicians' Report on Smoking and Health." *Lancet,* 1972, *1,* 243–248.

SHADER, R. I., AND DIMASCIO, A. *Psychotropic Drug Side Effects,* Baltimore: Williams and Wilkins, 1970.

SHARPLESS, S. K. "Hypnotics and Sedatives." In L. S. Goodman, and A. Gilman (Eds.), *The Pharmacological Basis of Therapeutics.* (3rd Ed.) New York: Macmillan, 1970.

SHEPHERD, M., COOPER, B., BROWN, A. C., AND KALTON, G. *Psychiatric Illness in General Practice.* London: Oxford University Press, 1966.

SIGG, B. W. "Le cannabisme chronique: Fruit de son developpement et du capitalisme." *Marrakesch and Algiers,* 1963.

SKOLNICK, J. *Justice Without Trial.* New York: Wiley, 1966.

SLOTKIN, J. S. *The Peyote Religion: A Study in Indian-White Relations.* New York: Free Press, 1956.

SMART, R. G. "Illicit Drug Use in Canada: A Review of Current Epidemiology with Clues for Prevention." *International Journal of the Addictions,* September 1971, *6* (3) 383–405.

SMART, R. G. *The Ethics and Efficacy of the Prevention of Drug Dependence.* Substudy 523. Toronto: Addiction Research Foundation, 1972.

SMART, R. G. *Addiction, Dependency, Abuse or Use: Which Are We Studying with Epidemiology?* Paper presented to the Columbia University Conference on Epidemiology of Drug Use, Puerto Rico, February 1973.

SMART, R. G., AND FEJER, D. "Extent of Illicit Drug Use in Canada: A Review of

Current Epidemiology." In C. L. Boydell, C. F. Boydell, and P. C. Whitehead (Eds.), *Critical Issues in Canadian Society.* Toronto: Holt, Rinehart & Winston, 1971.

SMART, R. G., AND JACKSON, D. *The Yorkville Subculture: A Study of the Life Styles and Interactions of Hippies and Non-Hippies.* Toronto: Addiction Research Foundation, 1969.

SMART, R. G., LA FOREST, L. AND WHITEHEAD, P. C. "The Epidemiology of Drug Use in Three Canadian Cities." *British Journal of Addiction,* 1971, *66,* 293–299.

SMART, R. G., AND WHITEHEAD, P. C. "The Consumption Patterns of Illicit Drugs and Their Implications for Prevention of Abuse." *UN Bulletin on Narcotics,* 1972, *24,* 39–47.

SMART, R. G., WHITEHEAD, P. C. AND LA FOREST, L. "The Prevention of Drug Abuse by Young People: An Argument Based on the Distribution of Drug Use. *UN Bulletin on Narcotics,* 1971, *23,* 11–15.

SMITH, A. J. "Self-Poisoning: A Worsening Situation." *British Medical Journal,* 1972 (5833), 157–159.

SMITH, D. E. "The Acute and Chronic Toxicity of Marijuana." *Journal of Psychedelic Drugs,* 1968, *2* (1), 37–47.

SMITH, J. P. "The Contents of Illicit Drugs." In R. H. Blum and Associates, *Drug Dealers—Taking Action,* San Francisco: Jossey-Bass, 1973.

SMITH, N. C. "Replication Studies: A Neglected Aspect of Psychological Research." *American Psychologist,* 1970, *25,* 970.

SMITH, R. "Traffic in Speed: Illegal Manufacture and Distribution." *Journal of Psychedelic Drugs,* 1969, *2* (2) 30–41.

SMITH, ROGER. *The Marketplace of Speed: Violence and Compulsive Methedrine Abuse.* Chicago: Aldine Press, 1971.

SMYTHIES, J. R., JOHNSTON, V. S., AND BRADLEY, R. J. "Behavioral Models of Psychosis." *British Journal of Psychiatry,* 1969, *115,* 55–68.

SNYDER, S. H., FAILLACE, L., AND HOLLISTER, L. E. "Two, Five-Dimethoxy-Four-Methyl-Amphetamine (STP): A New Hallucinogenic Drug." *Science,* 1967, *158,* 669–670.

SONNENREICH, M. In C. C. Brown and C. Savage (Eds.), *The Drug Abuse Controversy.* Baltimore: National Educational Consultants, 1971.

SOSKIN, W. F., AND KORCHIN, S. J. (with ROSS, N. W., STEIN, K. B., AND SOMERS, R. H.). *Children of the Good Life.* Second Interim Report on Project Community. Berkeley, Calif.: Psychological Clinic, Psychology Department, University of California, Berkeley, March 1972.

SOUEIF, M. I. "The Social Psychology of Cannabis Consumption: Myth, Mystery and Fact." *UN Bulletin on Narcotics,* 1972, *24,* 1–10.

SPEAR, H. B. "The Growth of Heroin Addiction in the United Kingdom." *British Journal of the Addictions,* 1969, *64,* 245.

SPIEGEL, D., AND SELLS, S. B. *Evaluation of Treatment for Drug Users in the DARP: 1969–71 Admissions.* Fort Worth: Texas Christian University Institute of Behavioral Research, 1973.

SPONG, W. *Report on the Psychotropic Convention to the U.S. Senate Foreign Relations Committee* (Sen. Fulbright, Chairman). Washington, D.C.: U.S. Government Printing Office, September 1972.

STERLING, J. W. "A Comparative Examination of Two Modes of Intoxication—An Exploratory Study of Glue Sniffing." *Journal of Criminal Law, Criminology and Police Science,* 1964, *55,* 95–99.

STEVENSON, G. H. *Drug Addiction in British Columbia.* (3 vols.) Manuscript. Vancouver: University of British Columbia, 1956.

STIMSON, G. V., AND OGBORNE, A. C. *A Survey of a Representative Sample of Addicts Prescribed Heroin at London Clinics.*" Paper read at the International Institute on the Prevention and Treatment of Drug Dependence, Lausanne, June 1970.

STOKINGER, H. E. "Toxicity of Airborne Chemicals: Air Quality Standards—A National and International View." *Annual Review of Pharmacology,* 1972, *12,* 407–422.

STOYVA, J., AND KAMIYA, J. "Electrophysiological Studies of Dreaming as the Prototype of a New Strategy in the Study of Consciousness." *Psychological Review,* 1968, *75,* 192–205.

STUART, R. B. "Drug Education Is Linked to Use." *New York Times,* December 3, 1972.

SZASZ, T. "The Ethics of Addiction." In C. C. Brown and C. Savage (Eds.), *The Drug Abuse Controversy.* Baltimore: National Education Consultants, 1971, 39–47.

TALALAY, P. (Ed.). *Drugs in Our Society.* Baltimore: Johns Hopkins Press, 1964.

TEDESCHI, D. H., AND TEDESCHI, R. E. *Importance of Fundamental Principles in Drug Evaluation.* New York: Raven Press, 1968.

TEMPKIN, O. In P. Talalay (Ed.) *Drugs in Our Society.* Baltimore: Johns Hopkins Press, 1964.

TERRIS, M. In B. Pasamanick (Ed.), *Epidemiology of Mental Disorder.* Washington, D.C.: American Association for the Advancement of Science, 1959.

TERRY, C. E., AND PELLENS, M. *The Opium Problem.* Publication 115. Montclair, N.J.: Patterson, Smith, 1970.

THOMPSON, T. "Drugs as Reinforcers: Experimental Addiction." *International Journal of the Addictions,* 1968, *3,* 199.

THUROW, L. C., AND RAPPAPORT, C. "Law Enforcement and Cost-Benefit Analysis." *Public Finance,* 1969, 48–54.

TINKLENBERG, J. "Marijuana and Alcohol." *Psychopharmacology Bulletin,* 1971, *7,* 8–9.

TINKLENBERG, J. "Corrections and Treatment." In R. H. Blum and Associates, *Drug Dealers—Taking Action,* San Francisco: Jossey-Bass, 1973.

TINKLENBERG, J. R., AND WOODROW, K. H. "Drug Use Among Assaultive Offenders." In S. H. Frazier (Ed.), *Aggression: Proceedings of the 1972 Annual Meeting of the Association for Research in Nervous and Mental Disease.* Baltimore: Williams and Wilkins, 1974.

TRAVIS, R. H., AND SAYER, G. "Insulin and Oral Hypoglycemic Drugs." In L. S. Goodman and A. Gilman (Eds.), *Pharmacological Basis of Therapeutics.* (4th ed.) New York: Macmillan, 1970.

TULLOCK, G. "Welfare Costs of Tariffs, Monopolies, and Theft." *Western Economic Journal,* June 1967, 224–233.

TULLOCK, G. "An Economic Approach to Crime." *Social Science Quarterly,* June 1969, 59–71.

"Twenty Years of Narcotics Control Under the United Nations." *Bulletin on Narcotics* (United Nations), 1966, *18* (1), 1–60.

UHLENHUTH, E. H., CANTER, A., NĿUSTADT, J. O., AND PAYSON, H. E. "Symptomatic Relief of Anxiety with Meprobamate, Phenobarbital and Placebo." *American Journal of Psychiatry*, 1959, *115*, 905–910.

UNITED NATIONS CONFERENCE FOR THE ADOPTION OF A PROTOCOL ON PSYCHOTROPIC SUBSTANCES. *Convention on Psychotropic Substances.* New York, February 19, 1971.

"United States Procedure for Screening Drugs." *UN Bulletin on Narcotics*, 1970, *22*, 11–17.

USDIN, E. "Classification of Psychopharmaca." In W. G. Clark and J. del Guidice (Eds.), *Principles of Psychopharmacology*, New York: Academic Press, 1970, 193–232.

VAILLANT, G. D., BRIGHTON, J., AND MC ARTHUR, C. "Physicians' Use of Mood-Altering Drugs." *New England Journal of Medicine,* 1970, *282*, 365–370.

VESSELL, E. S. (Ed.). "Drug Metabolism in Man." *Annals of the New York Academy of Science,* 1971, *179*.

VESSELL, E. S. "Advances in Pharmacogenetics." *Progress in Medical Genetics*, 1973, *9*, 291–367.

VESSEY, M. P. "Some Methodological Problems in the Investigation of Rare Adverse Reactions to Oral Contraceptives." *American Journal of Epidemiology,* 1971, *94*, 202.

VILLARREAL, J. E., AND SEEVERS, M. H. "Evaluations of New Compounds for Morphine-like Physical Dependence in the Rhesus Monkey." *Report of the Thirty-Fourth Annual Scientific Meeting, Committee on Problems of Drug Dependence,* 1972, *34*, 1040–1053.

WAALER, H. T., AND PIOT, M. A. "Use of an Epidemiological Model for Estimating the Effectiveness of Tuberculosis Control Measures." *Bulletin World Health Organization,* 1970, *43*, 1–16.

WADE, N. "Drug Regulation: FDA Replies to Charges by Economists and Industry." *Science,* 1973, *179*, 775–777.

WAY, E. "Contemporary Classification, Pharmacology and Abuse Potential of Psychotropic Substances." In J. R. Wittenborn, H. Brill, J. P. Smith, and S. Wittenborn (Eds.), *Drugs and Youth.* Springfield, Ill.: Thomas, 1969, 27–36.

WAY, E. L., MO, B. P. N., QUOCK, C. P., YAP, P. M., DU, G., CHAN, S. C., AND CHENG, J. "Evaluation of the Nalorphine Pupil Diagnostic Test for Narcotic Usage in Long-Term Heroin and Opium Addicts." *Clinical Pharmacology and Therapeutics,* 1966, *7*, 300–311.

WAY, E. L., ELLIOTT, H. W., NOMOF, N., AND FIELDS, T. "Comparaisons des tests chimiques et de la methode pupillaire pour le diagnostic de l'emploi de stupefiants." *Bulletin on Narcotics* (United Nations), 1963, *15*, 29–33.

WEIL, A. T. "Adverse Reactions to Marijuana." *New England Journal of Medicine,* 1970, *282* (18), 997–1000.

WEIL, A. T. *The Natural Mind,* Boston: Houghton Mifflin, 1972a.

WEIL, A. T. "The Pharmacology of Consciousness-Altering Drugs." In Patricia M. Wald and P. B. Hutt (Eds.), *Dealing with Drug Abuse,* New York: Praeger, 1972b, 329–344.

WEINGARTNER, H., AND FAILLACE, L. A. "Alcohol State-Dependent Learning in Man." *Journal of Nervous and Mental Disease,* 1971, *153* (6), 395–406.

WEISS, B., AND SIMON, W. "Quantitative Perspectives on the Long Term Toxicity of Methylmercury and Similar Poisons." In B. Weiss and V. Laties (Eds.), *Behavioral Toxicology.* In preparation, 1973.

WHITEHEAD, PAUL C. "The Epidemiology of Drug Use in a Canadian City at Two Points in Time: Halifax, 1961–1970." *The British Journal of Addiction,* 1971, *66,* 301–314.

WHITEHEAD, P., AND SMART, R. "Validity and Reliability of Self-reported Drug Use." *Canadian Journal of Criminology and Correction,* 1972, *14* (1), 1–8.

WHITFIELD, J. W. "The Imaginary Questionnaire." *Quarterly Journal of Experimental Psychology,* 1950, *2,* 76–87.

WIKLER, A. *Opiate Addiction: Psychological and Neurological Aspects in Relation to Clinical Problems.* Springfield, Ill.: Thomas, 1953.

WIKLER, A. "Clinical and Social Aspects of Marijuana Intoxication." *Archives of General Psychiatry,* 1970, *23,* 320–325.

WILLIS, J. H. "Drug Dependence—Some Demographic and Psychiatric Aspects in U.K. and U.S. Subjects." *British Journal of the Addictions,* 1964, *58,* 135–146.

WINICK, C. "Epidemiology of Narcotic Use." In D. M. Wilner and G. G. Kassebaum (Eds.), *Narcotics.* New York: McGraw-Hill, 1965.

WISSMAN, H., VON WOLF, L., FRANCOIS, C., AND VON MUELLER, H. In *Inneren Afrikas: ein Erforschung des Kassai Wahrend der Jahre.* Leipzig: Brockhaus, 1883.

WITTENBORN, J. R. "Reliability, Validity, and Objectivity of Symptom-Rating Scales." *Journal of Nervous and Mental Diseases,* 1972, *154,* 79.

WOODBURY, D. M. "Analgesics and Antipyretics." Goodman, L. S., Gilman A. (Eds.) "The Pharmacological Basis of Therapeutics." 3rd Edition. New York: McMillan Co., 1968.

WOODCOCK, J. "Action in the Schools." In Richard H. Blum and Associates, *Drug Dealers—Taking Action: Options for International Response.* San Francisco: Jossey-Bass, 1973.

YABLONSKY, L. "The Anticriminal Society: Synanon." *Federal Probation,* 1962, *26,* (3), 50–57.

YANAGITA, T. "An Experimental Framework for Evaluation of Dependence Liability of Various Types of Drug in Monkeys." *Fifth International Congress on Pharmacology,* 1973, *1,* 99–109.

YANAGITA, T., AND TAKAHASHI, S. "Development of Tolerence to and Physical Dependence on Barbiturates in Rhesus Monkeys." *Journal of Pharmacology and Experimental Therapeutics,* 1970, *172,* 163–169.

YANAGITA, T., AND TAKAHASHI, S. "Dependence Liability of Several Sedative Hypnotic Agents Evaluated in Monkeys." *Journal of Pharmacology and Experimental Therapeutics,* 1973.

YOUNG, J. *The Drug Takers.* London: MacGibbon and Kee, 1971.

YOUNGKEN, H. W. "Rauwolfia Serpentina." *The Herbalist,* 1957, *23,* 35–43.

ZACUNE, J. "A comparison of Canadian narcotics addicts in Great Britain and in Canada." *UN Bulletin on Narcotics,* 1971, *23,* 41–49.

ZACUNE, J. "What's in a name?" *Drugs and Society,* 1972, 28–29.

ZACUNE, J., AND EDWARDS, G. "Heroin Use in a Provincial Town." *Lancet,* 1968, *1,* 1189–1192.

ZACUNE, J., AND HENSMAN, C. (Eds). *Drugs, Alcohol and Tobacco in Britain.* London: Wm. Heineman Medical Books, 1971.

ZACUNE, J., MITCHESON, M. C., AND MALONE, S. "Heroin Use in a Provincial Town— One Year Later." *International Journal of the Addictions,* 1969, *4,* 537–570.

ZAKUSOV, V. V. *Farmakologiia.* Moskva: Meditsina, 1966.

ZINBERG, N. E. *Rehabilitation of Heroin Users in Vietnam.* Unpublished manuscript, 1971, 47.

ZINBERG, N., AND ROBERTSON, J. *Drugs and the Public.* New York: Simon and Schuster, 1972.

ZINBERG, N. E., AND WEIL, A. T. "A Comparison of Marijuana Users and Non-users." *Nature,* April 1970, *226.*

ZOLA, I. K. "Illness behavior of the working class." In A. B. Shastak and W. Bomberg (Eds.), *Blue Collar World: Studies of the American Worker.* New York: Prentice-Hall, 1964.

ZYLMAN, R. "Accidents, Alcohol and Single-Cause Explanation." *Quarterly Journal of Studies on Alcohol,* 1968, Supplement 4, 212–233.

Indexes

NAME INDEX

SUBJECT INDEX